THE COMPLETE
FLORAL HEALER

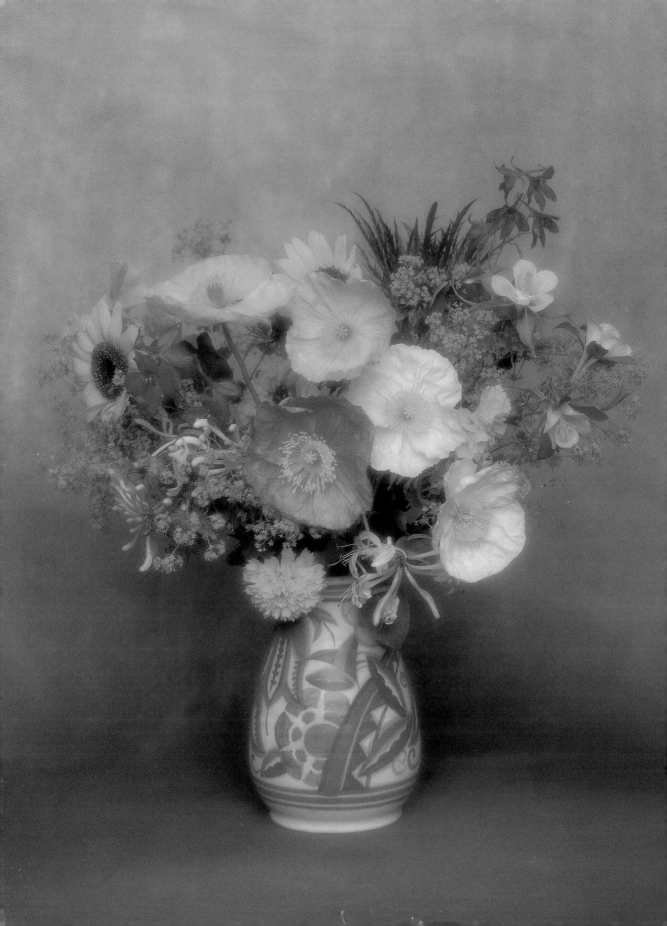

The Complete
FLORAL
HEALER

ANNE McINTYRE

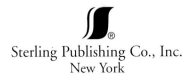

Sterling Publishing Co., Inc.
New York

Gaia Staff:

EDITOR Caroline Sheldrick

DESIGNER Bridget Morley

PICTURE RESEARCH Gill Smith

ILLUSTRATIONS Richard Bonson

SPECIAL PHOTOGRAPHY Philip Dowell

MANAGING EDITOR Pip Morgan

DIRECTION Joss Pearson, Patrick Nugent

The publishers have made every effort to trace the copyright holders of the poetry extracts in the text and apologize to anyone who has not been acknowledged.

Library of Congress Cataloging-in-Publication Data Available

1 0 9 8 7 6 5 4 3 2 1

Published in 2002 by Sterling Publishing Co., Inc.
387 Park Avenue South, New York, NY 10016
First published in the United Kingdom in 1996
by Gaia Books Limited, 66 Charlotte St., London W1P 1LR
and 20 High St., Stroud, Glos GL5 1AS
Copyright © 1996 by Gaia Books Limited, London
Text Copyright © 1996 by Anne McIntyre
Distributed in Canada by Sterling Publishing
c/o Canadian Manda Group, One Atlantic Avenue, Suite 105
Toronto, Ontario, Canada M6K 3E7

Sterling ISBN 0-8069-8689-1

Foreword

True healing involves treating the very base of the cause of the suffering. Therefore no effort directed to the body alone can do more than superficially repair damage. Treat people for their emotional unhappiness, allow them to be happy, and they will become well.
DR EDWARD BACH

The Complete Floral Healer is a unique book written by a skilled and articulate practitioner who has gained mastery of many ways of using plants in healing. It resonates with a depth of compassion that can only come when real experience blends with the consciousness of a green wise woman. The result is a practical, empowering book blending the science of medical herbalism with that of homeopathy, aromatherapy and the subtle art of flower essences.

The use of flowers in health care is becoming increasingly common and the practice of Phytotherapy is rapidly gaining legitimacy. However, there are many ways to view plant therapies. At one extreme they may be seen as natural 'drug delivery systems', whilst at the other they might be seen in esoteric terms of patterns in the healing journey. My feeling is that both standpoints are valid, and both equally limited. Anne McIntyre has done an admirable job of building meaningful bridges between such diverse perspectives.

The relationship between people and healing plants is an example of Gaia, the goddess of the earth, in action. Whether your focus is on the chemistry of secondary plant products or the energy fields of plants, the context is one of ecological embrace. A unique opportunity is created by the simple act of taking herbal medicines; in making a practical link with Gaia, ecological cycles for healing are activated. The door is opened to the possibility of a miracle of healing way beyond the removal of disease. There can be a direct experience of ecological flow and integration, a feeling of belonging, in the deepest sense, and of knowing that one is home, healed and whole. Such healing goes beyond the treatment of pathologies and the alleviation of bodily suffering that herbal remedies do so well. Rather, it is in the realm of the transcendent, it is the touch of the luminous, the transformation that comes about through divine touch.

Such profound experience has little to do with specific herbs or health care programs. It results from a healing of the separation from the embrace of both nature and soul that plagues humanity. Such experience cannot be created or predicted, but there are times when the use of green herbs touches us in an experience of 'the green'. The medieval herbalist and mystic Hildegard of Bingen talks of Viridatas, the greening power. By this I interpret her to mean a vital energy that is life, the spirit of the planet, the divine in form, that heals and transforms humanity. The healing offered so abundantly and freely by the plant kingdom is indeed a greening of the human condition, pointing to the reality of a new springtime.

Herbalism abounds with opportunities to experience the reality of the healing presence of nature, whether in treating disease or in hugging a tree. Approaching herbalism from any of its diverse components illuminates a field of human endeavour that is a wonderful weaving of the miraculous and the mundane. It is a therapy that encompasses anthraquinone laxatives, the spiritual ecstasy of the Amazonian shaman and the beauty of a flower. The limits to what might be called the path of the herbalist are only those imposed by parochial vision and constipated imagination!

It has been said that without vision the people die. Without a personal vision, life becomes a slow process of degeneration and decay, and without some social vision civilization rapidly disintegrates. Such life-affirming vision is different to taking on a dogmatic belief system. It is an expression of meaning in an individual's life and must come from the core. A green vision of humanity's places within the family of Gaia is rapidly illuminating our culture. Herbalism with its reverence for life is building bridges between plants and people, and is at the heart of this transformation.

From my herbalist's perspective it seems self-evident that Viridatas, the greening power, is a driving force behind changes touching humanity. It is an aspect of what has been called the paradigm shift, a profound change in our cultural world view and the context within which we live and envision. It is reminding us of who we are, where we live, and what embraces us.

DAVID HOFFMANN
Sonoma County, Shasta Bioregion, North America   1996

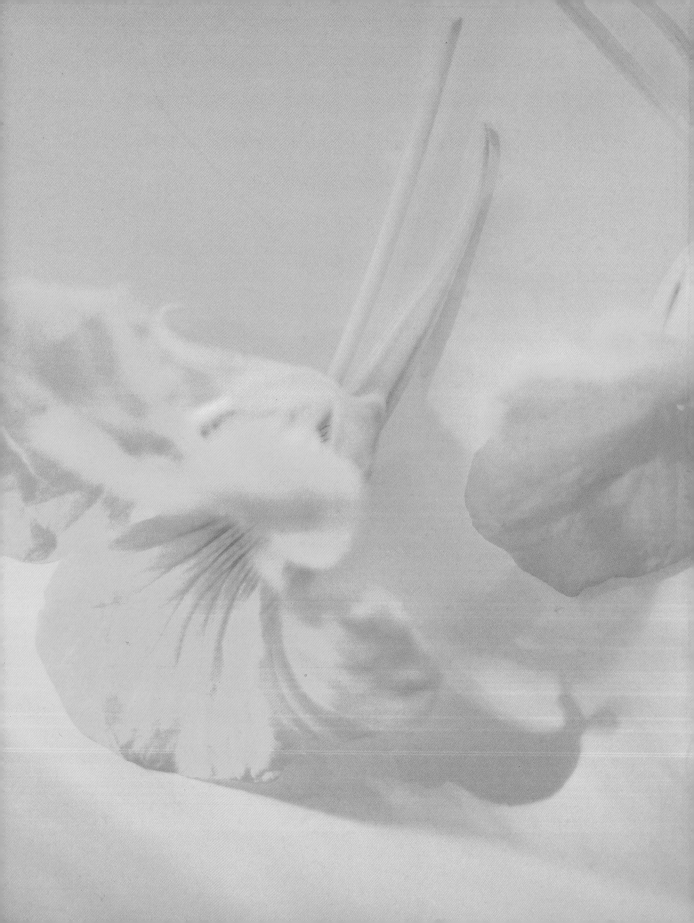

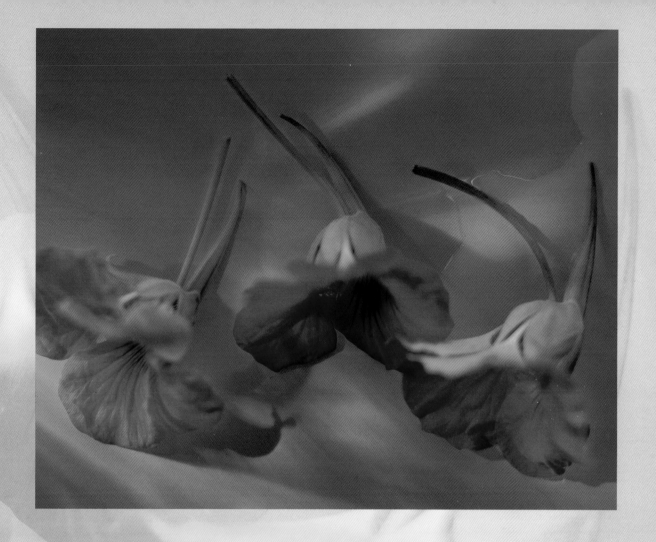

Contents

Introduction

The rose that with your earthly eyes you see
Has flowered in god from all eternity
ANGELUS SILESIUS

Exuberant red peonies, sweet-smelling primroses, exotic lilies, cheerful calendulas, delicate anemones and wonderfully perfumed roses – just some of the flowers that we all know and cannot help but love. All over the world such flowers are part of human life, marking every important occasion, every change and ritual from the cradle to the grave. Today, as thousands of years ago, flowers are able to express what we often cannot find the words to say. As Wordsworth so aptly wrote, inspired by flowers as many a poet before and after him,

'To me the meanest flower that blows can give,
thoughts that do often lie too deep for tears.'

THE INSPIRATION OF FLOWERS

Flowers express joy at the birth of a child, and adorn ceremonies in every religion. They are exchanged between men and women as tokens of love, are presented on birthdays, and given to family and friends, hosts and honoured guests as a gesture of appreciation. It is hard to imagine visiting a relative or friend in hospital without bearing flowers to lift their spirits and speed them to health, or picture a wedding without flowers woven into bridal crowns and bouquets to enhance the beauty and romance of the occasion. Flowers grace our tables at celebratory meals and banquets, they brighten the house through every season and warm the heart, even on cold winter days when the rest of nature apparently sleeps. Flowers in garlands and wreaths at funerals comfort the bereaved and pay respect to the departed. They give universal pleasure, inspiring us to grow them to delight us in our gardens, pots and window-boxes.

Similarly, they have inspired artists and poets through the ages. Our soft furnishings, cosmetics, soaps and perfumes will invariably incorporate floral motifs or flowers. So will many of our medicines, for since the beginning of time we have used flowering plants to heal our ills.

Given the deep bond that exists between flowers and humankind, we may yet be unaware how they came to play such an important part in our lives. We appreciate their aesthetic beauty, their perfect form and often heavenly smell, but often forget the history of the flowers around us which dates back to antiquity. Flowers have featured in the beliefs, art and medicine of our ancestors for thousands of years. All over the world flowers have been part of myth and legend, worship and religion. They have become symbols of a whole range of human and spiritual experience, including love and remembrance, purity and fidelity, fertility and abundance, joy and sorrow, death and rebirth, mortality and immortality.

Since earliest times, when people lived so much closer to nature than we do now, flowers have been endowed with magical, supernatural or divine properties, and often with natures and temperaments much like their own. Just as human life was imbued with the divine spirit, so too flowers were seen to possess an in-dwelling spirit or soul which determined each shape and form, way or habit of growth, and purpose in the world in relation to human life.

The Ancient Greek myths are a vast storehouse of flower legend and symbolism, and we can look to them for the origin of many of our own floral customs and traditions. Classical Greece of about 2000 to 3000 years ago was the intellectual and literary centre of Europe and the land richest in flowers. The Ancient Greeks were also responsible for the origins of western medicine, the inspiration of which has survived in the writings of great physicians such as Hippocrates and Dioscorides, and those of their followers.

THE GREEK MYTHS

Anyone who visits the Greek countryside in spring today will witness the extraordinary wealth of native flowers. It is not hard to imagine the days when the mythical gods and

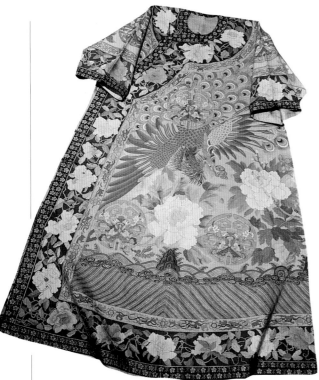

The silk phoenix robe of the 19th century Empress Dowager Tz'u hsi is decorated with peonies. In China the peony is considered the emperor of flowers, and has been grown there since around 900BC.

goddesses played on Mount Olympus and flowers were born into creation. The diversity and beauty of flowers and trees was an integral part of the spiritual lives of the Ancient Greeks. Their heroes, nymphs and deities were created alongside them as expressions of human archetypes and spiritual truths. To the Greeks nature itself was a religious symbol. The healing power of plants was a gift from the gods, and their beauty an inspiration to art. The innate character of specific plants leant meaning to and understanding of the reality of human and divine life. Temples and sacred places to worship and sacrifice to their gods were built in places of outstanding beauty, as ancient remains will testify. Flowers gave expression to a great deal of unconscious human and spiritual experience which would otherwise be difficult to communicate.

In those ancient days the Greeks would 'say it with flowers', and ever since those times flowers have been used to convey secret meanings, love and intimate messages, healing powers and religious significance.

A closer look at Greek mythology will reveal the symbolic meaning of some of the plants with which we are familiar today. Chloris (from chloe, meaning first green shoot and equivalent to the Latin Flora) was the goddess of flowers and personified spring. She carried out the wishes of Hera, and made plants grow with the help of Horae, daughters of Zeus and Themis, who reigned over the seasons and the cycle of growth. Chloris' lover was Zephyr, the god of the West wind who reawakened nature each spring. The nymphs of the springs took care of the plants and made sure they received vitalizing moisture from Oceanus, father of streams and rivers. Artemis, the moon goddess, revived the flowers each night with her refreshing dew, and her twin brother Apollo, the sun god, sent the sun's rays to make the plants live and grow in the daytime.

The fields and crops were the responsibility of Demeter, whose daughter Persephone was carried off by Hades, god of the underworld, to be his queen. She was imprisoned under the ground for half the year, throughout the winter, and returned to earth each spring. When Persephone was first captured, Demeter was inconsolable and searched for her daughter high and low until, exhausted, she sat down on a stone, where she stayed for nine days and nights.

During that time the gods caused poppies to grow up around her feet and Demeter breathed their heady scent and ate their narcotic seeds until she forgot her pain in the oblivion of sleep. Persephone symbolizes the corn seed hidden under ground, or in the earth, during winter, germinating in the spring, and then disappearing again with the coming of winter. She is sought by Demeter, goddess of harvest and agriculture. The poppies represent winter and sleep and their seeds represent fertility. When we eat bread decorated with poppy seeds we might bring to mind the allegorical story of Persephone and Demeter and the continual cycles of the seasons in earthly life.

Another story tells of the narcissus, which Gaia made grow to please Hades so that its sweet scent would entice Persephone into the underworld. Since the underworld symbolizes death, this relates to the custom of decorating graves with the bright daffodil in modern times. The name narcissus derives from the son of Cephisus, the river god, and Liriope, a forest nymph, called Narcissus. He was so beautiful that many a nymph fell in love with him, but he loved only himself. Aphrodite decided to punish him for this and made him fall in love with his reflection in a spring. He either slipped in and drowned, or pined away and died by the side of the water. Narcissus remained as a sweet-smelling spring flower crowned with gold which still leans over streams and rivers in search of its reflection in the water.

Daphne was a beautiful, shy young nymph, the daughter of Ladon the river god. Apollo, the sun god, was in love with her and amorously pursued her. So to escape him Daphne fled to her mother Gaia, who changed her into a laurel tree (*Laurus nobilis*). From then onward, the laurel was sacred to Apollo. When he killed the dragon Python he went into Delphi crowned as the conqueror with laurel branches, and thus the laurel became a symbol of respect, victory and fame, from which story originated the term laureate we commonly use today.

The elegant white myrtle flower with its lovely perfume and evergreen leaves was sacred to Aphrodite, the goddess of love, who hid her naked beauty behind a myrtle when she rose from the sea near Paphos in Cyprus. Myrtle thus became a symbol of beauty and youth, and is still commonly used today in wreaths and crowns to adorn brides.

Many of the flowers used for thousands of years for their medicinal virtues featured in the Greek legends, each story providing insight into their wonderful healing powers. Some of these legends are retold in the profiles of individual flowers in Chapter 2.

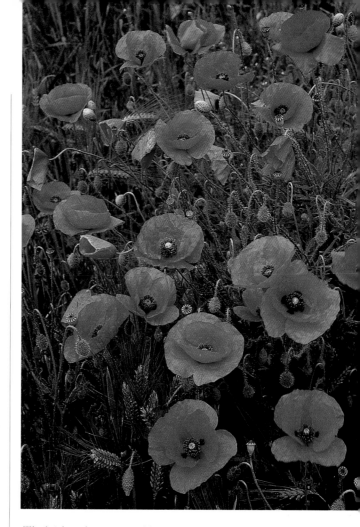

The bright red corn poppy likes to grow on disturbed land and according to a soldier's song, poppies appeared on the battle-fields of Flanders after the First World War. The British annually commemorate their war dead by wearing red poppies.

FLOWERS AND THE CYCLE OF LIFE

Flowers were also closely intertwined with the ancient concepts of life after death. In the gloomy regions of the Elysian fields presided over by Hades, the vast plains were covered with asphodels. These were planted on graves by the Greeks and Romans to symbolize eternal life. Flowers were believed in many cultures to grow in profusion in paradise or heaven; being spiritual in nature they were impervious to the destructive workings of time. Flowers were planted on tombs to aid the journey of the departed to the afterlife and symbolized the victory of the soul over earthly life. The dead were often buried in groves of sacred trees as the Greeks believed the souls delighted to walk amongst them. We still pay tribute to the dead with floral wreaths in the shape of a circle, designed originally to enclose the soul of the dead. The Ancient Egyptians crowned their dead with chaplets of flowers as a farewell gift and to ensure a safe journey. Graves of loved ones were also strewed with flowers such as myrtle, polyanthus and amaranth. Spring and summer flowers were placed on graves of those who had died in the bloom of youth and ancient trees and aromatic herbs were grown by graves of the elderly. White roses were planted on virgins' graves, while red roses were placed on graves of those who had led untarnished lives. Favourite funereal flowers included hyssop, sweet william, carnations and rosemary, as well as evergreens such as laurel and bay signifying eternal life.

Today mourners still favour rosemary, as well as roses, winter-flowering heather and aubretia. The snowdrop is an emblem of death, derived from the fact it appears to wear a shroud or burial robe. However, the snowdrop has also been seen as a symbol of life and hope. The story goes that when Adam and Eve were banished from the Garden of Eden, Eve stood sorrowfully looking at the flowerless earth around her covered with snow. An angel appeared, and catching a falling snowflake, blew on it and it was transformed into a snowdrop. As the angel handed the flower to Eve he told her to have hope as the summer was on its way, and as he left a ring of snowdrops appeared on the ground. Certainly as the first flowers to appear after the cold and apparent death of winter, the snowdrop is a very welcome sight.

I've brought some snowdrops; only just a few
But quite enough to prove the world awake,
Cheerful and hopeful in the frosty dew
And for the pale sun's sake.
CHRISTINA ROSSETTI (1830–1894)

Despite their apparent frailty and ephemeral nature, the beauty of flowers impart a lasting happiness. For a brief moment they seem to bring a touch of eternity, of joy that lies beyond the cares of the physical, mortal world.

The world's senseless beauty mirrors God's delight,
That rapture's smile is secret everywhere;
It flows in the wind's breath, in the tree's sap,
Its hued magnificence blooms in leaves and flower.
AUROBINDO GHOSE (1872–1950)

The poignancy of the brief life of the flower has influenced poets and artists alike, and has been used as a symbol of the transience of physical life, with a wider message to seize the hour before it passes. As the poet Robert Herrick said, 'Gather ye rosebuds while ye may, Old Time is still a flying.' At the same time flowers have represented a sense of eternity to others who have been inspired by this message from the flower world.

Though storms may break the Primrose on its stalk
Though frosts may blight the freshness of its bloom,
Yet spring's awakening breath will woo the earth
To feed with kindliest dews its favourite flower
That blooms in mossy banks and darksome glens,
Lighting the greenwood with its sunny smile;
Fear not then, spirit, Death's disrobing hand.
PERCY BYSSHE SHELLEY (1792–1822)

This is also expressed by Aurobindo Ghose: 'Earth's flowers spring up and laugh at time and death'.

To the Ancient Greeks the continual renewal of life in nature was seen as a manifestation of the mystery of the gods or the divine, and this gave sacred meaning to many plants and trees. The oak, the most majestic of all trees, was sacred to Zeus, whose wisdom was consulted at Dodona beneath a sacred oak. When the prayers of the believers were heard by Zeus, the tree was said to acknowledge this by rustling its leaves. The white poplar or aspen with its two-coloured leaves, was seen to symbolize the two worlds of the underworld and the living. Evergreens such as privet, laurel and olive were used in offerings to the Greek gods as symbols of permanence of the divine order.

FLOWERS AND THE LIFE OF THE SPIRIT

Since these classical times flowers have provided a perfect vehicle for the expression of religious ideas, concepts so intangible as to escape verbal communication. Throughout history they have expressed religious truths hidden within the great mysteries, and hinted at the divine nature of God. In the days of Christian persecution, floral emblems were used in art, literature or architecture as a secret form of communication.

In Ancient Egypt the lotus was a symbol of new life, while in Europe it represented the mystical centre of things. In the East the lotus was depicted springing from the navel of Vishnu, representing the universe evolving from a central sun. The lotus was the dwelling place of Brahma and the manifestation of his great power. With the coming of Christianity, flowers originally dedicated to Greek or Roman gods were assigned to saints, and churches were often built on the sites of pagan worship. Many flowers originally said to be ruled by Aphrodite or Venus became emblems of the Virgin Mary, the Christian symbol of female divinity or the goddess within.

The madonna lily is the flower most famously used in religious symbolism. It was originally used to illustrate the marvels of paradise; later it was frequently depicted in paintings in the hands of the Virgin Mary, where it signified purity and chastity, and does to this day. An angel carrying an olive branch in his hand represented a peacemaker; the rose originally and still is a symbol of earthly love, and was also an emblem of heavenly delight and the heart or mystic centre of being.

The rose
was not searching for the sunrise:
almost eternal on its branch,
it was searching for something else.
The rose
was not searching for darkness or science:
borderline of flesh and dream,
it was searching for something else.
    FEDERICO GARCIA LORCA (1899-1936)

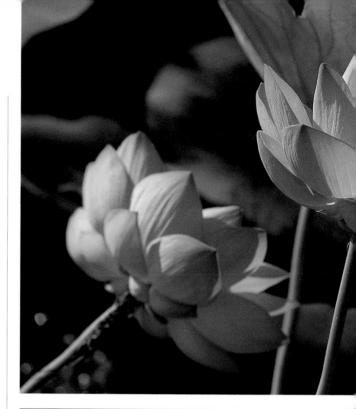

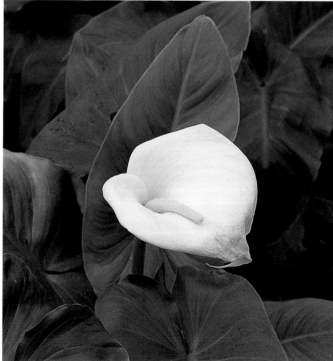

In Ancient Egypt the lotus (top) symbolized new life, while in the East it was said to be the dwelling place of Brahma and the manifestation of his great power. The madonna lily (bottom) was to early Christian artists a symbol of the marvels of paradise and the purity of the Virgin Mary.

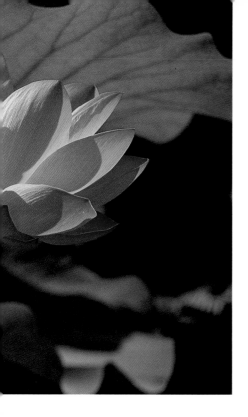

Flowers have been closely associated with the world of dreams. The ancients believed that dreams were communication from the world of spirits or of God's divine will, and their symbolic meaning was interpreted by magicians and diviners. The Ancient Egyptians believed that dreams were inspired by the goddess Isis. To dream of lavender, for example, meant a reunion, while calendula meant you will do well. Jasmine signified romance, daisy a birth and cowslip meant unexpected love.

FLOWERS ARE LOVE IN SEARCH OF A WORD

And what of flowers and love? Today, as ever, flowers express what we may not find the words to convey to the ones we love. The beautiful rose springs to mind as the flower most closely associated with love in most minds, whether of artist, poet or lover. 'My luve is like a red red rose' said Robert Burns, and Yeats wrote:

With the earth and the sky and the water
remade like a casket of gold
For my dreams of your image that blossoms
a rose in the depths of my heart.

When a medieval lady was called a 'rose' by her knight it was to convey that he considered her an exotically perfumed goddess of love, a delight to the eye and heart. The rose was the symbol of love, beauty and perfection, an emblem of the mystic heart of things. It was adopted by poets and artists to symbolize the perfect world – an ideal, or paradise. To ancient magicians a rose had other special meanings. If seven-petalled it represented the seven degrees of absolute perfection and if eight-petalled it meant regeneration or rebirth.

A posy was originally the name given to a poem which accompanied a bouquet of flowers given as a token of love. Several of the flowers commonly found in such bouquets were traditionally associated with love, since their mythical origins derived from love stories. Some flowers were said to grow from the blood or teardrops of sad lovers, or from beautiful girls fleeing

The trefoil, or shamrock, represented the Holy Trinity, and was used by St Patrick to illustrate the meaning of the true Godhead to the pagan Irish. The iris was a symbol of purity and majesty, the pink a flower of holy love, while jasmine was an emblem of the Virgin, also known as the star of divine hope. In a similar way flowers were used to represent evil and the forces of darkness and were used by witches and magicians in their spells.

The mystery of the flowers' growth and ephemeral yet continuous existence meant that flowers were believed to have many magical and supernatural qualities. Flowers such as hawthorn, clover, St John's wort, lavender and heather were believed, as they are today, to bring luck. Others, including anemone, peony, lily and St John's wort were used to protect against evil and the forces of darkness. Dandelions, daisies and calendulas, still a delight to children, were used not only as floral clocks, as their petals opened and closed at certain times each day, but also as love oracles. They revealed whether 'she loves me' or 'she loves me not' in a tradition that remains in many places today.

from advances of over-amorous lovers. Apollo fell in love with Hyacinthus, thereby arousing the jealousy of Zephyr, the wind god. One day when Apollo and Hyacinthus were playing quoits, Zephyr, in a jealous rage, threw one of the quoits and killed Hyacinthus. From his blood arose the flower that bears his name.

The rose, the most beautiful symbol of love, was created when Chloris, the Greek goddess of flowers, found the body of a beautiful nymph one day and asked the Three Graces to help her to make a special flower in honour of his beauty and her love. The tulip was once a young Dalmatian girl who was turned into a flower to avoid the advances of Vertuminus, the Roman god of the seasons. The forget-me-not, long an emblem of love and remembrance, derives its name from the German legend which tells of a knight and his lady walking along the banks of the river Danube. The lady caught sight of the pretty blue flower and as the knight leant by the water to pick it he lost his footing and fell into the river. As he drifted away to his death he was heard to say, 'forget me not'.

Flowers associated with courtship and marriage are designed to win the favour of the desired person and to symbolize the joy of their union. These were often plants associated with fertility, and aphrodisiacs for 'stirring up the passions'. Orchids, for example, were dedicated to Venus, the goddess of love and ruled by her. Satyrs of classical mythology were said to gorge themselves on the roots of orchids to excite the passions. In fact, one of the old names for orchids is satyrion. Such flowers were tradition-ally used in love potions or philtres to conquer the hearts of the desired man or woman. Pansies were a favourite; often they would be placed over the eyes of the loved one while asleep, to make him fall for the first person he saw on waking. Vervain was given by young girls to their lovers to keep their affections. Jasmine, roses and orange flowers were symbols of love and fertility, often used in garlands for the bride's head. Marjoram, basil, carnations, myrtle, and rosemary were similarly associated with love, weddings and fidelity. Many of the

flowers associated with marital union were climbing plants like jasmine, honeysuckle, clematis and ivy, which entwine themselves like a lover's arms.

THE LANGUAGE OF FLOWERS

The use of flower meanings or the language of flowers was a common form of communication in China, Egypt and India. It further developed in the harems of Turkey for illicit communica-tion between lovers and to idle away the hours. By the Elizabethan era Shakespeare was well versed in the significance of floral messages and obviously most of his audiences would have been familiar with his references and hidden meanings. In *A Midsummer Night's Dream* Oberon describes where Titania sleeps, using the symbolism of flowers to describe more than just a place of natural beauty.

I know a bank where the wild thyme blows
where oxslips and the nodding violet grows
Quite over-canopied with luscious woodbine
with sweet musk roses and with eglantine.

Thyme symbolized sweetness, oxslips meant comeliness, the violet 'love in idleness'; the rose represented love and eglantine (honeysuckle) meant united in love. In *Hamlet*, Ophelia says, 'There's rosemary, that's for remembrance; pray love remember; and there's pansies, that's for thoughts'.

The language of flowers was further developed in England by Lady Mary Wortley Montagu, an 18th century writer who during her extensive travels in Asia discovered some of the secrets of the harem. Around the same time Aubrey de la Mottraie, who accompanied Charles XII of Sweden during his exile in Turkey, popularized flower language in France. He wrote, 'fruit, flowers, and gold and silver thread ... have each of them their particular meaning explained by certain Turkish verses, which young girls learn by tradition of one another'. Writings in France were translated into German and the language of flowers gradually found its way to other parts of the world. It was

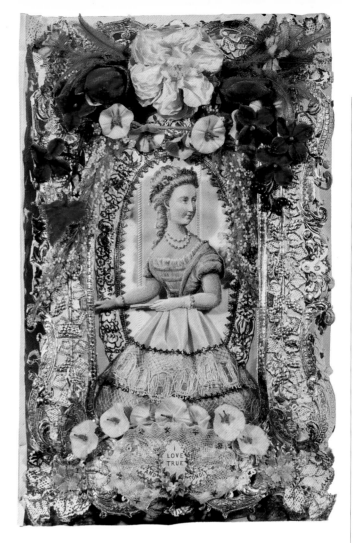

VICTORIAN LANGUAGE OF FLOWERS

Camellia: *perfect loveliness*
Candytuft: *indifference*
Gentian: *you are unjust*
Daffodil: *regard*
Passionflower: *faith*
Wallflower: *fidelity in adversity*
Hawthorn: *hope*
Broom: *ardour*
Clover: *happiness*
Carnation: *pure love*
Geranium: *comfort*
Hollyhock: *ambition*

A Victorian Valentine card conveying many hidden meanings through the popular language of flowers. The wallflowers here were often used in affairs of the heart to represent 'fidelity in adversity' and 'always true'.

developed into a popular art by the Victorians in Great Britain who expressed meaning in the colour and arrangement of the flowers as well as the choice of species. This was a source of great amusement and relief to many in the days when codes of courtship were extremely rigid, their reticence almost contrived. According to the rules, a gentleman was supposed to make the first move, although in reality this was prompted by a subtle indication of interest from the lady. Certain gestures accompanying floral gifts further detailed their messages. If the romantic young man wanted to convey thoughts about himself, he would pass the plant inclined to the left. If he wished to say something about her, he would incline the flower to the right. The answer to a floral question depended on the hand used. A flower presented with the right was positive, while if given with the left meant a refusal. A flower worn in the hair meant caution, but if worn across the heart it meant love. The language of flowers was beautifully expressed in Valentine cards fashionable in the Victorian era, which were a wonderful means of secret communication between sweethearts.

FLOWERS AND THE SOUL

There is something very healing about being with flowers which explains the worldwide love of growing flowers in gardens. A garden represents an enclosure, separate from the wildness of nature, a place of peace, a sanctuary. It is a symbol of the feminine in nature, a specially-devised womb for the conception and growth of living forces. Some might say it contains the secret of life itself. Many flowers were depicted in religious art in representations of the Garden of Eden, including the rose, the lily and the

15

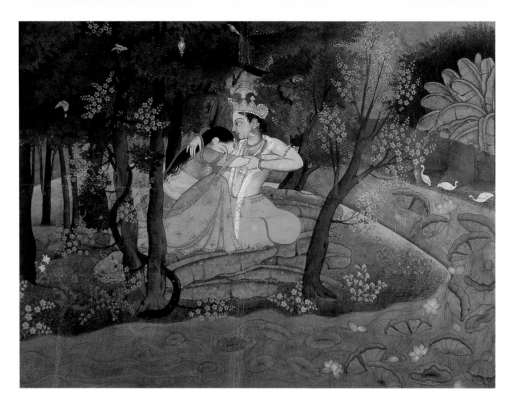

This 13th-century painting of Radhu and Krishna depicts an Indian idea of paradise – the Garden of Indra – where the gods relaxed among miraculous trees.

pink. Gardens in such art often represented sacred enclosures and feminine secrets.

A garden locked is my sister, my bride,
A garden locked is a fountain sealed.
Song of Solomon

Our ancestors planted certain flowers and trees to ward off intrusion by inharmonious spirits that threatened the garden's safety and tranquillity. Elder, apple, medlar and almond trees served such purposes, while flowers such as St John's wort, yarrow and angelica would protect against evil. To the psychologist the garden represents a sanctuary. It is a symbol of the unconscious mind, a sanctified enclosure, while a forest represents the primordial instinct struggling to overtake our efforts to be in control of our destiny. Those who enjoy their gardens will know a serenity that is hard to describe, a sense of joy and peace, a release from the trials and tensions of the working day, or everyday life. The garden can give us a glimpse of paradise. In fact the notion of paradise, or the Garden of Delight, is

to be found in nearly all ancient cultures. The Garden of Eden was in Judaism the first abode of the parents of mankind; Mount Olympus was the home of the Greek gods; while paradise or heaven is the place of peace in Christianity for the spirits of the blessed dead. The Garden of Indra is where Indian gods relaxed among miraculous trees, bright-coloured flowers and fruits that conferred immortality.

Paradise is a word in ancient Persian meaning garden or park, and poets and artists have made use of this image to conjure up a sense of heaven, supreme bliss, the divine. In China and Japan, from the times of the ancient civilizations to the present day, gardens have been developed to great heights of artistic creation and tranquillity. They are famous for their planting of exotic flowers, quiet pools and streams, bridges, fountains and pagodas to provide refreshment and inspiration. Enjoyed today by young and old, *hanami* or flower-viewing is an integral part of Japanese people's appreciation of beauty in nature, as well as being an important aspect of their social life. Cherry blossom time is the most favoured by the Japanese but they also find symbolic beauty in many other flowers and trees, such as the pine, maple, bamboo, plum, narcissus, willow, peony and iris. By their exquisite painting and flower arranging the Japanese capture, with a few seasonal blossoms, the essence of nature at a particular time of year and bring into their homes the flavour of beauty outside that is not always possible to see in its natural habitat. Thus, their everyday life is enhanced by living with the spirit of the season, and depending on the flowers used, flower arrangement is a mystical rite which confers upon the arranger special powers and virtues.

Flowers have I seen and honey have I tasted
and heard the cuckoo's song through to the end.
Now in this world or in the next, dear friend,
I shall forever know life was not wasted.
17TH CENTURY JAPANESE POEM

In Japan, a bride is given the name 'flower daughter' by her husband's family. In other traditions, gardens and flower lore have deeply influenced our language and thinking. We talk about the seeds of love, the budding of romances, a family tree, the blossoming of a child into adulthood, or of a girl into a woman. The word flower has frequently been used to describe places – the ancient Middle Kingdom of China was called the flowery kingdom, while great historical figures have also been referred to in floral language. The legendary King Arthur of England was the flower of kings, Geoffrey Chaucer was the flower of poets. Flowers are also used to describe personalities: the wallflower, the shrinking violet, or someone who is narcissistic – all epithets springing from the ancient symbolism of flowers.

Flowers touch our lives in ways that bring healing of infinite and indefinable measure. Imbued with philosophical, religious and symbolic meaning, they unite us with the rest of humanity, which has gazed upon the same flowers from which we derive meaning and pleasure today. They connect us to true beauty which is infinite, and enable us to become part

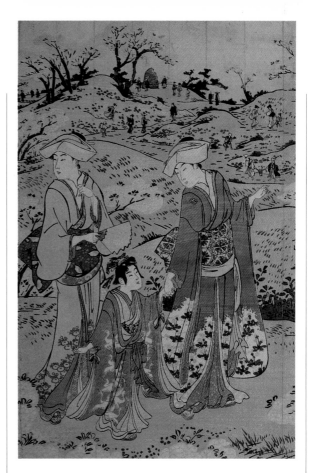

VIEWING THE CHERRY BLOSSOM AT ASUKAYAMA by Torii Kiyinaga (1753–1815). Flower-viewing, or hanami, *is an integral part of the Japanese people's appreciation of beauty.*

of this infinitude through our connection with flowers in everyday life. A flower contains all the elements of nature: ether, air, water, fire and earth. It has form, colour, texture and fragrance and still something more – an indefinable and mysterious quality, the vibrations of something that is abstract, pure and perfect. It is the form behind which is pure consciousness, the sound, the all-powerful creative mantra, the word, the womb of creation. It is for these almost inexplicable reasons that flowers are loved by men, women and children alike, and have the power to heal us on all levels of our being.

Little flower – but if I could understand
What you are, root and all, and all in all,
I should know what God is and man is.
ALFRED, LORD TENNYSON (1809–92)

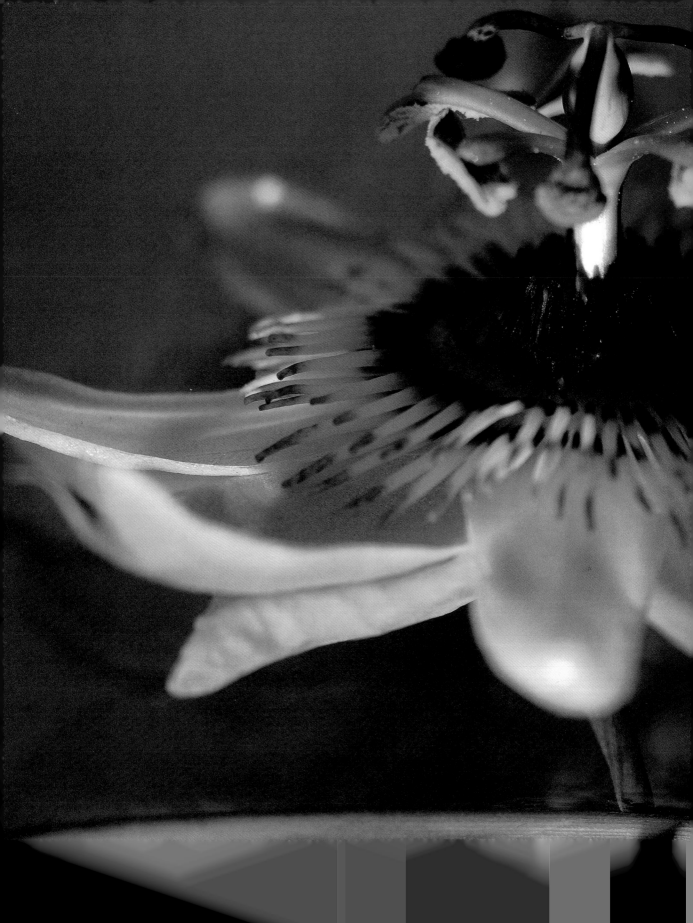

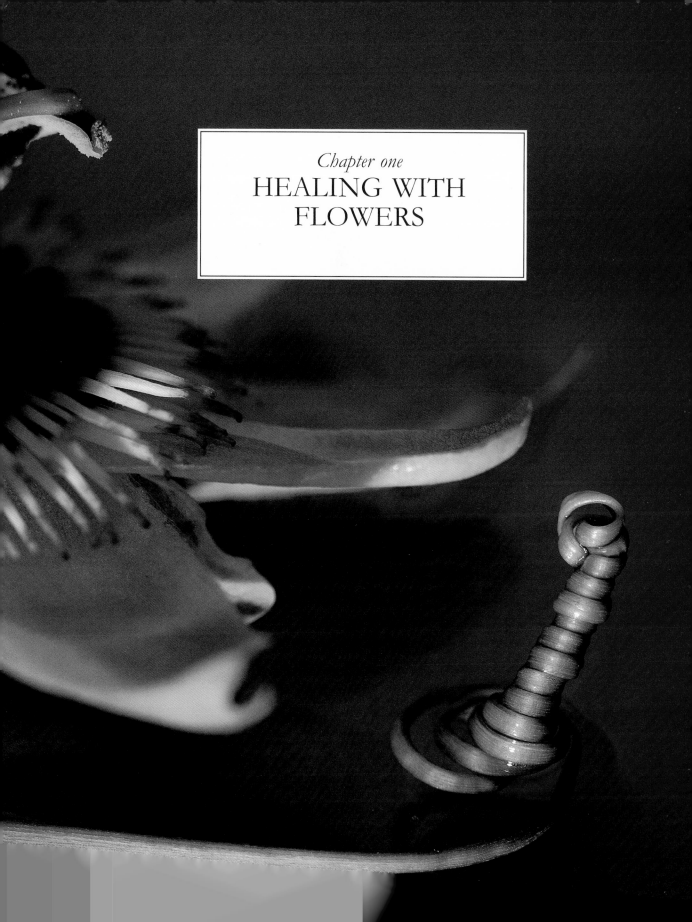

Chapter one
HEALING WITH
FLOWERS

Healing with Flowers

*If a man would pass through Paradise in a dream
and have a flower presented to him as a pledge
that his soul had really been there, if he
found that flower in his hand when he awoke.
Aye, and what then?*
    SAMUEL TAYLOR COLERIDGE (1772–1834)

The world of flowers with its extraordinary
repertoire of vibrant colour, beautiful intricate
patterns, and alluring scent brings more than a
touch of paradise to our earthly lives. It also
brings the possibility of healing on both physical
and non-physical levels of existence. True health
depends on the harmony of body, mind and
spirit, and is (as defined by the World Health
Organization) 'the condition of perfect bodily,
spiritual and social wellbeing and not solely the
absence of illness and injury'.

Plants and flowers have long been associated
with healing, not only for our physical ills but
also imbalances in the realms of the mind and
the spirit that may give rise to bodily symptoms.
As Dr Bach said, 'disease of the body itself is
nothing but the result of the disharmony
between the soul and mind'... 'health is
therefore the true realisation of what we are;
we are perfect; we are children of God.'

THE UNITY OF ALL THINGS

People throughout the world have always
associated flowers with spirituality, irrespective
of their religion. Mystics have referred to the
spiritual forces of flowers and trees and often
described them as angels, beings of light, or
devas, responsible along with the creator for
human existence and continued growth. May
Day celebrations, with dancing round the maypole, are pagan rituals performed yearly in honour of the spirit of trees and the fertile blooming of nature in spring. Native Americans have
always believed in the spirit of the earth and the
world of plants. In 1855, Young Chief of the

Cayuses said, 'the Ground says, it is the
Great Spirit that placed me here. The Great
Spirit tells me to take care of the Indians, to
feed them aright'. And Chief Luther Standing
Bear said, 'the man who sat on the ground in
his tipi meditating on life and its meaning,
accepting the kinship of all creatures and
acknowledging unity with the universe of
things was infusing into his being the true
essence of civilization.' Likewise the holistic
approach to healing is based on the concept of
this perfect unity of all things.

THE EARTH AS GAIA

The idea that nature was alive, animated by the
same spirit or vital force as humans and everything in creation, was in fact the standard
accepted view until the scientific revolution in
the 17th century. Subsequently, people began to
regard nature as completely inanimate and
unconscious, made solely of matter in motion.

Now, in the latter part of the 20th century,
'new' hypotheses and perceptions from the scientific world are seeing nature as alive and ani-
mate, even conscious. James Lovelock in his
Gaia hypothesis perceives the earth as an
infinitely complex living and evolving entity,
'involving the earth's biosphere, oceans and
soils, the totality constituting a feedback or
cybernetic system, which seeks an optimal physical or chemical environment for life on this
planet.' Just like the human organism, it possesses the inherent power to protect, regulate, adjust
and heal itself and thereby maintain 'homeostasis'. Gaia was the Greek goddess of the earth,
who created the universe and gave birth to the
race of gods and the first human beings.

New theories of quantum physics are now
recognizing that all forms of existence have the
same nature and that although they may appear
solid and separate from each other, they are in
fact simply energy vibrating at different frequen-
cies. Mind energy which vibrates so fast that it

*The evening primrose opens its fragrant flowers at
dusk, attracting night-flying moths which pollinate
them. The flowers' opening and closing symbolized
inconstancy and silent love in the language of flowers.*

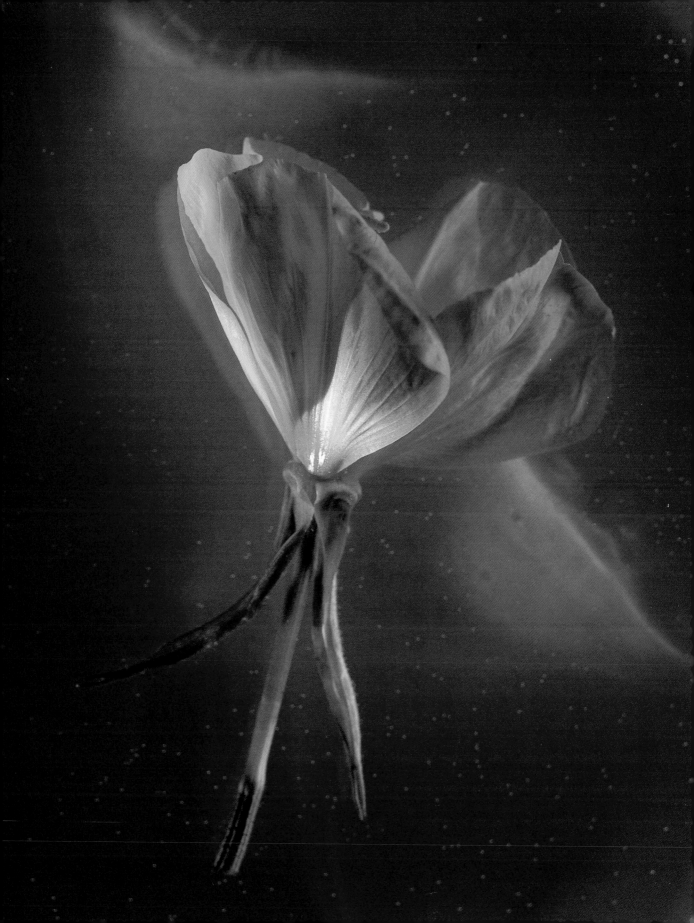

appears invisible is therefore not so different from a flower, or a tree, or even a rock that vibrates so slowly we may not recognize its essential dynamism. This may go a long way to explaining the deep connection we feel to the plant world. It is not to be wondered at, because we have lived side by side with plants since the dawning of our existence, been fed and clothed by them, sheltered and housed by them. They provide the oxygen we breathe and for thousands of years have given us medicines for almost every ill. By trapping the sun's energy through photosynthesis, they enable solar or life energy, on which all life depends, to be accessible to every inhabitant of the earth.

By resonating with us at all speeds of vibration, from the spiritual to the material, plants have the potential to heal us on every level of our being. Yet this is not all; something about flowers is particularly special, as if they express the essential nature of all flowering plants and convey their messages to us in all their variation of purpose. They are vital to the plant's survival and represent the peak of plants' evolution.

THE ROLE OF FLOWERING PLANTS

The first organisms were single-celled bacteria living in the sea. Then came algae, which are believed to be the ancestors of all other plants, followed by fungi, mosses and lichens. Ferns, taller plants and then trees such as giant horsetails came next, followed about 200 million years ago by plants bearing seeds known as gymnosperms – of which the wonderful ginkgo tree is a living example, as are conifers.

Flowering plants, botanically known as angiosperms, evolved about 140 million years ago, the earliest of them probably resembling a magnolia tree. In botanical terms a flower represents a reproductive structure made up of modified leaves which attract insects and a variety of other small creatures in order to ensure their cross-fertilization and reproduction, and hence their survival. This was a far more sophisticated means of reproduction than had gone before. The cones of conifers have sperm cells packed tightly in pollen grains relying on the wind to blow them to the ovules of female cones. Spores of fungi and mosses are also vulnerable to the vagaries of the wind. More than 80 per cent of all green plants are flowering plants and every flower has the same purpose, to ensure that male pollen grains from the stamens of one flower come into contact with the stigma of a female pistil.

The intricacies of nature are amazing in their perfection. The stigma produces special secretions making sure that no pollen from other species than its own germinates, and once the right pollen has germinated it extends a tube into the stigma down its style and makes contact with the ovary below, where two male pollen cells fertilize three female cells. An embryo is thereby produced with a food store wrapped up neatly in a seed capsule, and primed to spark into life once in favourable conditions.

The beautiful colours and shades of flowers, their enormous variety of shape, size and pattern, as well as their wonderful perfumes, are all developed to attract specific pollinators – insects, birds, moths, beetles, even snails. The evolutionary links between the form, colour, nectar and scent of flowers and the sensory perceptions of their pollinators is truly fascinating. One of the earliest pollinators was the beetle, which crawled into primitive flowers to eat pollen, distributing grains around the area and enabling self-pollination. More evolved species of flowers developed nectar-secreting glands to attract flying insects that would brush against the pollen and so carry it to other flowers.

Flowers with tubular shapes developed simultaneously with those insects and birds with a sucking proboscis sufficiently long to reach the nectar. Some flowers, such as antirrhinums, will only open when the right size pollinator lands on its lower lip. In some flowers patterns such as lines or spots on the petals, as seen in horse chestnut and eyebright, point the way to the nectar to the hungry insect. Scents wafting through the air will attract pollinating insects from huge distances, as will bright colours to those with good sight. Some flowers only emit their scents at night when their colour fades;

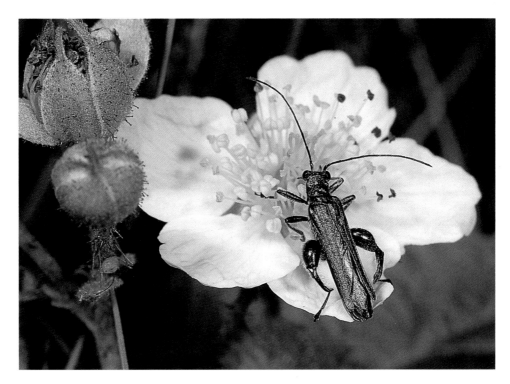

The beautiful colours and shapes of flowers, their size, patterning and perfumes, have evolved to attract specific pollinators. This beetle is eating wild raspberry pollen.

many, including evening primrose, open only at night to attract night-flying moths.

Flowers ensure the continuation of their species and therefore their survival. Flowering plants make up 80 per cent of all plants on the planet, and we depend on plants for our survival. So flowers are absolutely essential to all human life. Not only do flowers convey messages to their pollinators, but the early herbalists believed that flowering plants had messages regarding their healing virtues in their shape, colour, form and pattern. Certainly the delicate drooping blooms of the purple pasque flower intimate the sad drooping head of the nymph Anemone, forsaken by her lover, Zephyr the Greek god of the West wind. This points towards the flower's famous healing ability in women feeling similarly forsaken and forlorn when taken as a homeopathic remedy. The bright blue star-shaped borage flower by contrast has a much more uplifting nature, gladdening the heart and bringing courage to those who take it or even look at it. Borage has been used by herbalists for thousands of years to help alleviate depression and protect the body from the effects of stress.

The healing potential of flowering plants is an integral part of the deep bond that exists between humans and nature. That flowers have the ability to heal us, not only physically but also emotionally and spiritually, is something that has been recognized and utilized as far back as we know. Now, in the 20th century, with evidence of the healing role of flowers going back 60,000 years, we are still striving to understand the totality of their significance in our lives.

Flowers have been used in many different ways, in various herbal preparations, as essential oils, homeopathic remedies and flower essences. Each system of medicine claims a certain mode of action or vibrational level of healing for its own. One thing is clear from the flowers' history of healing, set out in the pages to come: the essence of the flower that permeates every remedy has the same healing potential that permeates the essence of our being.

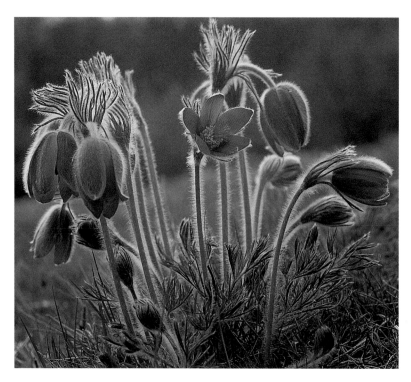

The delicate purple pasque flower with its drooping silken head intimates that of the sad nymph Anemone, when forsaken by her lover, Zephyr the Greek god of the West wind.

The history of floral healing

A brief journey through the history of the use of flowering plants in healing will serve to clarify our debt to nature and the circle which this evolutionary journey is forming. The story starts long ago on Mount Olympus where the Greek gods played among the vegetation that was the green canopy of the world, creating flowers and trees to be of service to both the gods and living mortals. Asclepius was the god of healing, symbolized by the image of the serpent, which itself represents the renewal of energy and renovation. The serpent had the power to discover healing plants as it slid along the undergrowth. Asclepius was the son of Apollo, the sun god, and had learnt his healing arts from Chiron the centaur in his cave. Chiron was the wise teacher of other famous Greek heroes, including Jason the Argonaut and Petenus, Achilles' father. So say the myths of classical Greece – when people believed that healing was a gift of the gods who alone understood the nature of plants.

The Ancient Greeks had many delightful stories in their mythology which explained how their healing plants came into being and how they could be used. These clearly illustrate the close relationship that has always existed between plants and human life and the great respect the ancients had for the plant world, so much so that many were held sacred and worshiped as attributes of the gods.

We can trace the link between human life and healing herbs and flowers to Neanderthal man. In 1963 archeologists opened a grave of a man in a cave made 60,000 years ago in Iraq. He had been buried along with many flowers. Grains of flower pollen there were analysed and found to include the distinctive pollen of cornflower, horsetail, hollyhock, St Barnaby's thistle, yarrow, grape hyacinth and ephedra. These flowers were no doubt present at the burial not only for their aesthetic value but also for their symbolic and healing virtues. Amongst these flowers there were diuretics, emetics, astringents, stimulants and pain relievers.

THE ORIGINS OF HERBAL MEDICINE

It is hard to know exactly how the ancients used flowers for healing in prehistoric times, before the time of writing and keeping records. However, we do know that as long ago as 3000BC schools of herbal medicine existed in Egypt. Imhotep was the first known physician there, who served Zoser, a 3rd dynasty pharaoh in around 2980BC. Imhotep was renowned as an astrologer, magician and healer and was elevated in the minds of people as the god of healing. Like the Greek gods, the Egyptian gods played an important role in early Egyptian medicine. Osiris was the god of vegetation and both his twin sister Isis and his mother had the power to renew life and gave their secrets of healing to mankind. The Ebers Papyrus, written around 2000BC, describes symptoms and their treatments using 85 herbs such as castor oil, dill, lettuce, senna, mint, gentian and poppy. Aromatic herbs such as myrrh, cumin, coriander and balm of Gilead were used for fumigation. The Egyptians placed flower wreaths in the tombs of mummies and planted flower gardens near the tombs.

Meanwhile in China, the *Pen T'sao* by Shan Xiang dating from 2800BC lists 366 plant medicines used at the time including ephedra. In Babylon, around 1800BC, King Hammurabi recorded on stone tablets information about plants used for healing, which included henbane, mint and licorice. Merodach Baladin, King of Babylon around 720BC, was known to have grown 70 different herbs in his garden including thyme, coriander and saffron. Tablets from the library of Assurbanipal, King of Assyria 668–626BC, show that 250 herbs were used for healing including turmeric, myrrh, poppy, almond, sesame and cumin.

The recorded use of herbs in the great civilizations including China, Egypt, Mesopotamia, Greece and India shows remarkable similarities, indicating considerable exchange of plants at this time. There was also a cross-fertilization of ideas, as the early herbalists sought answers to questions about the workings of the human body and the mysteries of the universe.

The first herbalists of every culture are known as shamans – men or women who had a particular gift for healing, whose instincts were raised to a highly intuitive level through years of training to develop their inner eye. This deeper perception enabled them to communicate directly with the plant world and the world of the spirit, which may explain some of the personification of plants or vice versa in Greek mythology and other ancient cults. These healers were also called priest physicians, since health of the body was not separated from that of mind and spirit as it was much later in the history of medicine.

Hallucinatory and mind-altering plants were traditionally used by the priest physicians. Incense and aromatic plants were also burned at religious rituals as tools of transformation to help transport the minds of the participants to another dimension – this was the origin of modern aromatherapy. The gods, on whom all human life was considered to depend, were honored in temples with incense and aromatic plants, since the gods were deemed particularly partial to fragrant smokes. In the cult of Asclepius priest physicians used recipes of therapeutic perfumes and incense to enhance the psychological and physical wellbeing of their patients. They used aromatic herbs such as rosemary, pine and thyme for fumigation to ward off infection and negative influences such as sorcery and evil.

THE ORIGINS OF GREEK MEDICINE

The celebrated Hippocrates (468–377BC) was the first important medical thinker that we know about, and is known as the 'father of medicine' (of the western tradition). In Greece, Hippocrates began to establish a scientific and yet holistic basis for medicine, relying less on magic and ritual and basing his treatments on results. He is recorded as using around 400 herbs as well as advocating the importance of fresh air, exercise and good diet. He saw that all matter could be explained by the five basic elements: ether, air, fire, water and earth. The individuality of people was explained by the four humours arising from these elements: blood, phlegm, choler and melancholy. The proportions of these humours in each person would determine his or her personality and body type.

The element water corresponded to phlegm and a phlegmatic temperament. Phlegm had a cold and damp nature, epitomized by the season of winter, and gave rise to illnesses such as catarrh, respiratory infections, overweight and fluid retention. Warming and drying herbs such as thyme, hyssop and ginger were used to clear cold and damp symptoms and thereby restore the balance of the humours.

Earth corresponded to the melancholic humour or temperament, black bile and the season of autumn. It had a cold and dry nature, giving rise to symptoms such as constipation, arthritis, depression or anxiety. Warming herbs such as ginger and senna would be used to clear black bile and restore balance.

The element air corresponded to blood and the sanguine temperament, epitomized by the season of spring. A sanguine type would be easy-going and good humoured, but prone to excesses and over-indulgence, giving rise to problems such as gout and diarrhoea. Cool, dry herbs such as burdock or figwort were used to balance the humours.

Lastly, fire corresponded to choler, or yellow bile, related to summer. A choleric type would be hot-tempered and prone to liver and digestive problems. Cooling and moistening herbs such as dandelion, violets and lettuce would help to balance the excess heat and dryness of the choleric temperament.

Hippocrates thus perceived that illness was not a punishment of the gods, as believed by his forefathers, but arose from imbalances of the elements that composed everything in nature. His humoral theory was paralleled in both China, which has a similar five-element theory, and in India's Ayurvedic medicine. In Ayurveda, the five elements of matter relate directly to the three basic constitutional types, or *doshas*. These are *vata* (air and ether), *pitta* (water and fire) and *kapha* (earth and water). In each system the foods and herbs used in treatments would be dictated by the predominant humour, element or *dosha*, so they became subject to the same classifications. (See pages 35–37.)

Another famous Greek physician was Theophrastus (372–286BC), who was both a friend and pupil of Aristotle. Theophrastus inherited Aristotle's garden and library, and wrote *Enquiry into Plants,* the first important herbal to survive until today. He listed 500 healing plants and describes the properties of oils and spices, basing much of his work on Aristotle's botanical writings which expanded much of Hippocrates' work. He established himself as a scientific botanist and his work has been referred to throughout history and remains an interesting and valuable source of information. We know from him, for example, that bay-laurel was used to produce a trance-like state and that roses, coriander and myrtle were used as aphrodisiacs.

A further great source of herbal knowledge derives from the Alexandrian school. Alexandria was named in honour of the Greek Emperor Alexander the Great, around 330BC. The school enabled Greek medicine to flourish – it drew on Greek herbal knowledge as well as Egyptian, Sumerian and Assyrian healing traditions and included knowledge brought back from the emperor's campaigns in Asia. The strong traditions developed here survived into medieval Europe through the writers and scholars of the Arab world.

Galen (131–201AD), another notable Greek physician, studied at the Alexandrian school and became renowned as surgeon to the gladiators in Rome, and personal physician to Emperor Marcus Aurelius (121–180AD). In his herbal *De Simplicibus* he expanded on Hippocrates' philosophy and his classification of herbs into the four humours. His works became the standard medical text of Rome and later of Arab physicians and medieval monks. His theories are still clearly to be found in Unani medicine today.

The famous herbal written by Dioscorides can still be seen today and this provided the major source of herbal knowledge for the next 1500 years. It has been copied and quoted in all the herbals that followed right up to the present day. Pedanius Dioscorides from Anazarb in Cilicia was a Greek physician serving with the Roman Emperor Nero's army, allowing him to travel extensively in Asia Minor. Around 60AD he set himself the enormous task of collating all the current knowledge on medicinal plants and healing substances in one work: *De Materia Medica*. It included discussion of the components of perfumes and their medicinal properties; aromatic herbs used for these included balm, basil, coriander, fennel, garlic, hyssop, marjoram, mint, myrtle, rosemary and violet.

The Roman armies were responsible for the spread of herb lore and plants around Europe – the madonna lily, for example, was taken from camp to camp and used as a wound herb. Garlic was similarly valued for its antiseptic and strengthening properties. The Romans also developed the use of aromatic flowers and herbs for perfumes and fragrant oils which played a central role in their bathing rituals – almonds, quinces and roses were among their favourites. As in Greece and Egypt, such perfumes and oils were commonly used for basic hygiene, to oil the skin and hair to keep it healthy, and to mask unpleasant odours when water was scarce and washing infrequent.

Pliny the Elder, also known as the 'worthy Pliny' (23–79AD), was a Roman naturalist who collected together herbal knowledge, often unreliably, for a sort of universal encyclopedia known as the *Naturalis Historia*. This appeared in Rome in 77AD.

Under the Romans, however, the attitude to herbs began to change. The Catholic papacy grew more powerful and the early Christians, feeling that the church rather than the physicians should be responsible for health of mind and soul, started to repress the use of many 'pagan' herbs. In 529AD, Pope Gregory the Great ruled that learning which was not in accordance with the political ambitions of the papacy should be forbidden. Thus, during the Dark Ages (roughly 200–800AD) knowledge of herbs and the use of the great herbals was pushed under ground, and scientific research and writing in Europe came to a halt.

GREEK AND ARAB TRADITIONS

However, the highly sophisticated Arab culture of the time happily maintained and developed the healing legacy of the Greeks, merging it with their ancient folk medicine and what survived of the Egyptian tradition. By 900AD all surviving Greek herbal and botanical texts were translated into Arabic in the cultural centres of Cairo, Damascus and Baghdad. When Arab armies invaded North Africa and Spain they took with them their knowledge of healing plants and medicine. A succession of renowned Arab physicians including Albucasis, Razis and Avicenna were particularly responsible for the development of medicine at this time, adding their own inventions and discoveries to the sum of herbal and botanical knowledge.

Avicenna (980–1037AD) brought together all that was available on the nature of disease, plant medicine, aromatics and medical theories in his *Canon Medicinae*. It was Avicenna who developed the process of distillation which had originated in the Alexandrian school in the 3rd century. He invented the apparatus and method of alembic distillation to extract essential oils from aromatic plants – a great landmark in the history of aromatherapy. Fragrant oils were particularly used for their purifying and restorative properties at this time, and were thought to make destructive emotions such as grief and fear have less of an impact on the health of the body.

The Greek and Arabic traditions were revived in medieval Europe through two major routes. In Toledo in Spain (Christian since 1085) a body of translators established a school and translated herbal texts from Arabic to Romance (old French) and then into Latin. In Italy, Constantine 'the African' (1020–1087) became a Benedictine monk and spent many of the last years of his life translating Arabic texts into Latin. The great medical schools of the Middle Ages blossomed from this time on. The famous school at Salerno, for example, made great use of Constantine's translations. The school at Montpelier was founded by Gerald of Cremona (1114–87), who had translated Avicenna's work which was used as a standard text for students.

Crusaders returning from the Middle East also brought back ancient knowledge that had been lost to Europe during the Dark Ages.

MEDIEVAL MONASTERIES

Throughout medieval Europe, the teachings of Hippocrates and Dioscorides in particular were kept safe and alive in Christian monasteries. Monks copied and recopied manuscripts in many languages, translating them from other languages including Arabic and exchanging their works with other monasteries and countries. However, throughout the medieval period observation and empirical knowledge and techniques were very limited. As in the days of the early Greeks, healing involved as much prayer as medicine, which was often administered with incantations and supplications.

Outside the monasteries, Anglo-Saxon healers, such as the renowned physicians of Myddfai, were still using herbs in traditional ways and some manuscripts from those times have survived, the best known being the *Leech Book of Bald*. This was compiled around 950 by a scribe Cild, under the direction of Bald, apparently a friend of King Alfred, and was one of the few texts not to be based on the Greek herbals. Herbs such as vervain, plantain, lungwort, wood betony and yarrow were popular in Anglo-Saxon times to remedy physical illnesses and to ward off the evil eye. The 'perfumes of Arabia' as essential oils were known were popular both for their aesthetic pleasure and to use in fragrant rubs for aches and pains, and for fumigation to protect against disease, particularly the plague. Pomanders, scent boxes and 'tussie mussies' (herb posies) were carried for this purpose. Fragrant herbs were strewn in halls of dwellings and castles, wherein, it must be remembered, as many animals as people lived.

Herb and flower gardens came into their own in the grounds of European abbeys and monasteries in the Middle Ages. Particularly memorable is the beautiful poem written by a monk called Walafrid Strabo around 840. He was tutor to Charles, the son of Charlemagne's

successor Louis the Pious and later Bishop of Richenau (the home of another famous medical school). 'Hortulus', meaning the little garden, tells of the changing seasons and serenity of the monastery garden and its herbs and flowers: *Who can describe the exceeding whiteness of the lily? The rose, it should be crowned with pearls of Arabia and Lydian gold. Better and sweeter are these flowers than all other plants and rightly called the flower of flowers.*

With the dawning of the Renaissance the Golden Age of Herbals began, originally with translations and adaptations of former great works, culminating in beautiful herbals adorned with botanical drawings. An increasing number of exotic herbs and spices were arriving from the East and the Americas. The arrival of William Caxton's printing press further revolutionized and spread the thinking of the time and increased the number of herbals available. Many new herbals were compiled, reflecting the theories not only of Hippocrates and Galen but also of Paracelsus. These included theories of planetary influence, current magic and superstition and the doctrine of signatures.

THE DOCTRINE OF SIGNATURES

The doctrine of signatures was first expounded by a German, Theophrastus Bombastus von Hohenheim, born in 1493 and better known by his alchemical name, Paracelsus. The theory probably originated much earlier as is indicated in early literature. It was based on the premise that the Creator had provided guidance for humans looking for remedies for their ills by imprinting on herbs certain outward signs.

The spotted leaves of lungwort, resembling the lungs, was therefore indicated for pulmonary ailments; walnuts looked like the head and the brain and were therefore considered good for enhancing mental activity; hepatica with leaves resembling the three lobes of the liver acquired a wide reputation for curing liver problems. Pilewort or lesser celandine has root tubers looking rather like haemorrhoids and was used to treat them; flowers with milky juice were considered to promote copious supply of breast-

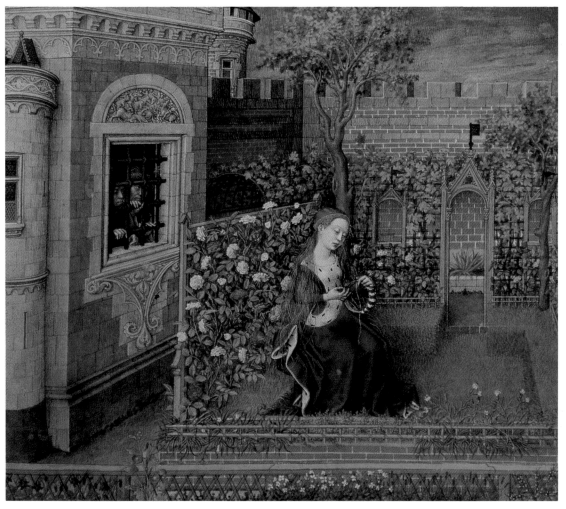

EMILIA IN HER GARDEN from the Hours of the Duke of Burgundy *(1454–55),*
illustrating the medieval walled garden which in early Christianity symbolized chastity.

milk in feeding mothers and plants containing red juice were used to purify the blood. The leaves of beetroot with their branching red veins signified a cure for the heart and circulation. Plants with yellow juice resembling bile were used to treat complaints of the liver.

In the late Middle Ages and early Renaissance herbalists searching for meaning and unifying principles between nature and humankind delighted in reading great significance into such resemblances. Paracelsus, despite his obscure way of writing, developed a large following. If any herb valued for its medicinal virtues was not imprinted with a clear sign from God, it would be considered the will of God intent on testing the skill of the herbalist in matching the plant to the complaint! Some of these apparently quaint ideas actually contained more than a grain of truth and have remained applicable to the present day. Many herbs with yellow juice, such as greater celandine and dock, make valuable remedies for the liver and gall-bladder. St John's wort, with little oil glands on the leaves that resemble tiny perforations and signify its use for cuts and wounds, is in fact a wonderful remedy for healing the skin and stopping bleeding.

In the 16th and 17th centuries, several herbalists supported the doctrine of signatures, notably William Cole, who was born in 1626 in Oxfordshire and educated at New College, Oxford. He took up the study of botany and became the most celebrated herbalist of his day. His books, *The Art of Simpling* and particularly *Adam in Eden or Nature's Paradise*, indicate his independent character and originality, and his repudiation of beliefs in any planetary influence. Another renowned work was that of Mattiolus, *Commentaries on the six books of Dioscorides* in 1565. Mattiolus was a flamboyant Italian scholar and physician who attended several European courts.

The classic century of herbals was really established with William Turner's *A New Herball* in 1551 and included the works of John Gerard, a barber-surgeon, John Parkinson and Nicolas Culpeper. Turner was the first Englishman to study and classify plants scientifically and like Theophrastus centuries before, he was known as the father of botany. He is memorable for having written in English so that his work was available to the apothecaries and women of the household who gathered herbs, and not simply the physicians who were educated in Latin.

More popular, however, is John Gerard's *The Herball* printed in 1597. Although much of his knowledge and writing derived from the Dutch physician to Maximilian II and Rudolf II, Rembert Dodoens (1517–1585), it is a large repository of knowledge of the time, quoted time and again in herbals of the 20th century. Gerard loved herbs and flowers and apparently grew 1000 varieties in his riverside garden in Holborn, London.

John Parkinson was also a great enthusiast and produced a vast and lovingly illustrated 'flower book' called *Paradisi in sole Paradisus Terrestris* in 1629. The title is a pun on his own name: Park-in-sun's Earthly Paradise. He had his own garden at Long Acre and was apothecary to James I of England and later wrote a less flowery book, a herbal called *Theatrum Botanicum* (1640) which dealt with 3800 plants.

Nicolas Culpeper, born 1616, the famous and controversial apothecary and herbalist, based much of his herbal treatment and classification of herbs on the laws of astrology. This was nothing new – since the time of Hippocrates physicians had studied astronomy and the influence of the stars. He was a colourful and revolutionary character, full of scorn for the money-grabbing tendencies of many contemporary doctors, and was daring enough to translate the Latin pharmacopeia into English, and provide free treatment for the poor. Even in his own time Culpeper was severely criticized by more orthodox writers such as Cole, but it will gratify many that Culpeper's *Herbal* has run and run since the 17th century and still appears in bookstores to this day.

THE DAWNING OF THE SCIENTIFIC AGE

After this period of medical history, things began to change. Paracelsus was one of those responsible for the sowing the seeds of this transformation. He publicly burned the books of Hippocrates and Galen, rejecting their ideas of humoral medicine and planetary influence. He preferred to use individual preparations, including small doses of metals, to treat specific diseases. Paracelsus then was a propounder of the 'like curing like' method of healing, perceiving that a poison that caused a disease could, in minute doses, become its cure. Together with Hippocrates many centuries earlier, who had also written about healing by 'similars' as well as by 'contraries', he founded the basis of homeopathy which was to be developed 200 years later by Hahnemann.

Paracelsus' vast pharmacopeia included almost every animal, vegetable and mineral medicine known at the time. Unfortunately, physicians following in his footsteps used metals and other substances in far larger doses than he ever advised, and medicines were sometimes more dangerous than the diseases for which they were prescribed. Paracelsus had also advocated that the active ingredient be extracted from a plant medicine and used in isolation, giving a much more potent medicine while, he

The title page of Gerard's Herball, *one of the most popular herbals from the 16th century.*

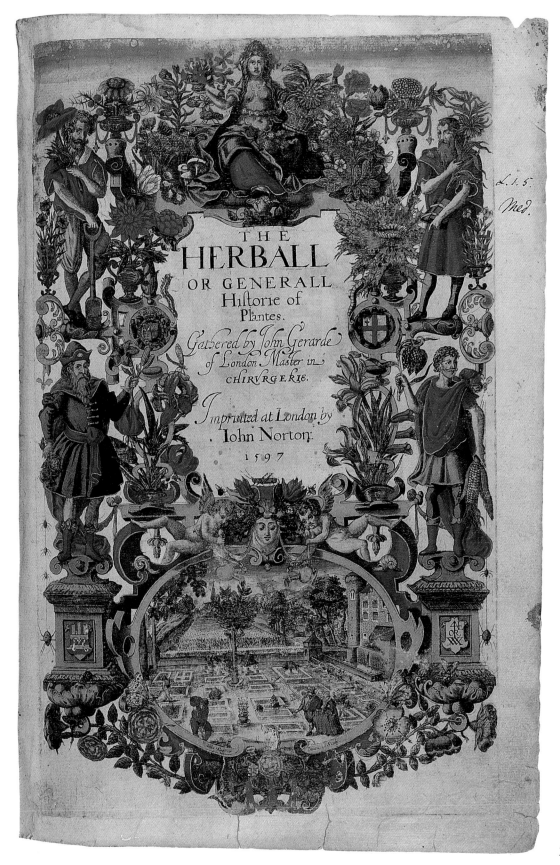

THE
HERBALL
OR GENERALL
Historie of
Plantes.

Gathered by John Gerarde
of London Master in
CHIRVRGERIE.

Imprinted at London by
Iohn Norton.
1597

purported, remaining as safe as in its whole form. In this way, the holistic approach to treatment of disease began to disintegrate. It was the start of allopathic medicine, which focussed on treating the disease rather than the patient, using powerful medicines that brought with them an array of side-effects. This approach was supported by great discoveries in the plant world. Peruvian bark (*Cinchona*) was found to be an excellent cure for malaria, and sarsaparilla (*Smilax ornata*) specific for syphilis.

The ideas of Rene Descartes (1596–1650) with his division of mind and body, nature and ideas, were taking hold. The dawn of the scientific age was bringing to light all kinds of exciting advances in medicine, botany and chemistry. For example, in 1628 William Harvey discovered the way the blood circulated around the body and the old idea of humours became obsolete. The body was beginning to be seen more as a machine and disease a breakdown in its mechanics. The sciences of anatomy and physiology, as separate disciplines from psychology and religion, was fast developing.

HOMEOPATHY

Against this backdrop emerged a doctor who was sorely disillusioned by the limits of the orthodox medical approach and by the cruel and often unsuccessful treatments of his day. These included blood letting, purging, and poisonous drugs with terrible side-effects. His name was Samuel Hahnemann, born in Saxony in 1755. He abandoned his practice, preferring to spend his time studying, writing and translating to support him during his research.

While translating Dr William Cullen's *A Treatise on Materia Medica* Hahnemann felt sceptical of Cullen's explanation of the effectiveness of Peruvian bark for treating malaria, and decided to test small amounts on himself. His experiments revealed that it produced the same symptoms in a healthy person as it was used to cure. This discovery was the instigator of the development of homeopathic medicine. Further experimentation proved that other substances produced the same symptoms in a healthy person that they were able to cure when used therapeutically. The system of healing that grew up as a result of this was named homoeopathy from the Greek word *homoios* meaning similar and *pathos* meaning suffering or disease, to differentiate it from orthodox medicine known as allopathy, meaning 'opposite suffering'. Up to this time any symptom such as constipation would have been treated with an opposite medicine or antidote, a laxative. During the next six years Hahnemann carried out move provings of a whole range of substances and eventually set up his medical practice again, armed with this new knowledge.

To prescribe the right remedy Hahnemann needed to take an accurate case history and establish a 'symptom picture' which he could use to match the symptoms caused by one of the remedies in his dispensary. Thus he could match the symptoms to the treatment, and despite the disbelief he witnessed from his contemporaries he began to achieve remarkable results. He also incurred the wrath of his local pharmacists, by not only prescribing only one remedy at a time, but also in smaller and smaller doses to minimize the risk of side-effects.

Hahnemann found that when diluting the strength of his remedies, if he shook the remedy in between each dilution (known as succussion) it had the effect of potentizing infinitesimal amounts of the remedy prescribed. Even more interesting, the more the remedy was diluted and succussed the more powerful and effective it became. He believed this was because the shaking released the energy of the healing substance and so made it more active. Remedies were numbered according to the number of times they were diluted, so one diluted six times would be called 6c and one diluted thirty times would be 30c.

In 1810, Hahnemann published *The Organon of Rational Medicine* which clearly described his homeopathic system; and between 1811 and 1821, he published six volumes of *Materia Medica Pura* containing his proving of 66 remedies. In 1828, he published *Chronic Diseases and their Homeopathic Cure*, containing more of his provings, use of remedies up to the 30th dilution and his theory of miasms to explain why some patients failed to respond to their indicated remedies. From his experience he saw that a history of diseases such as syphilis, gonorrhea or tuberculosis were linked to certain conditions and that specific homeopathic remedies could remove these often inherited blocks to health, which he called miasms.

After Hahnemann's death in 1843, homeopathy continued to survive and flourish both in Europe and North America, developed by many notable homeopaths who followed in his footsteps. Constantine Hering (1800–80) continued to prove remedies and to take further Hahnemann's theories, such as that of miasms. James Kent (1849–1916) was an American who advocated the use of much higher potencies and published his famous *Repertory*, his *Philosophy* and *Materia Medica*. He further developed Hahnemann's and Hering's symptom pictures into 'constitutional types', describing more fully the emotional and mental tendencies of each type. In 1844 a Dr Frederick Quin with a highly successful homeopathic practice established the British Homeopathic Society (later to become the Faculty of Homeopathy) and founded the London Homeopathic Hospital in 1849.

Towards the end of the 19th century, however, orthodox medicine was growing from strength to strength. The existence of microbes had been established, and the dangerous drugs detested by the herbalists and homeopaths alike were being replaced by powerful new ones with less apparent side-effects. Gradually, with the emergence of pharmacology and biochemistry, the value of homeopathy and plant remedies diminished rapidly in the public and scientific mind. Herbal remedies began to be lumped together with old wives' tales, homeopathy was considered too unscientific, while scientists developed the means to isolate and then synthesize constituents of certain plants. The famous heart medicine digitalis (foxglove) later yielded digoxin, the poppy produced morphine (1803), the wild yam provided steroids, and willow bark provided the chemical base for aspirin.

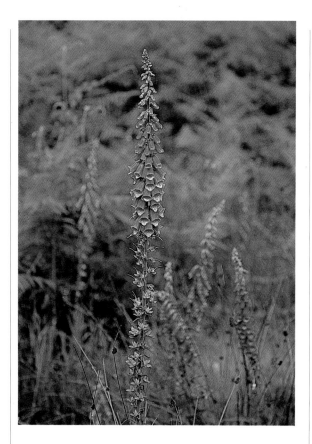

The medicinal value of the foxglove was discovered by William Withering (1741–79) who noted the improvement in dropsy patients given extracts of foxglove by the local wise woman.

THE HEALING TRADITION IN AMERICA

A handful of traditional herbalists remained, maintaining their holistic outlook, basing their treatments on the person rather than the disease and the use of whole plant medicines as opposed to the more potent isolated or synthetically made chemical constituents with their accompanying risk of side-effects.

In the mid-19th century, the National Association of Medical Herbalists (now the National Institute of Medical Herbalists) was set up in the UK to represent the small body of professional herbalists. This was inspired by a similar small body of herbalists in North America, known as Physiomedicalists, who blended together the traditions of European herbalism brought to America by the Pilgrim

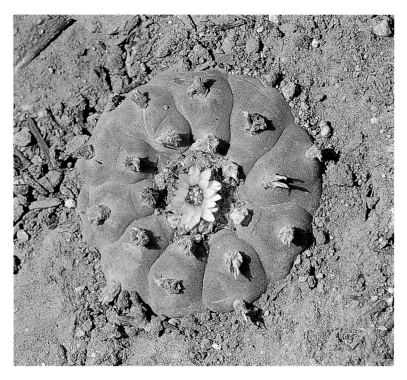

Peyote, a mind-altering plant used by shamen in North and South America.

Fathers with the herbal wisdom of the people then called the North American Indians.

Native American, like South American, herbalism was a shamanic tradition. Ritualistic dances, playing of drums and rattles and the use of mind-altering plants such as peyote and datura were used to enable the shaman or medicine man or woman to enter a trance-like visionary state. This enabled communication with the plant world and the soul of the ill person to bring about healing. Plants were revered not only for their ability to cure diseases of the body, but also imbalances in the mind, emotions and spirit. They were an inextricable part of native religion and mythology, used in ceremonies and rituals. Disease was seen to be caused by human, supernatural or natural causes and the medicine man or woman was called upon to administer herbs for anything from wounds and broken bones to unfulfilled dreams, spiritual intrusion and soul loss.

Everything that the native North American did was in a circle, and according to Black Elk of the Teton Dakato, the 'Power of the World'

always worked in circles. 'All our power came to us from the sacred loop of the nation', he said and his people flourished as long as the circle was unbroken. 'The flowering circle of the four quarters nourished it. The east gave peace and light, the south gave warmth, the west gave rain and the north with its cold and mighty wind gave strength and endurance.'

The renowned physiomedicalist Dr Samuel Thomson (1769–1843) was the first to bring the Indian remedy lobelia to the attention of the medical world. He kept alive traditional ideas, such as that of allowing the body to heal itself and helping to create the ideal conditions for this with the use of herbs. He mixed these traditions with knowledge he had gained by observation of the North American native medicine men such as the value of sweating for clearing toxins from the body.

Thomson, like ancient as well as modern herbalists, recognized the presence of the vital force, the energy which flows throughout nature and animates all in existence. The same wisdom described as the spirit in plants by the Ancient

Greeks and American cultures, the Qi of China's medicine and philosophy, and Prana of Ayurveda, is our innate healing energy that manifests itself daily in the amazing feats of the body. The cough to clear the airways of phlegm, the sneeze to shift irritants from the nose, vomiting to clear the stomach of infection, diarrhoea to remove toxins from the bowel are all examples. This self-healing mechanism is called homeostasis by modern science.

Thomson also held that all bodies were composed of the four elements: earth, air, fire and water, and health derived from their harmonious interplay. Herbs were used primarily to maintain or correct this balance, and prescriptions were designed to do one of four things: astringe (tone) or relax, stimulate or sedate. Toning herbs include shepherd's purse, agrimony and beth root, relaxing herbs include cramp bark and lemon balm. Ginger and cayenne are stimulating while chamomile and yellow jasmine are sedating.

Thomson's model led to the founding of Physiomedicalism by physicians such as Dr Curtis and Dr Cook. It was followed in America by other botanic schools, notably the Eclectics founded by Dr Wooster Beech in the 1830s. The Eclectics were the dominant group in both numbers and their legacy today. Beech also used native American traditions mixed with European knowledge as well as orthodox practices. Physiomedicalism was brought to England in 1838 by Dr Albert Coffin, and Wooster Beech arrived in the 1850s to bring Eclectic medicine to Europe.

Flower healing in modern times

Despite the enormous advances in modern scientific medicine, and the emergence of powerful drugs and the miracles of microsurgery, there is something that still draws many of us to these more ancient holistic systems of medicine. Herbal medicine is again enjoying enormous popular benefit from the marriage of ancient wisdom and modern scientific development and discovery. These have served not to bring herbal

medicine into disrepute after all, but rather to prove through pharmacological analysis of the constituents involved a scientific explanation of their ability to heal.

So much has herbal medicine earned respect and recognition that the first degree course in the subject was established in 1994 at Middlesex University in London, England. With the enormous interchange of cultural ideas possible nowadays, the old systems of the east, whose ancient medical traditions have never been broken as they have here in the west, are beginning to become more integrated into modern healing methods.

AYURVEDIC MEDICINE

The name Ayurveda derives from two Indian words, *ayur* meaning life and *veda* meaning knowledge or science. So Ayurveda is the knowledge or science of life; more than a system of healing, it is a way of life, encompassing science, religion and philosophy, intended to enhance wellbeing, and to enable achievement of longevity and eventually self-realization.

Ayurvedic medicine evolved in India over 5000 years ago from the deep understanding of creation of spiritually enlightened beings known as Rishis, in the far reaches of the Himalayas. It has survived largely as an oral tradition until the present day, one of its greatest values being its timelessness and its application to every facet of daily living now as it was all those centuries ago.

According to Ayurveda, the origin of all aspects of existence is the field of pure intellect or consciousness. This appeals to those influenced by the theories of modern quantum physics which locate the basis of the physical universe in a single unified field that directs and orchestrates the continuous flow of matter. Energy and matter are one. Ayurveda does not separate the external world from the inner world. Everything that exists in the macrocosm has its counterpart in the microcosm of the inner universe of the human being. Cosmic energy manifests in the five elements that are the basis of all matter: ether, air, fire, water and earth. In the body ether is present in the spaces

THE THREE *DOSHAS*

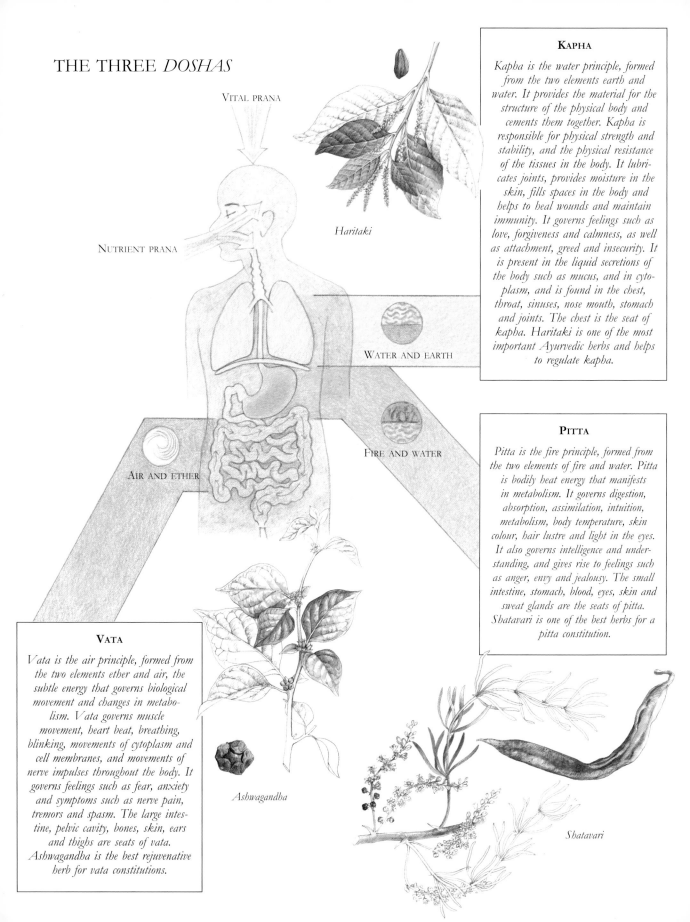

VITAL PRANA

NUTRIENT PRANA

Haritaki

WATER AND EARTH

FIRE AND WATER

AIR AND ETHER

Ashwagandha

Shatavari

KAPHA

Kapha is the water principle, formed from the two elements earth and water. It provides the material for the structure of the physical body and cements them together. Kapha is responsible for physical strength and stability, and the physical resistance of the tissues in the body. It lubricates joints, provides moisture in the skin, fills spaces in the body and helps to heal wounds and maintain immunity. It governs feelings such as love, forgiveness and calmness, as well as attachment, greed and insecurity. It is present in the liquid secretions of the body such as mucus, and in cytoplasm, and is found in the chest, throat, sinuses, nose mouth, stomach and joints. The chest is the seat of kapha. Haritaki is one of the most important Ayurvedic herbs and helps to regulate kapha.

PITTA

Pitta is the fire principle, formed from the two elements of fire and water. Pitta is bodily heat energy that manifests in metabolism. It governs digestion, absorption, assimilation, intuition, metabolism, body temperature, skin colour, hair lustre and light in the eyes. It also governs intelligence and understanding, and gives rise to feelings such as anger, envy and jealousy. The small intestine, stomach, blood, eyes, skin and sweat glands are the seats of pitta. Shatavari is one of the best herbs for a pitta constitution.

VATA

Vata is the air principle, formed from the two elements ether and air, the subtle energy that governs biological movement and changes in metabolism. Vata governs muscle movement, heart beat, breathing, blinking, movements of cytoplasm and cell membranes, and movements of nerve impulses throughout the body. It governs feelings such as fear, anxiety and symptoms such as nerve pain, tremors and spasm. The large intestine, pelvic cavity, bones, skin, ears and thighs are seats of vata. Ashwagandha is the best rejuvenative herb for vata constitutions.

such as the mouth, the abdomen, the thorax, the capillaries and cells. Movement of space is air, manifest in movements of, for example, muscles, the pulsation of the heart, peristalsis of the digestive tract and nervous impulses. Fire is present in the digestive system, governing enzyme systems and metabolism, as well as body temperature, vision and the light of the mind, intelligence. Water is present in secretions like the digestive juices, saliva, mucous membranes, plasma and cytoplasm. Earth is responsible for the solid structures holding the body together, bones, cartilage, muscles and tendons and skin.

The five elements manifest also in the functioning of the five senses: hearing, touch, vision, taste and smell, so they are closely related to our ability to perceive and interact with our environment. From the five elements derive three basic forces, the *tridoshas*, that exist in everything and influence all mental and physical processes. From ether and air, *vata*, the air principle is created, from fire and water comes *pitta*, the fire principle, and from earth and water derives the water principle, *kapha*.

The balance of the *doshas* in each person will promote health and wellbeing, while imbalance leads to ill-health and disease. We are all born with a certain balance of *doshas* bought about mainly by the *dosha* balance in our parents at the time of conception. This is our basic constitution (*Prakruti*) that remains unchanged throughout our lives. The dominant *dosha* determines body type, temperament and those illnesses to which we may be susceptible. Our *Vkruti*, our present *dosha* balance, reflects the effect that lifestyle has on *Prakruti* to cause further imbalances that predispose to ill-health.

Both *Prakruti* and *Vkruti* can be ascertained by careful diagnosis which includes a detailed case history, observation of the body, tongue and pulse diagnosis. Once *dosha* balance has been correctly diagnosed, then the correct treatment and lifestyle advice may be given. Initial treatment consists usually of cleansing methods to eliminate toxins that have contributed to imbalance. Then medicines from plant or miner-al sources will be prescribed, and diet and lifestyle advised which is appropriate to the individual and their *dosha* balance.

CHINESE MEDICINE

Traditional Chinese medicine is an equally ancient system of healing that can be traced back to around 2500BC. As in Ayurveda, the early texts, such as the *Yellow Emperor's Canon of Internal Medicine* dated around 1000BC, are still studied, and their precepts adhered to by modern practitioners.

The Chinese, like the Indians, regard the human body and all its functions as a microcosm of the macrocosm. All forms of life are seen to be animated by the same essential life force called Qi. By breathing we take in Qi from the air and pass it into the lungs, and by digesting we extract Qi from food and drink and pass it into the body. When these Qis meet in the bloodstream they become what is known as Human Qi which circulates around the body as vital energy.

The quality, quantity and balance of Qi in each person influences their state of health and lifespan and this in turn is affected by factors such as the season, climate, lifestyle, diet and air breathed. Qi flows through a network of channels or meridians throughout the body and can be stimulated and balanced using acupuncture, acupressure, diet and herbal medicine.

The principles of Chinese medicine originate in traditional Taoist philosophy, China's most ancient school of thought. Central to this philosophy is the idea of fluctuation and mutability, explaining natural phenomena in terms of the constant ebb and flow of cosmic forces. Yin and yang, the two primordial cosmic forces, are concepts that are familiar to many.

Yin symbolizes passive yielding force that is cold, dark, negative, contractive and female, represented by water. Yang is active, positive, hot, light, expansive and male, symbolized by fire. The constant interplay between these opposite and mutually dependent forces produces all the change and movement in the universe. Different parts of the body are described as being

THE FIVE ELEMENTS
and the network of relationships they form

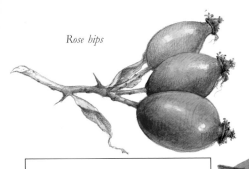

Rose hips

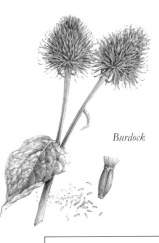

Burdock

FIRE
SEASON: summer
TASTE: bitter
EMOTION: joy
BODY PART: heart, blood vessels, tongue, small intestine
COLOUR: red

Fire gives rise to bitterness, and bitter herbs are yin, cooling, draining and drying. They have detoxifying and anti-inflammatory properties and are often antibiotic, antiparasitic and antiviral. The bitter taste stimulates the secretion of digestive juices throughout the gastro-intestinal system, and the flow of bile from the liver, stimulating appetite, enhancing digestion and absorption, and aiding elimination of toxins via the bowels. Burdock, dandelion and tree peony are examples of such bitter herbs.

EARTH
SEASON: Indian summer
TASTE: sweet
EMOTION: desire, worry
BODY PART: stomach, spleen, muscles, mouth
COLOUR: yellow

Earth gives rise to sweetness, and sweet tasting herbs are yang, warming, soothing, nourishing, body-building and tonic. Most foods are classified as sweet, and they are obviously nourishing – whole grains, beans, dairy products and meat are called 'full' sweet, while foods with an abundance of simple sugars such as honey, sugar, sweet fruits and juices are 'empty' sweet as they tend to intensify rather than satisfy a craving for sweet taste. Herbs with a sweet taste include rehmania, ginseng and Chinese angelica.

WOOD
SEASON: spring
TASTE: sour
EMOTION: anger
BODY PART: liver, gall-bladder, eyes, tendons
COLOUR: green

Wood gives rise to the sour taste, and sour herbs nourish the yin and astringe, preventing unwanted loss of body fluids or Qi, by contracting flaccid tissues and stopping abnormal secretions. The sour taste is cooling and refreshing, and promotes digestion, enzyme secretion and liver function. Sour-flavoured herbs include rose hips, hawthorn berries, and Chinese dogwood berries.

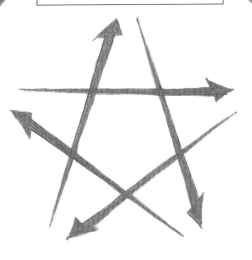

WATER
SEASON: winter
TASTE: salty
EMOTION: fear
BODY PART: kidneys, bladder, ears, bones, nails
COLOUR: black

Water gives rise to saltiness, and salty herbs are classified as yin, cooling and moistening. They nourish the kidneys and help to maintain fluid balance. Most seaweeds and barley are salty.

METAL
SEASON: autumn
TASTE: pungent
EMOTION: grief
BODY PART: lungs, large intestine, skin, nose
COLOUR: white

Metal gives rise to the spicy or pungent taste and spicy herbs are yang, warming, dispersing and drying. They tend to move energy from the interior to the surface of the body, improving circulation, dispelling cold, stimulating energy and improving digestion. Cinnamon, ginger, peppers and cloves are all warming spices which can be used to increase warmth, relieve mucous congestion, cold and flu, pain of arthritis and rheumatism and regulate menstruation.

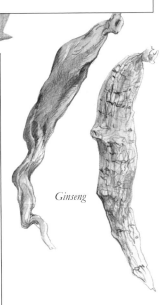

Ginseng

Barley

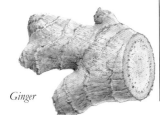

Ginger

predominantly yin or yang. Yin is found in the internal, lower and front part of the body, in the body fluids and blood, and governs innate instincts. Yang governs Qi, vital energy and learned skills, and presides in the upper, external and back parts of the body. To maintain health yin and yang need to be in balance.

As in Ayurveda, the theory of five elements is vital to the Chinese understanding of life in all its variety. Wood, fire, earth, metal and water are the elements that compose and relate to all aspects of life, including parts of the body, vital organs, emotions, seasons, colours and tastes. To illustrate, wood relates to spring, the colour green, the liver and gall-bladder, anger and the sour taste. Fire corresponds to summer, the heart and small intestine, joy and the bitter taste.

The constant interplay of the five elements along with that of yin and yang sparks off all change and activity in nature. The fundamental relationships among the five elements are the key to understanding how our bodies and the environment interact and influence each other. To maintain good health the elements need to be in harmony – if one element becomes over-dominant, imbalance and illness can result.

Using diet, herbs and sometimes acupuncture it is possible to manipulate these natural relationships to adjust energy imbalances caused by excess or deficiency of these forces in the body. Before this is possible a clear diagnosis needs to be made, which involves reading of the basic indicators of health and disease such as the complexion, lustre of the eyes and hair, colour and texture of the tongue and its coating, and the pulse. Neither diagnosis nor treatment remain static; the practitioner regularly reviews the situation throughout a course of treatment.

Aromatherapy

Today, amid the flurry of natural healing methods that have grown up as alternative or complementary to orthodox medicine, the use of essential oils distilled from flowers as well as herbs and trees is enormously popular. This is only natural, given that people have enjoyed the perfumes of plants as far back as we can remember. What could feel more luxurious than soaking in a warm bath breathing in the delicate fragrance of orange blossom, or being massaged with that most sensuous of fragrances, rose?

Most ancient civilizations have used fragrant oils and plants; herbs, flowers and aromatic woods were burned in temples to purify the atmosphere and to please the gods. Their perfumes were believed to rise higher than the temple ceilings to the heavens where they scented the realms of paradise. In Biblical times aromatic oils were used for anointing and as temple incense – we read of the smell of spikenard, smoke perfumed with myrrh and frankincense, camphor and cinnamon to perfume rooms. Myrrh and frankincense were obviously so highly valued that they were considered by the Magi as worthy gifts for the infant Jesus.

The Ancient Egyptians used aromatic oils skilfully in their healing ointments and in the mummification process and used perfumes just as we do today in courtship. Queen Cleopatra's royal barge apparently emitted the most exotic perfumes as it sailed down the Nile to meet Mark Anthony. Cleopatra is said to have bathed several times daily with essence of rose and orange blossom.

The Romans loved aromatic oils, favouring rose above all for wine-making, perfumes and their famous baths. Roman emperors used to fill their swimming baths and fountains with rose water and sat on carpets of rose petals for their feasts and orgies. When the fashion for bathing died out or when water was short aromatic oils would be applied to skin and clothes to mask more unpleasant smells – they were particularly popular in Tudor and Elizabethan times in England. In Queen Elizabeth I's reign perfumed gloves were the height of fashion, and in fact the queen possessed her own stillroom for distilling oils, for the making of the royal floral perfumes.

So powerful was the effect of scent with its sensual, often mind-altering properties, that when the Crusaders returned from the Holy Land laden with perfumes of the Orient, the medieval clergy were greatly alarmed and associ-

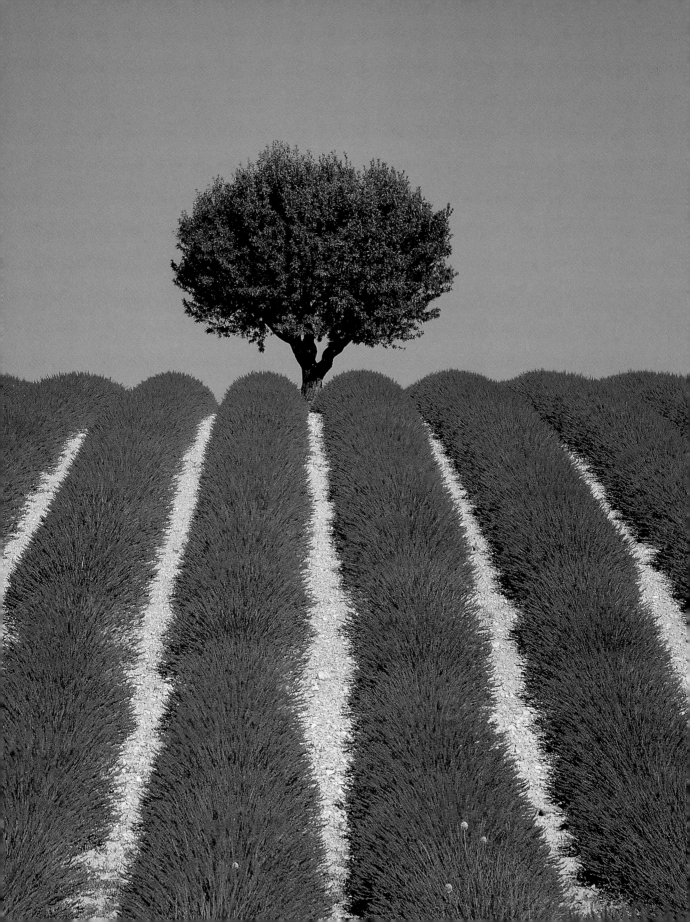

ated it with the forces of evil. Later in the 18th century the British parliament considered applying the laws of witchcraft against women who tried to seduce any of His Majesty's subjects into marriage with the aid of scent! Certainly the fragrances of plants have always been associated with the supernatural, used in magical or religious ceremonies to heighten perception, for divination and love potions.

Fragrant oils have long been associated with healing, too. From Hippocrates onwards we know that aromatic baths, massages and inhalations have been employed to remedy all kinds of health problems. Throughout history aromatic herbs have been used to combat disease during epidemics, even of the plague. Herbs such as rosemary, pine and juniper were burned and pomanders were worn to keep contagion away.

With the development of scientific analysis of plants and their constituents, more has become known about the amazing range of biochemical constituents that make up the volatile oils producing such wonderful aromas. In the 1920s a French chemist, Rene Gattefosse, brought the healing benefits of oils to the attention of the orthodox scientific world. By this time much of the benefit to be derived from the plant world was ignored, and preference given to the synthesis of more powerful drugs in the laboratory. Gattefosse had a family perfume business, and while experimenting in his laboratory he burned his arm badly and plunged it into a vat of lavender oil. The result was, to his great delight, that the arm healed quickly with no scarring. Gattefosse was thereby inspired to devote much time researching essential oils and their medical application, particularly in relation to their benefit on the skin.

In 1937 he published a book entitled *Aromatherapy* – the name he coined for describing the healing benefits of essential oils used to this day. Gattefosse's research papers were read by a French army doctor, Jean Valnet, who was so interested in the subject he began his own clinical research. He used oils on soldiers as

Lavender fields in Provence, France.
The plant has a wonderful aroma with
calming and balancing effects on the
emotions, and also antiseptic properties.

antiseptics and wound healers, and was greatly impressed by their efficacy. He then began to experiment with treating the emotional or psychological problems of war veterans, and to write extensively about aromatherapy. Valnet's *Practice of Aromatherapy*, published in 1964, is a standard text now for all professional aromatherapists.

However, the practice of aromatherapy as it exists today, using essential oils with massage for health and wellbeing, was popularized by an Austrian biochemist, Marguerite Maury, who was married to a homeopath. Dr Maury was particularly interested in the healing and rejuvenating properties of essential oils and carried out an extensive research programme on the effectiveness of oils when absorbed through the skin. She went on to write about essential oils, and published *La Capital Jeunesse* in 1961 which has been reprinted and translated into English as *The Secret of Life and Youth*.

Dr Maury opened several clinics for aromatherapy as have many practitioners since, offering massage using essential oils to treat a wide range of physical problems. At the same time she viewed the use of oils in a holistic way, using them to address many underlying emotional and mental imbalances. Massage gives the benefit of the comfort of touch, which is of great therapeutic value, as well as the great versatility of the effects of the essential oils.

FLOWER REMEDIES AND ESSENCES

Homeopathy has now regained much of its popularity and more besides, flourishing throughout Europe, North and South America, Australia and New Zealand and over much of Asia. Meanwhile, further developments have taken place in the realm of 'vibrational' medicine, that is, in healing methods which act on a subtle or vibrational level as opposed to the purely physiological level perceived by orthodox medicine. The story of flower remedies really begins with Dr Bach.

Dr Edward Bach (1886–1936) had a deep compassion for all living things, particularly those suffering pain or distress. He was led to train in medicine, at which he excelled and in the first years of his practice he was a respected immunologist, pathologist and bacteriologist. Dissatisfied, however, with medicine's palliative rather than curative effect on illness, he was driven to continue his studies.

He knew like Hippocrates, Paracelsus and Hahnemann before him that true health and wellbeing come from within and depend on harmony of body, mind, emotion and spirit. His research as a bacteriologist led to his discovery of the relationship between the bacterial population of the gut and chronic illness and the use of vaccines from these bacteria.

In 1919, working in the London Homeopathic Hospital, he discovered the work and philosophy of Dr Samuel Hahnemann which echoed much of his own approach to medicine – the treatment of the person not the disease. He began to prepare his vaccines homeopathically and used them, now referred to as nosodes, with great success. However, he still felt that he was working in the area of physical disease and not addressing the underlying causes. His understanding was that disease resulted from inner disharmony, negative thoughts and feelings, which were frequently manifested on a physical level. He saw that stresses arising from fear, anxiety, panic, anger, intolerance and impatience put a strain on the individual, depleting general vitality and resistance to disease.

Dr Bach had a great love of nature and intuitively understood, like so many before him, that remedies to unhappy thoughts and feelings were to be found among flowers, herbs and trees. So, at the height of his medical career, he left to spend the rest of his life travelling in Wales and Southern England in search of such remedies to restore peace of mind and happiness which he believed to be the essential nature of our being.

During this time he discovered 38 plants which provided answers to the many sufferings of people, derived (with the exception of one) from flowering trees and plants. Among nature Dr Bach's intuition developed and his senses became more refined. The intense physical and mental disharmony he experienced led him to find the right flower in the fields or hills around him within a few days of the onset of the symptoms, for he could touch a flower with his hand or place it on his tongue and experience its healing effect on both mind and body. He also discovered that the early morning dew on plants exposed to sunlight had absorbed the properties of that plant far better than on those growing in the shade. So he devised a method of extracting the properties of the plants that anybody could employ, and which would not damage the plant.

The sun method involves placing the picked flower heads in a glass bowl to float on top of the spring water that fills it. The bowl is placed on the ground near the parent plants and exposed to sunlight for a few hours, after which time the flowers are removed carefully with a twig or leaf. The essence is then poured into bottles half full of brandy as a preservative. The alternative, boiling method, involves placing the plant in an enamel pan of spring water and simmering it for half an hour. Once cool the essence is filtered and preserved in equal parts of brandy.

Dr Bach said it was 'our fears, our cares, our anxieties and such like that open the path to the invasion of illness.' By using the flower remedies he discovered, he said, that we could treat our cares and our worries and thereby 'not only free ourselves from our illness, but the Herbs given unto us by the Grace of the creator of all, in addition take away our fears and worries and leave us happier and better in ourselves.' He published his discoveries in the main homeopathic journals and produced several booklets for lay people so that his remedies would be accessible to everyone. These included *Heal Thyself, Free Thyself* and *The 12 Healers.*

Although flower remedies soon became associated with Dr Bach in people's minds as they gained in popularity, they had actually been described in the 1500s by Paracelsus. He had prepared remedies from dew collected from flowers to treat his patients' emotional problems. In the early 1970s 'flower power'

Hibiscus rosa-sinensis. *As a flower essence hibiscus helps women feel comfortable with their sexuality, particularly those who have suffered trauma in the past and are unable to express warmth and love.*

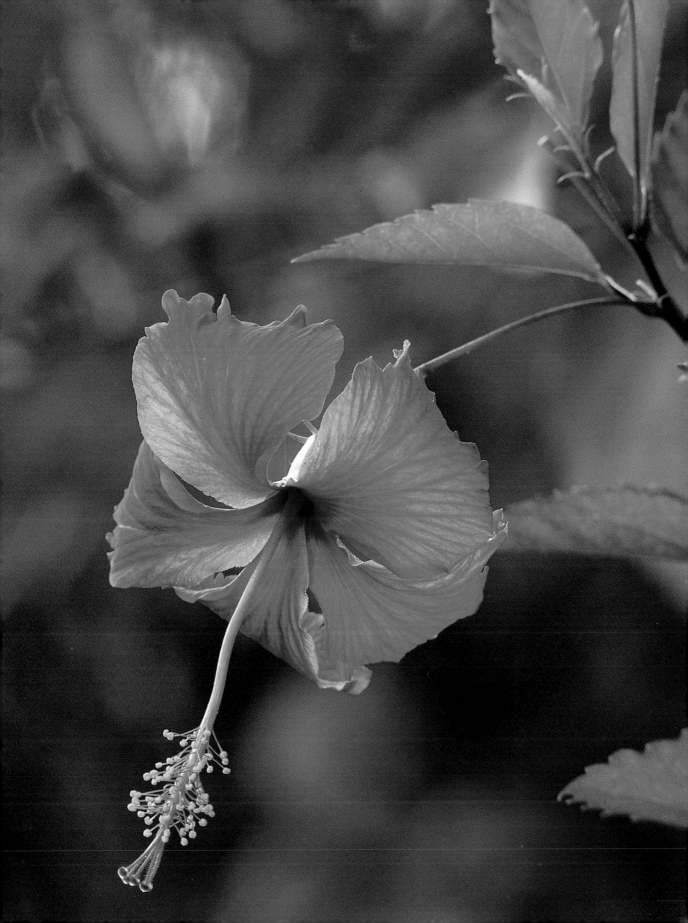

were the words on many people's lips, particularly in California, and such people would refer to 'good vibrations', the wisdom of the East, the power of love and meditation. Flowers were in vogue, and not surprisingly various people in the healing and psychic world began to discover intuitively a cornucopia of new flower essences.

Within the context of mind-altering substances and popular New Age concepts, the profusion of flower remedies led to doubts about their healing abilities. Richard Katz and Patricia Kaminski were among those who were developing flower essences, having worked with the Bach Flower Remedies for many years. They were concerned that charlatans in the area would bring flower healing into disrepute. In 1979, they set up the Flower Essence Society to separate the sound from the speculative, to gather case studies from practitioners around the world, and to confirm the genuine effects of flower essences. They also ran training courses for students and seminars for practitioners.

After extensive testing of their remedies on health practitioners, the Flower Essence Society (FES) produced a range of flower essences called Quintessentials, made from organically grown flowers cultivated around the Californian Sierra Nevada. While Dr Bach's remedies reflected the spirit of his era, during the Depression, with flowers for negative emotions such as fear, anger, resentment, depression and discouragement, the Californian Flower Essences were affected by California in the 1970s. Their remedies include flowers for enhancing spiritual development, for sexual inhibitions, blocks to creativity and problems in relationships. From that time onward the world of flower essences has continued to blossom with ranges of flower essences originating from many parts of the world – New Zealand, Hawaii, Alaska, Scotland, the Himalayas, Africa, the Amazon and Australia.

The Australian Bush Flower Essences were evolved by a naturopath, Ian White, who had used the Bach remedies and wanted to explore the healing potential of flowers closer to home. As a boy he had grown up in the Australian bush and there his appreciation and respect for nature developed as he accompanied his herbalist grandmother on walks searching for medicinal herbs. As an adult, information about bush essences, a picture of the flower, where it could be found and often its name, was channelled to Ian White during meditation.

Working with other practitioners who were excited by this new discovery, he set about verifying the effects of the remedies, not only by working with patients but also testing them with Kirlian photography, kinesiology and vega machines, and with other mediums. His book *Bush Flower Essences* describes 50 Australian essences and their applications; since its publication twelve more remedies have been discovered and researched. (See pages 260–265.)

Flower remedies are highly dilute from a physical or chemical perspective, effective not because of their chemical constituents but for the life force derived from the flower contained within the water-based fluid. Like homeopathic remedies their presence is more subtle than physical. They address profound issues of spiritual wellbeing, emotional and mental harmony, and the healing of emotional and mental difficulties creating blocks to spiritual development and realization of our full potential. They can provide catalysts for helping people to heal themselves, to understand their purpose and direction in life, and free themselves from mental or emotional suffering that may be hindering them on their path. Dr Bach said that flower essences 'raise our vibrations and open up our channels for the reception of our spiritual self. They are able, like beautiful music or any gloriously uplifting thing which gives us inspiration, to raise our very natures and bring us nearer to ourselves and by that very act to bring us peace and relieve our suffering'.

These words echo the words and experience of so many others who have glimpsed the deeper significance of the world of flowers. The essential nature of flowers inspires healing of every dimension in us simply by being in their presence. The world of writing and poetry offers many illustrations of this.

Yes! in the poor man's garden grow
far more than herbs and flowers
kind thoughts, contentment, peace of mind
And joy for wary hours.
    MARY HOWITT

Flowers ... have a mysterious and subtle influence
upon the feelings, not unlike some strains of music.
They relax the tenseness of the mind.
    HENRY WARD BEECHER (1813–87)

O, see a world in a grain of sand,
and heaven in a wild flower.
    WILLIAM BLAKE (1757–1827)

The kiss of the sun for pardon
The song of the birds for mirth
One is nearer God's Heart in the garden
Then anywhere else on earth.
    DOROTHY FRANCES GURNEY

That same vital force of subtle energy that was recognized as the spirit of the flower by the Ancient Greeks, as Qi by the Chinese, Prana by the Indians, is central to the story of medicine since its ancient beginnings. The same healing power that exists in a flower, whether used as a flower itself, a herbal maceration of the flower, a distilled oil of the flower, a potentized homeopathic remedy from the flowers or a flower essence, is clear to see as one looks closer at individual flowers and their healing potential. In Chapter 2, The Flowers, each flower's healing properties are described according to the different ways it is used, but it is the story of the flower itself which binds all together.

Take yarrow, for example, the famous wound remedy of the Greek warrior Achilles. It is a great astringent and healing herb, with its main influence observed on the blood and circulation, an essential oil with astringent properties and to enhance the circulation, a homeopathic remedy for venous haemorrhages, and a flower remedy to astringe the boundaries around a person and prevent their energy from bleeding into their environment. Mugwort, whose Latin name Artemisia comes from the Greek moon goddess,

the patron and protector of women, is an excellent female herb, for enhancing their inner strength, their receptive quality and used by the ancients in dream pillows to help gain important spiritual insights. As a homeopathic remedy mugwort is an excellent female remedy for menstrual problems and threatened miscarriage as well as spasms and epilepsy brought on by extremes of emotion. As a flower essence mugwort also enhances the moon-like receptive quality of the psyche, allowing greater awareness of the dream world, and is predominantly a women's remedy, useful for a whole range of physical imbalances of the cycle, as well as in pregnancy and childbirth.

It may be believed by some that herbs and essential oils have an impact on the physical and emotional world, while homeopathy and flower remedies affect the deeper emotional and spiritual realms. However, one only has to look at the flower in all its simplicity to know that its very presence is healing. Certainly, flowers as herbal remedies and essential oils have their often powerful physical effects partly explained by their amazing range of biochemical constituents. However, their more subtle attributes live within their physical forms, just as our soul animates us in our human bodies. In the various healing methods different parts of a flowering plant may be employed – sometimes the root, other times the stem, or the bark or the seed, but these are only parts of the whole, of which the flower is its vital expression. It is the flower that displays itself in all its magnificence, not only to attract pollinating insects, but also to bring its healing nature to the attention of mankind who has such need of its gifts. Flowers, their beauty, their scent, said Pope:

All are but parts of one stupendous whole
whose body Nature is, and God the soul:
look around our World, behold the chain of love
combining all below and all above.

Night-flying moths and hungry insects, as well as the whole of mankind, continue to gaze on their beauty in wonder.

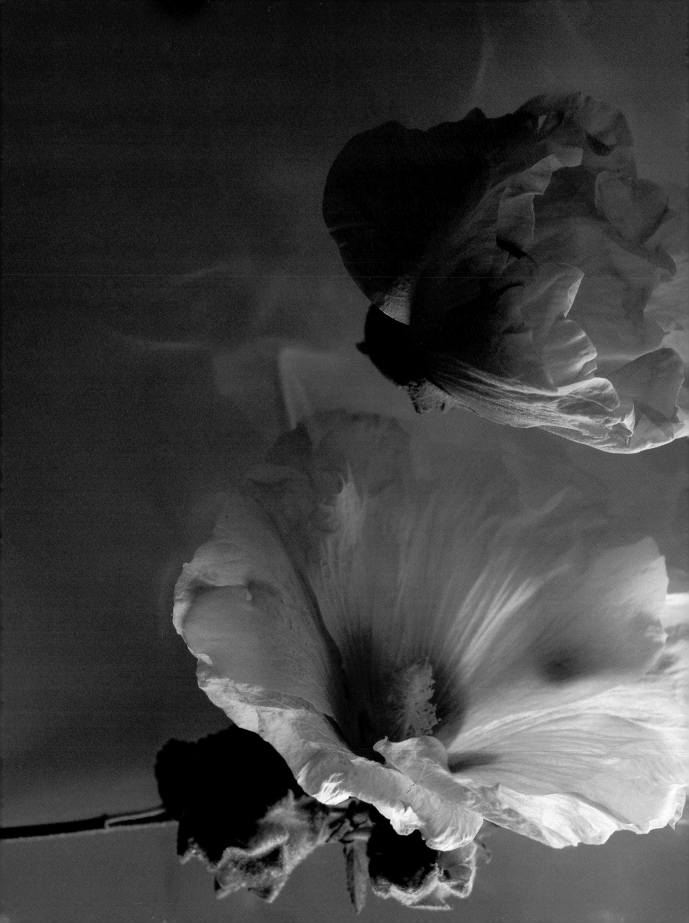

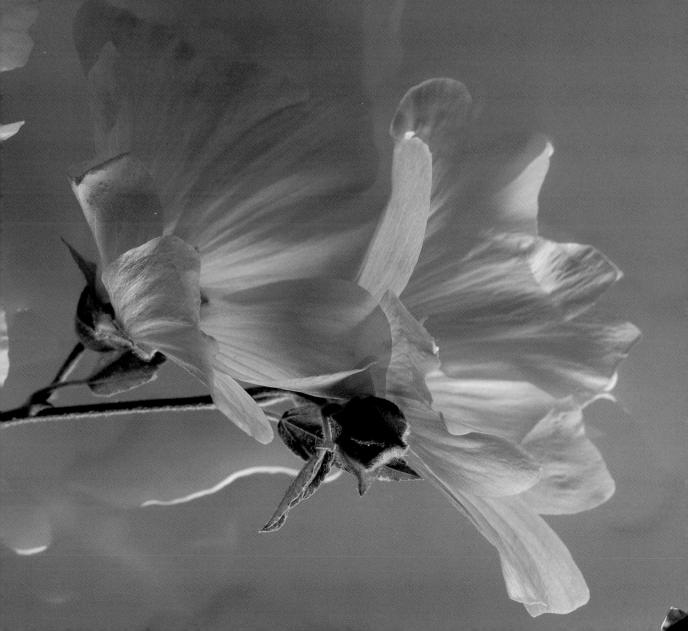

Chapter two

THE FLOWERS

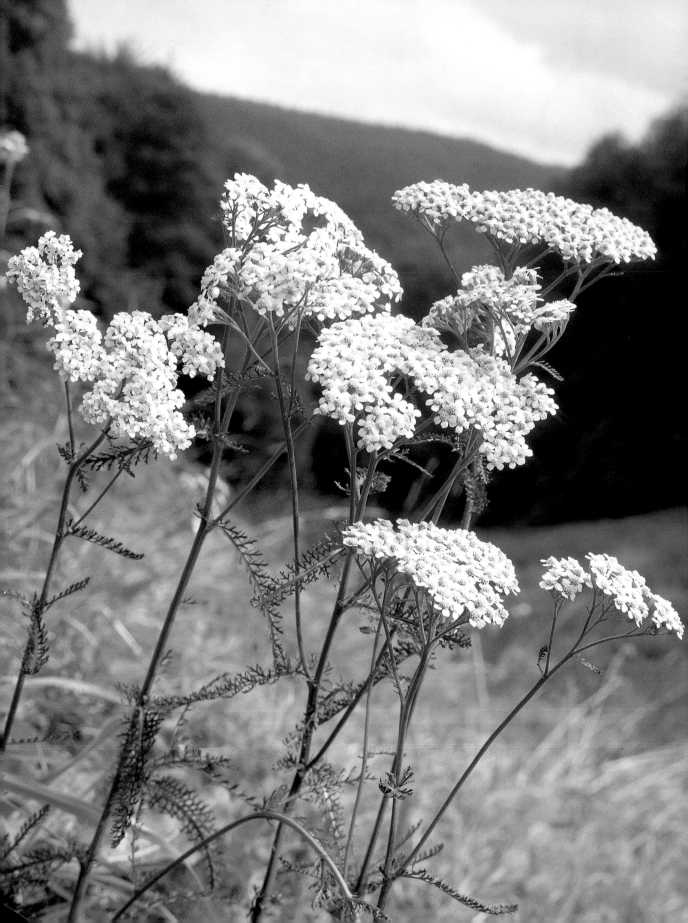

Yarrow

The flower of invulnerability

Thou pretty herb of Venus Tree
Thy true name is Yarrow
Now who my bosom friend must be
Pray tell thou me tomorrow.
HALLIWELL

Yarrow is a member of the Compositae family, cousin to dandelion and daisy, a perennial with aromatic leaves. It is found all over the globe in hedgerows, lanes and fields, preferring light sandy soils. Yarrow is one of the finest and most versatile healing plants, and respected as such since at least the time of the Ancient Greeks and Egyptians. Dioscorides, the Greek physician, writing in the 1st century AD referred to the healing properties of yarrow for battle wounds. The name Achillea commemorates the Greek hero Achilles, who used yarrow to heal the wounds of his friends. Achilles was renowned for his invulnerability. Throughout history until the First World War, yarrow has been used for treating wounds, hence its common names soldiers' woundwort and staunchweed.

The name yarrow is apparently derived from *hieros* which means sacred, because of the plant's association with ceremonial magic. Yarrow was thought to be richly endowed with spiritual properties, so it was preserved in temples and treated with special reverence. Its healing effect upon the blood was seen as an ability to influence the 'life-blood', the essence or ego that is carried in the blood. It was used as an amulet, a charm to protect against negative energy and evil, capable of overcoming the forces of darkness and being a conductor of benevolent powers. It was also believed to be a love charm and to be ruled by the planet Venus. In folklore, a maiden who places yarrow under her pillow and repeats the rhyme (above) will dream of her future husband.

In China yarrow stalks were used to reawaken the spiritual forces of the superconscious mind during ritual divination using the *I Ching*.

Herbal remedy

The contemporary use of yarrow in healing relates back to its religious, mythological and folkloric history with the primary effect on the blood and circulation. It makes an excellent remedy for wounds; the volatile oils are anti-inflammatory and antiseptic, the tannins are astringent and stop bleeding, the resins are also astringent and antiseptic, while the silica promotes tissue repair. An infusion makes a good vaginal douche, an eyebath, and a skin lotion for varicose veins and haemorrhoids. Yarrow's astringent effect is felt throughout the body, staunching bleeding from the nose, the digestive system and the uterus. It regulates the menstrual cycle and acts as a tonic to the nervous system. Yarrow is an excellent remedy for the digestive tract, stimulating the appetite, enhancing digestion and absorption. An infusion stimulates the circulation and promotes perspiration. It reduces fevers and clears toxins, heat and congestion by aiding elimination via the skin and the kidneys through its diuretic effect.

Aromatherapy oil

The essential oil of yarrow is used in aromatherapy for much the same range of problems. Its anti-inflammatory and detoxifying properties are useful in relief of arthritis and gout. As an antispasmodic it relieves cramps, colic and painful periods. As an astringent, it stimulates the circulation and enhances digestion, also regulating heavy periods.

Homeopathic remedy: YARROW

Homeopathically yarrow is used predominantly for venous haemorrhages and varicose veins which tend to occur in ruddy-complexioned people, after vigorous exercise or exertion, strains or injuries.

The flower essence

As a flower essence yarrow is used to protect against negative outside influences and for psychic shielding, bestowing the invulnerability of Achilles. It helps to clarify boundaries between people: particularly useful for those who are easily influenced and depleted by others and their environment. It is for those who easily absorb negative influences, and may be prone to allergies and environmental illness. By 'astringing' the boundaries around a person and preventing their energies from 'bleeding' into their environment, it acts to strengthen and solidify the self, the essence, allowing and enhancing their ability to heal, teach, counsel or follow their chosen path.

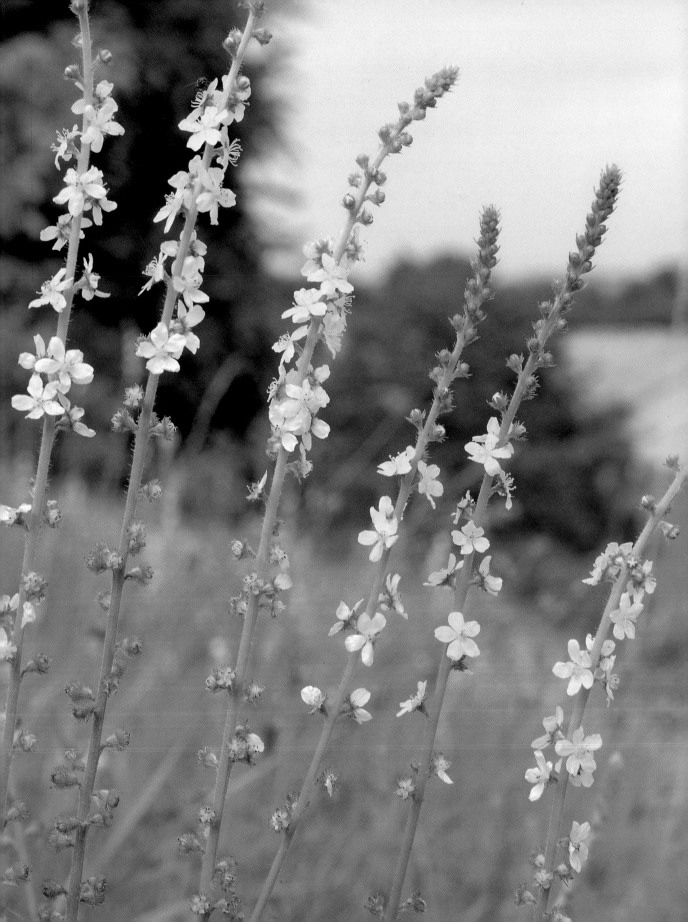

Agrimony
The flower of perception

Next these here Egremony is,
That helps the serpent's biting.
MICHAEL DRAYTON (1563–1631)

Found in summer hedgerows, fields and waste ground, agrimony is easily recognized by its delicate long spike of yellow flowers smelling of apricots, and its beautifully shaped leaves. Its country name, church steeples, refers to its rising spire of yellow flowers, while names such as cockleburr and sticklewort refer to the seed which attaches itself to passers-by, both animal and human.

Agrimony was praised by the Ancient Greeks and Romans for its healing properties. The name agrimony comes from the Greek *argemone*, a white speck in the eye, because of its ability to heal the eyes; the Greeks apparently used it for cataracts. Eupatoria is derived from Mithridates IV Eupator, King of Pontus 120–63BC, a skilled herbalist who was the first to employ agrimony for liver complaints and also to counteract poisons.

In Anglo-Saxon times agrimony was used to heal wounds and treat snakebites and was one of the 57 herbs in the Anglo-Saxon Holy Salve believed to protect one from goblins, evil and poison. Chaucer refers to its use for 'alle wounds' and medieval monks grew agrimony in their monastery gardens as a cure for stomach aches and open wounds. Culpeper recommended it to be taken internally and applied externally for gout, as well as for bruises, sprains, wounds and snakebites. Gerard said it was 'good for naughty livers'. In North America agrimony was a fever remedy for native Americans and Canadians and it has been likened to Peruvian bark for its ability to relieve fever and malaria. The French drink agrimony *tisanes* and use on sprains and bruises in their famous *eau de arquebusade*, made originally for battle wounds in the 15th century. In the language of flowers agrimony symbolizes gratitude.

Herbal remedy
Today, agrimony is still important as a digestive tonic and an astringent. The tannins act to tone the mucous membranes of the gut, improving their secretion and absorption while protecting against irritation and infection. It helps to prevent and to reme-

dy peptic ulcers and colitis and makes a good remedy for diarrhoea. The bitters stimulate the secretion of digestive juices and bile from the liver and gall-bladder, enhancing digestion and absorption as well as bowel function. In Germany agrimony has been used to treat gallstones and cirrhosis of the liver. It is also a good remedy for gout and arthritis, as it acts as a diuretic, clearing excess uric acid.

You can also use agrimony as an excellent astringent for heavy periods, and externally for stemming bleeding and speeding healing of cuts and wounds. As a gargle or mouthwash you can use it for sore throats and inflamed gums. It makes a good eyewash for inflammatory eye problems and a douche for vaginal discharges and infections.

Homeopathic remedy: AGRIMONIA
Agrimonia is also used for menstrual and digestive problems. It helps to clear catarrh throughout the digestive, respiratory, and genito-urinary systems.

The flower essence
Agrimony is particularly for those who appear carefree and cheerful; they are popular and have a good sense of humour. However, their brave face masks inner torture or turbulence which they are careful not to inflict on others. They are concerned to keep peace and harmony, so do not like to upset other people and are distressed by tension and conflict. They will go out of their way to avoid confrontation and to keep other people happy. When ill they make light of their symptoms. Generally they hate to sit still or to be alone, for fear their suppressed emotions may come to the fore and they may have to face their darker side or their problems. Agrimony people keep their rose-tinted spectacles firmly on. Such people may indulge in alcohol, drugs or a wide range of exciting activities to distract them from their inner selves.

Agrimony helps such people to acknowledge the real, sometimes darker side of themselves or others. It engenders inner strength to face the problems of everyday life and from the past. In this sense, agrimony is a remedy for perception. The Greeks used it as a remedy to heal the eyes. As a flower remedy it helps one to see things as they truly are.

Horse-chestnut

The flower of Jupiter

O chestnut tree, great-rooted blossomer,
Are you the leaf, the blossom or the bole?
O body swayed to music, O brightening glance,
How can we know the dancer from the dance?
  W B YEATS (1865–1939)

The magnificent horse-chestnut tree with its pyramidal flowers in white, pink or yellow, is a native of India and was brought to Europe in the mid-17th century. It is also found all over North America and is popular not only for its handsome floral spikes but also for its bright shiny fruit, called conkers, which children so love to play with. Their rich colour has given its name to a shade of dark auburn hair.

The name horse-chestnut comes from the tree's ancient use in Turkey. Flour of the fruit was mixed with oats and fed to broken-winded horses and is apparently still so used today. Also, all over the smaller branches of the tree are horseshoe-shaped scars from fallen leaves.

The fruit and their capsules contain the toxin aescine which is poisonous when raw. The Native Americans cooked them and washed the flesh to render the toxin harmless. During wartime 'conkers' were roasted in parts of Europe and ground to make a rather bitter coffee substitute. The flower buds flavoured drinks and replaced hops in beer. The fruit are rich in saponins, which make a lather in water. They were used in the past for washing clothes and to store with clothes to prevent mould and infestation. The fruit were also carried in the pockets of country women to ward off rheumatism, piles, giddiness, chills and backache. They were also carried to bring money and success as they were said to be under the dominion of Jupiter.

Herbal remedy

The bark of the tree is rich in tannins and has been used for diarrhoea and to bring down fevers. It was often given as a substitute for Peruvian bark for malaria and intermittent fevers. The bark influences the portal circulation, and relieves congestion in the venous system which causes piles and varicose veins.

The buds of the flowers, the bark and the nuts all make excellent ointments, creams and lotions for strengthening veins. They are good for varicose veins, ulcers, and a first rate remedy for haemorrhoids. Horse-chestnut extracts also relieve neuralgia, sunburn, bruises and sprains.

Homeopathic remedy: A. HIPPOCASTANUM

Aesculus hippocastanum is a great pile remedy. It has a particular affinity for the lower bowel area, relieving painful engorged haemorrhoidal veins, backache, weak legs, constipation and a feeling of prolapse in the rectum. It is also excellent for varicose veins, venous stasis, and congestion in the digestive tract.

The flower essences

Chestnut bud is for those who tend to make the same mistakes over and again and never seem to learn from the experience. They tend to enter the same kind of relationships which fail, or experience the same physical symptoms over and again without analysing the reason – such as gastric pain after eating cheese, or migraines when becoming stressed. Their inability to learn from their mistakes may be because of indifference, or lack of attention and observation. It is often due to their wish to escape from themselves, to block out the past and avoid the responsibility of learning the lessons of life. Chestnut bud is a good remedy for children who are absent-minded and inattentive. It helps people to be more observant and aware of the present, to see their mistakes and remember them and to gain knowledge and wisdom. It helps to see oneself more clearly.

White chestnut is a wonderful remedy for those who suffer from recurrent thoughts that go round and round in the head. It may occur after an argument or when something has upset or worried you. The thoughts can be so all-pervading that they prevent you from attending to the present even to the extent of not listening when spoken to. If the interest in the present is strong the thoughts may quieten temporarily, only to return to wake one from sleep, or ruin one's relaxation time. In severe cases the persistent unwanted thoughts can feel like mental torture, and lead to exhaustion and depression. White chestnut helps to calm the mind, to control thoughts and imaginings and put mental energy to constructive use. It enables you to allow thoughts to enter but not monopolize your mind.

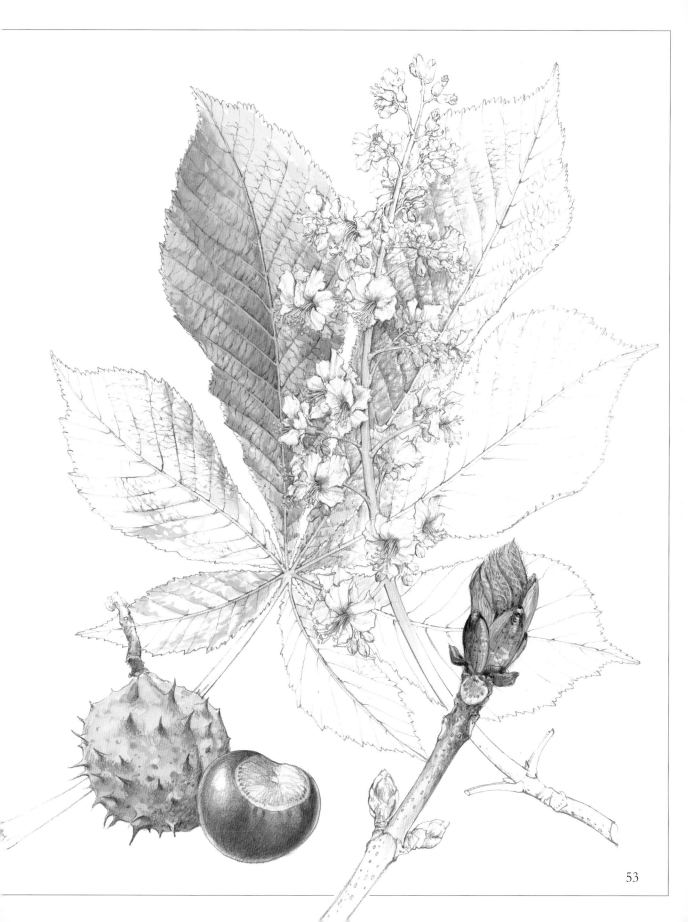

53

Garlic

The flower of power

A feast is not a feast unless to begin
Each guest is given ample Toes of Garlic,
That finest aphrodisiac
To whet his appetite for later revelry.
    QUINTUS HORACE (65–8BC)

Garlic is a member of the lily family and a wonderfully impressive remedy used in healing for thousands of years. An Egyptian medical papyrus dating as far back as around 1500BC included over 200 prescriptions using garlic for problems such as headaches, physical weakness and throat infections. The Ancient Greeks apparently ate large amounts of garlic, Galen saw it as a panacea for all ills while Dioscorides used it as a remedy for asthma, jaundice, toothache, skin problems, worms and as an antidote to poisons. In 1st century India, Ayurvedic physicians employed garlic for preventing heart disease and rheumatism and for centuries in China and Japan it has been taken for high blood pressure.

Throughout garlic's use in healing there run three main themes – it is strengthening and energy-giving, detoxifying and an antidote to poisoning, and it lends protection against a whole host of evil influences both physical and metaphysical.

The Ancient Egyptians were well aware of garlic's stimulating and energy-giving properties; the builders of the great pyramid at Giza are said to have eaten garlic to give them strength. The Romans gave it to their workmen and soldiers to give them strength and courage. The Ancient Greeks also saw garlic as a symbol of strength – athletes at the Olympic Games chewed it before taking part to improve their chances of victory. Culpeper said that garlic was ruled by Mars, and the name is said to come from the Anglo Saxon *gar* meaning spear and *lac* meaning plant, referring either to the shape of the leaves or the fact that garlic imparts warlike properties.

Garlic has also been seen as rejuvenative and aphrodisiac, and when considering the wonderful array of therapeutic actions that garlic possesses this is hardly surprising. It has been used for centuries as an invigorating tonic and used in many an elixir of youth. The fact that garlic imparts energy and vitality may explain its reputation as an aphrodisiac. It was sold in taverns and on street corners as such, and in Greece during the 5th century BC street vendors apparently hawked garlic by chanting, 'It is truth, Garlic gives men youth.' Garlic is famous for its powerful defense against infection. Galen described it as the rustic's theriac, meaning heal-all or antidote to poison. (It has since become known as poor man's treacle.) It has been used for poisoning, diarrhoea, dysentery, cholera and typhoid. It was the principal ingredient in the famous four thieves' vinegar used very successfully at Marseilles against the plague. Apparently four thieves confessed that while protected by covering themselves with garlic vinegar, they plundered bodies of the dead in complete safety.

At the turn of this century garlic preparations were still a major remedy for TB. In the First World War garlic was used to combat dysentery, typhus and to treat suppurating wounds; in the Second World War British doctors successfully warded off septic poisoning and gangrene of battle wounds with garlic.

Perhaps the ability of garlic to drive away infection is linked to its reputation for shielding one from evil and driving away vampires. For like many other strong-smelling herbs, garlic was believed to possess occult magic. In Ancient China it was used to ward off the evil eye and in many traditions garlic was hung in strings from roofs of houses and sterns of boats to prevent attack by witches, sorcerers, demons and evil spirits. It was garlic in Homer's *Odyssey* that Hermes recommended to Ulysses to protect him against the sorceress Circe who turned men into swine. Garlic was dedicated to Hecate, the Greek goddess of witchcraft, famous for her knowledge of plants and her magical garden in Colchis on the shore of the Black Sea. Garlic was placed by the Ancient Greeks on piles of stones at crossroads as supper for Hecate. There is a Mohammedan legend that tells, 'when Satan stepped out of the Garden of Eden after the fall of man, garlic sprang up from the spot where he placed his left foot and onion from that where his right foot touched'.

Herbal remedy

The humble garlic bulb, maligned for its powerful and lingering odour, is a wonderful medicine. As recognized centuries ago, it is an effective antibacterial, antifungal, antiviral and antiparasitic remedy.

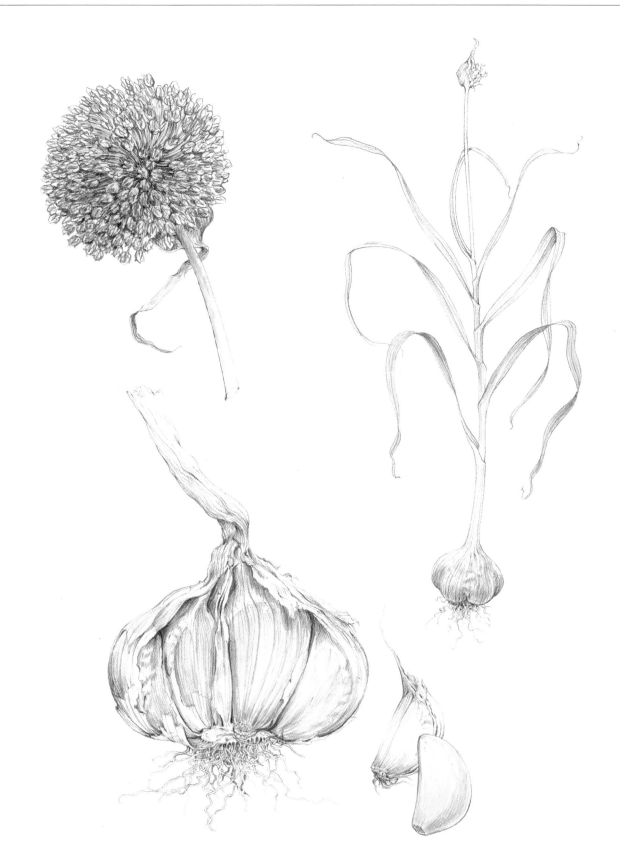

Raw garlic when crushed releases allicin, which has been shown to be more powerfully antibiotic than penicillin and tetracycline. Garlic exerts its antimicrobial effects throughout the body. When absorbed from the digestive tract it circulates in the bloodstream and is excreted via the lungs, bowels, skin and urinary system, all of which are disinfected in the process. Garlic can be used for sore throats, colds, flu, bronchial and lung infections, infections in the gut and to help re-establish beneficial bacterial population after an infection or orthodox antibiotics. It is an effective remedy for worms when taken on an empty stomach, as well as for candidiasis, and thrush in the mouth or vagina when used locally.

Like other pungent remedies, garlic acts as a decongestant, helping to clear catarrh, and augmenting its antiseptic action in the respiratory tract. Its expectorant properties make garlic an excellent remedy for acute and chronic bronchitis, whooping cough and bronchial asthma, as well as sinusitis, chronic catarrh, hay fever and rhinitis. By causing sweating it helps resolve fevers.

Garlic has a beneficial effect on the digestion, stimulating secretion of digestive enzymes and bile, and enhancing the movement of food through the gut. With its antiseptic action, this has the effect of cleansing the liver and digestive system, eliminating harmful bacteria and thereby improving general health, since the origin of many diseases is the accumulation of toxins in the digestive tract. Garlic improves digestion, relieves wind and distension, and enhances absorption and assimilation of food. It also benefits the pancreas, enhancing the production of insulin, making it an excellent remedy to lower blood sugar in diabetics.

Recent research has shown that garlic acts as a powerful antioxidant and its sulphur compounds have anti-tumour activities, while it is also said to protect the body against the effects of pollution and nicotine. Thus garlic helps to slow down the ageing process, verifying our ancestors' use of garlic as a rejuvenative tonic. By clearing the body of toxins and diseases it helps to maintain a youthful vigour, and with such energy one is able not only to fend off disease but also a whole range of negative influences.

In confirmation of the ancients' use of garlic for heart disease and high blood pressure, recent research into the heart and circulation has shown that garlic can significantly lower the level of harmful blood cholesterol – particularly important for those suffering from arteriosclerosis and high blood pressure. Garlic also reduces blood pressure and a tendency to clotting, thereby helping to prevent heart attacks and strokes. It has a vasodilatory action, opening up the blood vessels and increasing the flow of blood to the tissues and to the periphery of the body. This not only reduces blood pressure, but also increases the circulation, relieving cramps and circulatory disorders, and promoting a feeling of warmth and wellbeing, especially welcome on cold winter days and nights.

Externally, garlic can be crushed and macerated in oil or made into an ointment to treat cuts and wounds, inflamed joints, gout and rheumatism, sprains, unbroken chilblains, athlete's foot, ringworm, stings, bites and warts. An oil infusion can be used as eardrops to relieve ear infections and earache, and rubbed into the chest for chest infections and coughs. Garlic vinegar can be used for disinfecting and dressing ulcers and septic wounds.

Homeopathic remedy: ALLIUM SATIVUM

Allium sativum suits those who are used to high living, who have voracious appetites and eat more than they drink. It acts on the intestinal mucosa, and will relieve colitis and diarrhoea with pathological flora in the gut, with dull pain in the lower abdomen. Garlic people tend to be anxious and impatient, full of fears, such as fear of not recovering, or fear of being poisoned. They may be sensitive and sad, weep during sleep, and have an impulse to run away.

Garlic also helps constipation, wind and flatus that burns as it is passed, and a sensitive stomach and bowel that is deranged from the least change of diet.

The flower essence

Garlic imparts strength and active resistance physically, emotionally and psychically. It is recommended particularly for those who are plagued by fears and anxieties and emotionally drained as a result. In a depleted state they are prone to chronic nervousness, insecurity, and are vulnerable to negative influences. This may manifest as a poor immune response with a tendency to parasitic or viral infection or a tendency to fall prey to emotional or psychic parasites in one's life. This leads inevitably to further draining of vital energy; the face may be pale, the eyes vacant, and there may be a feeling of being scattered. Garlic helps to restore wholeness and strength, imparts courage to help overcome fears, and increases resistance to parasitic entities and poisonous influences. Garlic has a stablizing and harmonious effect.

Mugwort

The flower of Artemis

Mugwort and the other Artemisias, southernwood and wormwood, are named after Artemis, the Greek moon goddess, identified with the Roman Diana. Artemis revived plants each night with her refreshing dew, while her twin brother Apollo, the sun god, sent the sun's rays, both essential to the growth and wellbeing of the plant world. As the moon goddess, Artemis was regarded as the patron and protector of women, to influence their fertility, regulate their menstrual cycles and to watch over them in childbirth. For thousands of years women giving birth have evoked her aid and given prayers and offerings to ensure a safe delivery, and given thanks to her afterwards.

The healing power of the plants named after Artemis reflects her influence in the sphere of women's health, and explains why ever since the time of Hippocrates, Pliny and Dioscorides mugwort has been considered the female remedy *par excellence*.

Throughout its applications in healing mugwort is used for balancing menstrual disorders and for treating a wide range of female problems. Not surprisingly Culpeper tells us that mugwort is under the dominion of the planet Venus, indicating the plant's connection to the emotional world of women, enhancing clarity and inner strength, and to the receptive quality of woman, the world of the psyche and dreams. It was used in making dream pillows, which were slept upon to gain visions of the future and important spiritual insights.

Since early times mugwort was believed to be a magical herb. It was used as a talisman against tiredness. Pliny in his *Naturalis Historia* recommended travellers to carry mugwort with them. There is an old French saying, 'He who carries artemisia on his travels will never feel weary'. Mugwort was also said to be a powerful herb for warding off danger and evil. It was used in spells against a whole range of mortal dangers including evil spirits, sunstroke, poison, wild beasts, fire and illness. It was placed in the entrance to houses to keep away infections, and inside the house to stop lightning from striking.

In the Middle Ages mugwort was called *cingulum sancti Johannis*, or St John's girdle, as it was said that John the Baptist wore a girdle of mugwort while in the wilderness. It was traditionally worn on St John's (midsummer's) Eve as a garland round the head or waist, when dancing round the fire. Afterwards it was thrown on to the fire to protect the wearer from danger and sickness in the following year.

Mugwort grows wild on wasteland, embankments, roadsides, among rubble and stony ground throughout America, Europe and North Asia.

Herbal remedy

Mugwort has been used since the time of the Ancient Greeks and Romans for menstrual problems, for irregular, heavy, painful or suppressed periods, and troubles associated with the menopause. It regulates the cycles and generally enhances health and wellbeing.

Mugwort was recommended to increase fertility, and as a remedy to facilitate childbirth. The first English gynaecological handbook recommended it for a difficult birth along with the other artemisias. 'Make her a bath of mallows, fenugreek, linseed, wormwood, southernwood, pellitory and mugwort, boiled in water and let her bathe in it for a good time'. Since it acts as an emmenagogue it should probably be avoided during pregnancy and only used just before or during the birth. However, in China mugwort is used to stop rather than bring on uterine bleeding and for some cases of threatened miscarriage, particularly for women who are deficient in energy and feel cold.

As a diuretic mugwort is useful for fluid retention, particularly around period time. It also helps elimination of toxins via the urine, thereby acting as a blood cleanser and making it helpful in treatment of arthritis and gout. Like wormwood, mugwort is an excellent bitter tonic, stimulating the appetite and enhancing digestion by increasing secretion of digestive enzymes and bile from the liver and gallbladder. It can be used to expel worms. It makes a good remedy for those with a weak, sluggish digestion, toxins and congestion in the gut, liver problems and those feeling run down and debilitated and during convalescence.

As an antispasmodic it relaxes spasm of the intestinal muscles and helps relieve colic, diarrhoea, constipation, intestinal spasm and indigestion. Mugwort has mildly sedative properties and has a beneficial effect generally on the nervous system. It has been used for centuries for epilepsy, nervousness, fright and convulsions. The 13th century physicians of Myddfai prescribed it for hysteria (it is interesting that this word relates to the womb; for instance, hysterectomy means removal of the womb). It was also used for problems of nervous origin, such as nausea, vomiting, colic, indigestion or diarrhoea.

By stimulating the circulation, mugwort is warming and strengthening. Taken hot it increases blood flow to the skin and thereby enhances perspiration, useful in bringing down fevers. Its antiseptic and blood cleansing properties make it a good remedy for treating febrile infections as well as more chronic infections such as pelvic inflammatory disease and thrush. It is also useful for cystitis, colds and coughs. In China mugwort leaves are rubbed together and bound in a cylindrical shape and burnt over certain acupuncture points to stimulate the circulation and warm the point.

Homeopathic remedy: ARTEMISIA

The root of *Artemisia vulgaris* is used mainly for spasms and epilepsy brought on by extremes of emotion or excitement, or fright. It is also prescribed for petit mal attacks (short losses of consciousness), for sleepwalking, catalepsy and dizziness caused by coloured lights when associated with nervousness. Artemisia is used mainly as a woman's remedy, in particular for irregular, scanty periods, painful periods, threatened miscarriage with violent cramps in the abdomen, and for uterine prolapse.

The flower essence

A close relative of *Artemisia vulgaris*, *Artemisia douglasiana*, a native of America also called mugwort, is used. Like the herbal remedy, it enhances the moon-like receptive quality of the psyche, allowing greater clarity and awareness of the dream world. It helps to integrate the insights gained from our dreams and our psychic awareness into our daily lives, and to understand their significance.

Mugwort is used to balance the transition from night to day consciousness, and to help those who have a tendency to an overactive psychic life, cutting them off from the physical world of 'reality', remain connected to the practical, earthy aspects of life. It is recommended for people who tend to be irrational, over-emotional and hysterical, prone to disturbed nights because of an overactive dream life.

Mugwort is predominantly a woman's remedy, assisting the 'flowing processes' in the body, such as menstruation and childbirth. It connects menstrual cycles more closely to the lunar cycle.

The flower remedy can be added to a herbal oil made from mugwort and used for massage to remedy menstrual problems and aid childbirth. It also stimulates the circulation giving a feeling of warmth.

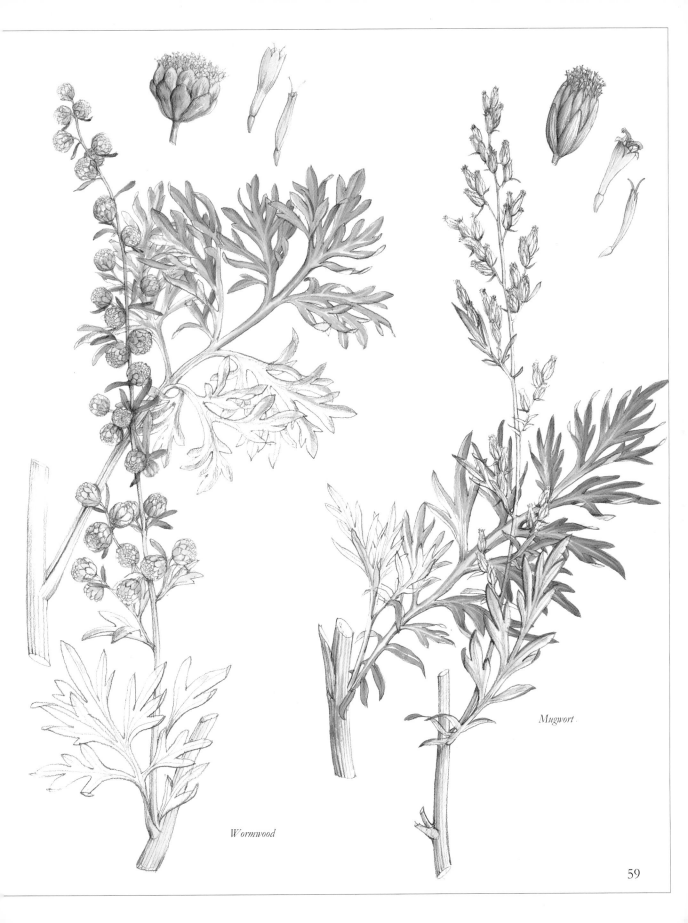

Wormwood

Mugwort

59

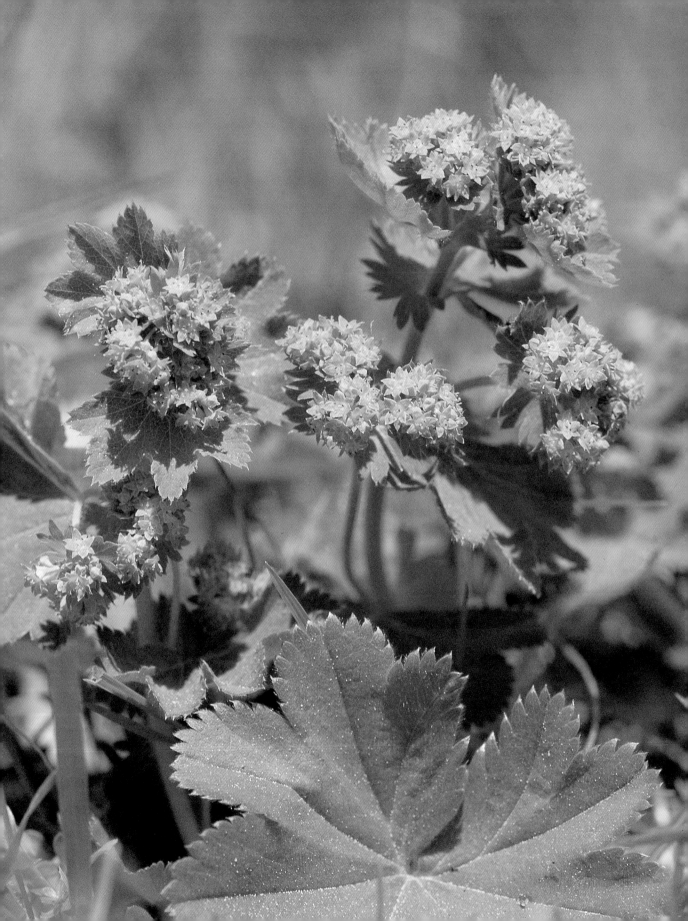

Lady's mantle

The flower of alchemy

The name Alchemilla derives from the Arabic word *alkemelych* meaning alchemy, for this attractive plant with its elegant foliage and lacy yellow flowers was a favourite of the medieval alchemists. Perhaps because of its wonderful healing powers, the alchemists considered it magical. In their search for the philosopher's stone, the magical way of turning baser metals into gold, they collected the pearly drops that form and sparkle on the leaves of lady's mantle, which they called 'water from heaven'. The dew drops, which are actually exuded from the plant itself, were thought to extract subtle healing and magical virtues from the leaf, and were used in many an alchemist's potion.

In the Middle Ages, lady's mantle was also dedicated to the Virgin Mary, and as its name suggests, the scalloped-edge leaves were thought to resemble Mary's cloak. In healing, the plant has a strong affinity with women and the female reproductive system. Culpeper said that it was ruled by Venus.

Lady's mantle can be propagated in spring or autumn by root division. It will grow in poor, slightly acidic soil, and likes full sun or partial shade.

Herbal remedy

The whole plant makes a remedy which lives up to its old name 'woman's best friend'. It has astringent tannins which help to reduce heavy periods, particularly useful around the menopause. As a uterine stimulant and emmenagogue it stimulates menstrual flow and can be used to stimulate contractions during childbirth. It will help to reduce period pains and regulate periods. Culpeper recommended drinking distilled lady's mantle water for 20 days to encourage conception.

As a general tonic to the reproductive tract it can be used after trauma such as abortion, miscarriage and childbirth, as well as for fibroids, pelvic inflammatory disease, post partum bleeding and genito-urinary infections. It helps normal involution of the uterus after childbirth and reduces risk of prolapse. It helps the breasts to regain their tone after breast-feeding.

The astringent properties, particularly in the fresh root, are excellent for treating diarrhoea and gastroenteritis, while the salicylic acid reduces inflammation in the digestive and reproductive systems. The diuretic properties are helpful in relieving fluid retention.

Externally, lady's mantle makes a douche or lotion for vaginal discharge, irritation and infection. An infusion is a good skin lotion for rashes, cuts and wounds, sores and insect bites. As a mouthwash or gargle it relieves bleeding gums, mouth ulcers and sore throats.

The sparkling dewdrops from the leaves were included in the past in cosmetic preparations for restoring female beauty.

The flower essence

The applications of lady's mantle continue along the same theme of alchemy and women. The alchemist's 'philosopher's stone' is that which can never be lost or dissolved, something eternal, the mystical experience of the divine within one's own soul. Lady's mantle is a remedy for those women who wish to be more in touch with the divine female power within them, and for those who seek the inspiration or protection of Mary, or the goddess within. It is particularly recommended for those who feel alienated from women or from their feminine side, perhaps because of negative experiences during childhood with women who had authority in their lives. Being an alchemic plant, lady's mantle helps to dissolve away those earthbound or superfluous elements which are concealing the 'stone' within. It aids transition in one's life, helps one move away from the past, and release ties that bind.

It is particularly useful during times of change that may bring fear, such as childbirth, moving home, the break up of a relationship, or a bereavement.

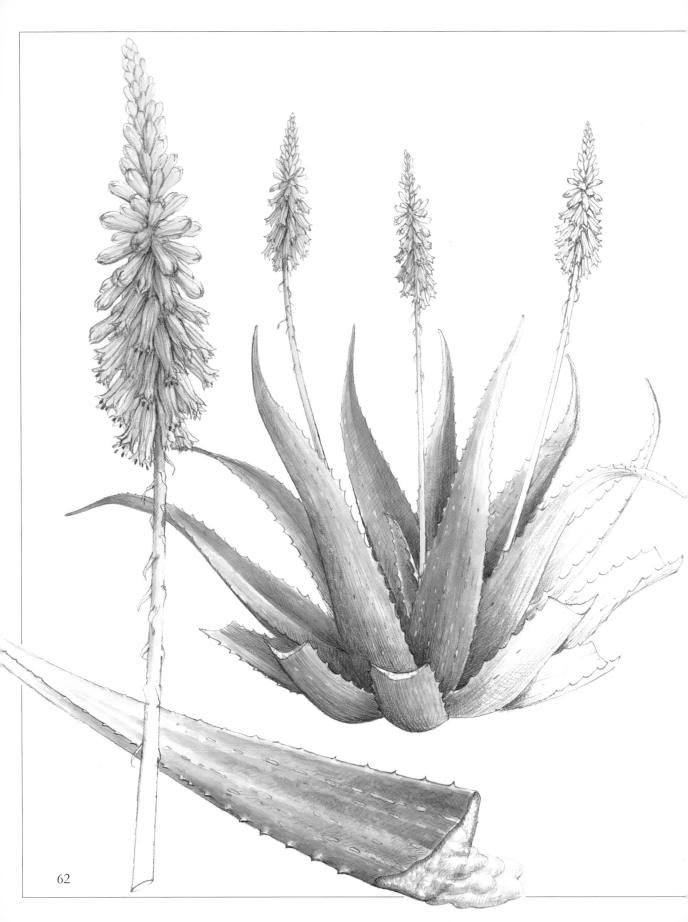

Aloe

The flower of regeneration

This succulent perennial of the lily family is indigenous to East and southern Africa, but grows happily in other tropical places. In temperate climates it grows as a houseplant. There are two distinct parts of *Aloe vera* used in healing: the juice, extracted from the base of the leaf (which can be dried to a powder) and the juicy gel from inside the leaves.

Aloe was known to the Ancient Greeks, and has been used medicinally since the 4th century BC as described by Dioscorides and Pliny. It grew on the island of Socotra. The aloe plant has been revered in Islam as a religious symbol. Pilgrims would carry it to the Prophet's shrine and then hang it over their own doorway at home for protection. One kind of aloe was traditionally planted at the foot of a grave to lend patience to the dead while they waited for resurrection.

In Sanskrit aloe's name *kumari* means a young girl or virgin, because the plant apparently imparts the energy of youth and brings about the renewal of female energy. *Aloe vera* is a remarkably resilient plant. It is protected against drought by its succulent leaves. Even if left with no water until shrivelled, a leaf once immersed in water for a few hours will become plump and fresh again. It also heals itself remarkably quickly if a leaf is damaged.

Herbal remedy

Aloe juice is a powerful laxative or purgative, and should be taken with a carminative such as ginger or turmeric otherwise it may cause severe griping. It helps control micro-organisms in the gut.

Aloe gel has a wide variety of therapeutic uses. It acts as a bitter tonic to the liver and the whole of the digestive tract. It enhances the secretion of digestive enzymes, balances acid in the stomach, aids digestion and regulates sugar and fat metabolism. Aloe gel has wonderful demulcent properties, soothing and protecting the lining of the gut. It can be used to treat colitis, peptic ulcers and irritable bowel syndrome. It has a generally cooling and moistening effect and can be used for problems associated with excess heat and inflammation. It is particularly useful for hot fiery people, who are prone to inflammatory problems and to feelings of anger, irritability and self-criticism.

Externally, aloe gel has remarkable healing powers. It is used for treating burns including sunburn, and after radiation therapy. It also relieves pain, soothes inflammation and has a mildly antibiotic effect. It is used in lotions to rejuvenate the skin and reduce wrinkles. Legend has it that Cleopatra used it to maintain her beauty. It is excellent for sensitive and allergic skin conditions. In shampoos it improves the condition of dry, brittle hair. Aloe gel is applied to haemorrhoids to soothe pain and irritation and speed healing. It makes a useful application to relieve irritating skin conditions.

Homeopathic remedy: ALOE SOCOTRINA

Aloe also has an affinity with the digestive tract, the liver and reproductive system. An aloe person tends to feel angry at themselves, and feel dissatisfied and ill humoured particularly on cloudy days. They feel exhausted, disinclined to work, anxious or restless, and are worse in heat and feel better when cool. Their physical symptoms are characterized by heat and congestion, and internal complaints are often expressed through inflammatory skin problems. They are generally worse in hot conditions, worse if constipated, and feel better in cool conditions or with cool applications, and they long for juicy things. There can be a feeling of fullness in the liver area, burning and irritating haemorrhoids, which may be so bad as to resemble a bunch of grapes. It can relieve painful periods, labour-like pains in the loins and groin which are worse on standing.

The flower essence

The theme of renewal of energy and rejuvenation continues through aloe's use as a flower essence. As in herbal medicine and homeopathy, aloe particularly suits those who have a fiery, creative constitution, who are suffering from lethargy or exhaustion having burnt themselves out. It is an excellent remedy for 'workaholics' who tend to drive themselves so hard that they neglect their physical and emotional needs in order to accomplish their goals. They may be driven by self-criticism and have strong willpower, but eventually deplete their inner energy. Aloe vera pours 'water' on excess 'fire'.

Marshmallow, Hollyhock

The flowers of softness

The Hollyhock distains the common size of
Herbs,
and like a Tree do's proudly rise;
Proud she appears, but try her and you'll find
No plant more mild or friendly in mankind
She gently all obstructions do's unbind.
    ABRAHAM COWLEY (1618–1667)

The marshmallow is an attractive mild plant that
grows in salt marshes and damp fertile places. The
leaves are as soft as velvet. It can be grown from
seed or root division and likes full sun. The flowers
are followed by a ring of seeds shaped like a cheese.
The tall hollyhock will grow in most soils. It originated in China where it was an emblem of fruitfulness.
In Victorian England it was a symbol of female
ambition, perhaps because it was said to be ruled by
Venus. It was believed to grow well only at the gates
of happy homes. The leaves were used to treat
horse's swollen heels, so it was originally called hock-
leaf, and since it was thought to come from the holy
land it became known as hollyhock.

Marshmallow and hollyhock are of the Malvaceae
family, the word malva coming from *malakos*, Greek
for soft or soothing, referring to the demulcent and
emollient properties of these plants. In fact
marshmallow is probably more soothing than any
other plant because of its high mucilage content.
Althaea comes from the Greek *althane*, to heal.

For the Ancient Greeks and Romans mallows
were vegetables and healing herbs. The Pythagorean
philosophers considered the mallow sacred because
the flowers always turned towards the sun. It was for
them the symbol of moderation and control of
human passions, which they considered necessary for
attainment of wisdom and health. Mallow is also the
symbol of sweetness and mildness, and it certainly
has a sugary flavour and smooth texture. The tender
leaves and young tops of marshmallow are edible and
can be added sparingly to salads. Mallows were eaten
by the poor in Ancient Greece. Marshmallow is the
origin of the soft sweets of the same name.

Herbal remedy

Marshmallow is a wonderful remedy for any kind of
irritation or inflammation inside or outside the body,
because of its great soothing and healing properties.
The demulcent mucilage soothes the digestive,
respiratory and urinary systems, while the tannins
heal inflammation and ulceration of the mucous
membranes. Marshmallow will help relieve heartburn
and indigestion. Both as a mild expectorant and an
immune enhancer it is helpful for dry, irritating
coughs and chest infections.

In the urinary system, marshmallow acts as a
soothing diuretic, useful in cystitis and irritable
bladder, and was a traditional remedy for easing
the passage of urinary gravel and stones.

Hollyhock has also been used for soothing
digestive, respiratory and urinary complaints. Both
plants have a cooling effect and should be thought
of whenever there is excess heat and inflammation.

Marshmallow was traditionally added to herbs to
ease childbirth and has also been used to improve
production of breastmilk. Teething babies were given
a marshmallow root to gnaw, to cool their inflamed
gums. Adults used the root as a tooth cleaner.

Externally, marshmallow and hollyhock can be
used in gargles for sore throats, mouth problems
and spongy gums. The leaves can be applied to wasp
and bee stings, and insect bites, scalds and burns,
sunburn and inflammatory skin problems such as
eczema and acne. They were used in the past for
bruises, sprains and strains, and joint and muscular
aches and pains. The leaves or pulverized root were
used to draw out thorns, or as a warm drawing
poultice for boils and carbuncles.

The flower essence

Mallow is used as a flower essence to engender
warmth and openness. The plant used is a different
mallow, *Sidalcea glauscens*, from the same Malvaceae
family. It is particularly useful for those who feel
isolated, lonely, cut off and unable to give or receive
warmth and friendship. This may stem from
insecurity, fear, or lack of trust related to incidents
in early life. The feelings may give rise to problems
making or keeping friends, or in making a commitment to a relationship.

Mallow helps to overcome such barriers to
friendship, and to warm and caring relationships,
and helps to soothe and ease communication.

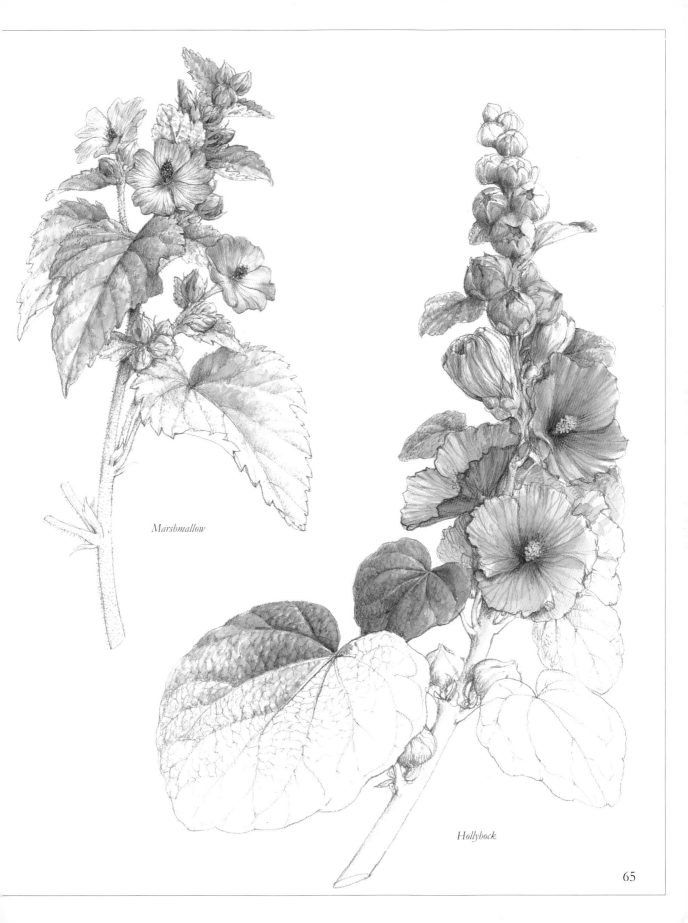

Marshmallow

Hollyhock

65

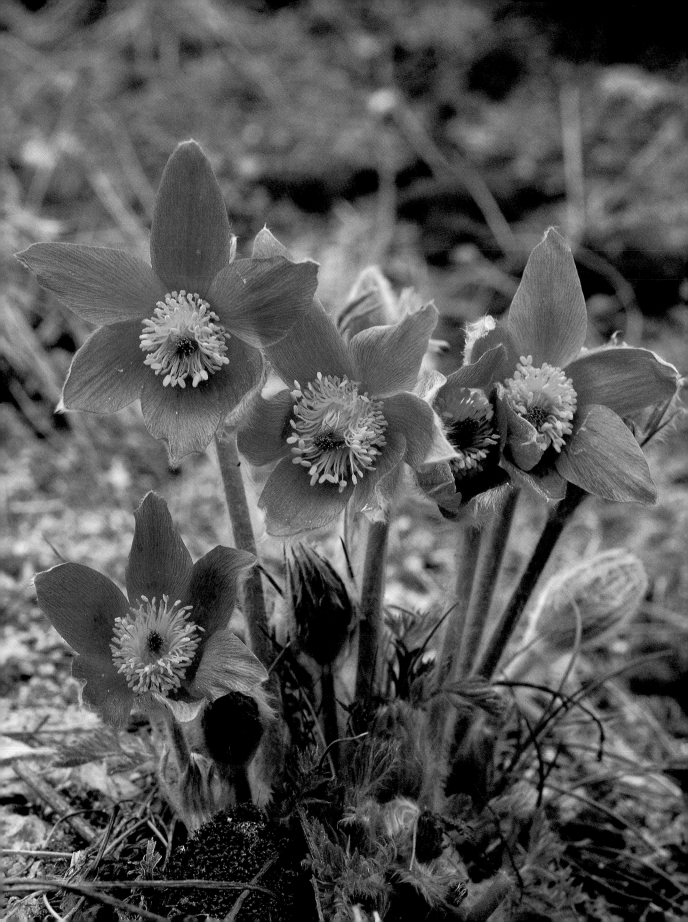

Pasque flower

The flower of forsakeness

Then came the wind-flower
In the valley left behind, pale
As a wounded maiden
with purple streaks of woe.
SYDNEY DORRELL (1824–74)

The beautiful pasque flower, also called pulsatilla, has silky purple flowers and is so named because it flowers in spring and often on Easter Day (*Pascha*) in the Northern hemisphere. It is also known as the wind flower as the word anemone comes from the Greek *anemos* meaning wind. In Greek mythology Anemone was a beautiful nymph beloved of Zephyr, the god of the West wind. The goddess Flora, his wife, became very jealous and transformed Anemone into the little wind flower and she was abandoned by Zephyr to Boreas, god of the North wind. He wooed her every spring and she would open only at his bidding. For this reason in the language of flowers anemone represents all those forsaken in love.

Pasque flower is ruled by the planet Venus and there is another story that tells that the flower sprang from the tears of Venus, the goddess of love, as she wept over the body of Adonis who had been slain, and for this reason also anemone means forsaken. However frail this flower may sound it resiliently withstands the cruel winds of the early spring and it does have remarkable healing powers. The first anemone of the year to be found, it is said, has special healing properties, and it used to be wrapped in red cloth and tied on the arms of the sick.

Herbal remedy

The dried pasque flowers and leaves make a wonderful tonic for the nervous system. By promoting relaxation and sleep it facilitates recovery by those nervously run down by conserving their nervous energy. It is particularly effective for women and children who are irritable and weep easily.

Pasque flower has a particular application to pain, spasm and inflammation in the reproductive system, both male and female. Its analgesic properties are useful during childbirth, while the relaxant and tonic action in the uterus helps to promote and facilitate the birth. After the birth it can be used for any kind of over-excitement, weepiness or depression.

Pasque flower also has an affinity to mucous membranes, particularly in the respiratory and digestive systems. Because it brings blood to the surface and increases sweating it will reduce fevers and can be used to treat eruptive infections.

Homeopathic remedy: PULSATILLA

Pulsatilla has similar applications although the pasque flower used is *A. pratensis*. The name wind flower is particularly in keeping with its homeopathic use, for a pulsatilla person is changeable, yielding and gentle, fickle and easily blown around by the wind. Physical symptoms tend to come and go and are all characterized by changeability.

Emotionally, pulsatilla types are like changeable weather – one moment sunshine, and showers the next – and they laugh and cry easily. Behind their fickleness is a deep fear of being alone, of being forsaken just like the nymph Anemone.

Pulsatilla has a particular affinity to the female reproductive tract and is used for a number of menstrual disorders, including late onset of periods. It also has applications during pregnancy and in childbirth, and for afterpains and postnatal depression.

Like the herbal remedy, homeopathic pulsatilla also has an affinity for mucous membranes and is used for thick, yellow-green catarrh.

Pulsatilla will help where there are varicose veins, sluggish venous circulation, chilliness, anaemia, nosebleeds, fever, measles with catarrh, lethargy and restless sleep with troubled dreams. The patient feels worse in a stuffy atmosphere and better in fresh air.

The flower essence

Like the windflower, blown about by the spring breezes, people needing the flower remedy tend to be changeable, happy then tearful, full of vitality one moment then exhausted the next. Like the frail-sounding anemone, one can be tearful, lonely and vulnerable and yet still essentially resilient.

The flower essence allows the gentle, emotional side of oneself to flourish while engendering a sense of inner security and groundedness. Pulsatilla enhances your inner strength and stability, allowing you better to express yourself emotionally and spiritually while balancing your vital energy.

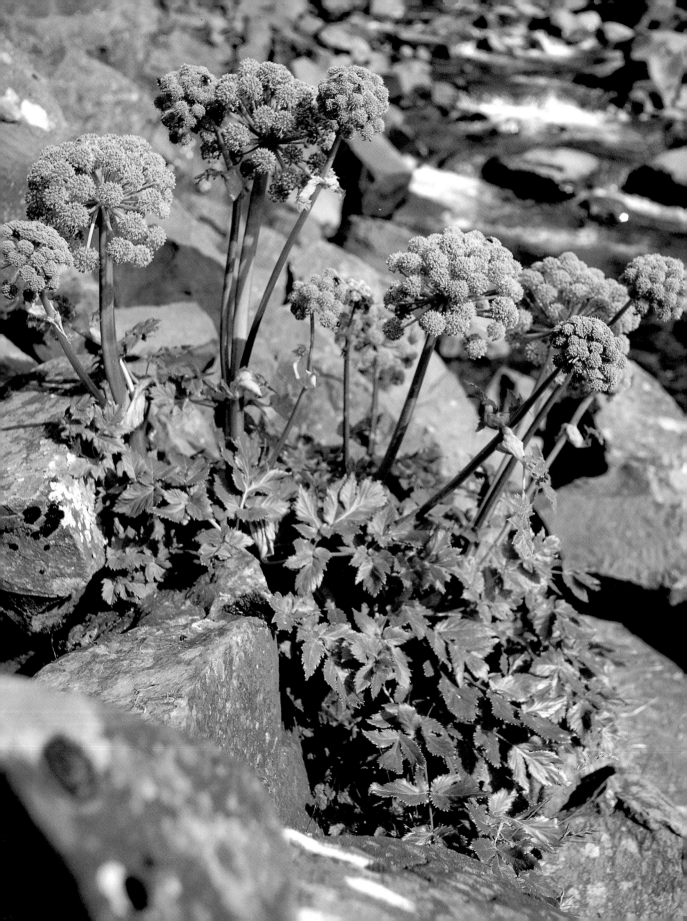

Angelica

The flower of inspiration

Contagious aire ingendring pestilence
Infects not those that in their mouth have ta'en,
Angelica, that happy counterbane,
sent down from heav'n by some Celestial scout,
As well the name and nature both avow't.
    DU BARTAS (1544–90) *(translated by Joshua Sylvester)*

Angelica is a large Umbellifer, growing up to 8–10 feet (3 metres). The whole plant is aromatic, with a pungent, sweet smell and taste. It is not to be confused with *A. sinensis*, Dong Qui, the Chinese species.

Angelica has an ancient history as a protective herb against contagion, poisons and illness as well as evil spirits and witchcraft. In several North European countries it was dedicated to pre-Christian gods and featured in pagan festivals.

In Christian times angelica became linked with the archangel Michael, as it was seen to flower on his day, 8 May. It was also associated with the springtime festival of the Annunciation. Some say it was given its name because a wise man or monk declared that St Michael appeared to him, saying the plant could be used to cure the plague, with instructions to hold a piece of root in the mouth to drive away 'pestilentiall aire'. Angelica was held in such high esteem that it was named 'root of the Holy Ghost'. It was also taken as an antidote to intoxicating drinks and was said to be the symbol of inspiration.

Angelica is most well-known now for its candied stalks that are used to decorate cakes and puddings. The fresh leaves stewed with rhubarb and gooseberries reduce their tart flavour, while the young stalks can be peeled and eaten sparingly in salads, or cooked as a vegetable like celery. The seeds have been used to make liqueurs such as Chartreuse and Benedictine and as a flavouring in gin.

Angelica can be grown from seed in late summer or autumn or propagated by root division. It likes damp soil and light shade. If prevented from flowering it will live for several years, but if it does flower it is biennial. Planted in companionship with angelica, nettles apparently increase angelica oil by 80 percent.

Herbal remedy

Angelica has a sweet pungent taste with a warming effect. Culpeper said it is ruled by the sun in Leo.

It stimulates the circulation, and is particularly suitable for people who feel the cold and whose conditions are aggravated by cold and damp. It warms and invigorates the stomach, and relieves wind, spasm and indigestion from lack of 'vital fire' in the stomach. It can be used for nausea, poor appetite and weak digestion. The stems used to be chewed to relieve flatulence. Its cleansing action in the digestive system helps to detoxify the body and thereby protect against illness and infection. The essential oil in the root has antibacterial and antifungal properties: the Lapps preserve fish by wrapping them in the similarly disinfectant leaves.

The whole plant is a warming expectorant and can be used for colds, catarrh, coughs, bronchitis and asthma. In hot infusion it increases perspiration and effectively reduces fevers. The warming effect extends to the reproductive system where angelica can be used to promote uterine circulation, relieve period pain and premenstrual syndrome. It helps to regulate the female cycle, and is considered a superior tonic for women.

Its tonic and stimulating effects extend to the nervous system, where it can be used for nervous exhaustion, tension and as an aid for students before exams. It was taken to impart strength to athletes and convalescents alike, and was considered to have rejuvenative powers. It was chewed by the Lapplanders to prolong life. Angelica has also been a treatment for several urinary problems, and for arthritis and rheumatism.

Externally, angelica is a helpful ingredient in lotions for cuts and wounds, arthritis, and skin problems such as boils and ulcers.

Homeopathic remedy: ANGELICA

Apparently Angelica, if taken regularly either herbally or homeopathically, will cause an aversion to alcohol, and is helpful for alcoholics.

The flower essence

Angelica the flower essence is for those people who tend to feel cut off from their inner selves, and from spiritual protection and guidance. This may occur particularly in difficult or transitional times in life or when approaching death.

Dill
The flower of slumber

Dill is an aromatic annual from the Mediterranean with an aniseed smell. The name dill may derive from the Saxon word *dilla*, meaning to lull, because of its ability to induce sleep in babies and children. The name Anethum is from the Greek *aitho*, to burn, as it was also used as a burning perfume. Dill was an ingredient in medieval love potions, and was hung at doors and windows to keep away the evil eye.

Herbal remedy The volatile oil in dill seeds and dill weed relaxes smooth muscle throughout the body. In the digestive system it soothes colic and indigestion and relieves nausea and vomiting. In the respiratory system dill acts as an antispasmodic and expectorant and is good for coughs and asthma. In the reproductive system dill will relieve painful periods and regulate menstruation. In the East dill is given to women prior to childbirth to ease the birth. It increases milk when breastfeeding, and as a tonic to the nervous system helps alleviate tiredness from disturbed nights. Culpeper said, 'Mercury has the dominion of this plant and therefore to be sure it strengthens the brain'. The leaves were often cooked with fish to add flavour and stimulate the brain. Dill also helps treat insomnia, and is good for stress-related digestive disorders. Recent research indicates that its volatile oils have anti-cancer properties.

Aromatherapy oil The essential oil has relaxant and digestive properties and has been used traditionally in the preparation of gripe water. The oils are ingredients in warming liniments and massage oils.

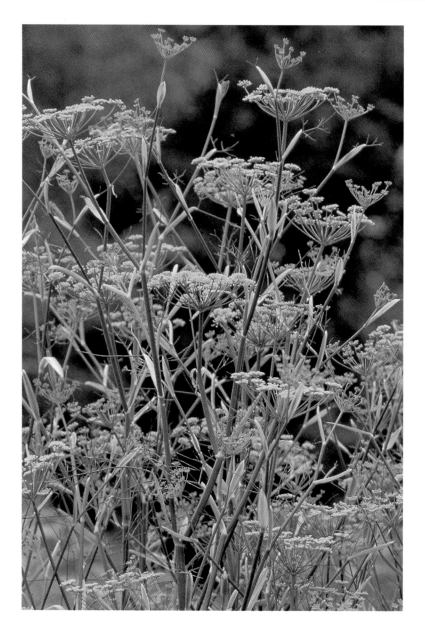

The flower essence Dill makes a good remedy for those who feel stressed and nervously overwrought by the hustle and bustle of life. Those who feel over-stimulated or overwhelmed by the world around them, who suffer a kind of 'sensory indigestion', may well have physical signs of stress such as digestive problems and for such people dill can engender a sense of relaxation and inner nourishment. Rather than seeking a remote place cut off from sensory stimulation and living as an ascetic to develop spiritually, dill is used to help us use the world of the senses as a vehicle for understanding our inner selves, rather than a distraction from our higher purpose.

Arnica
The flower of recovery

Arnica grows wild in the peaty soil of high meadows in Europe, the slopes of the Andes, in Northern Asia and Siberia. It also grows throughout the mountains of the western United States and Canada. The plant was first mentioned in the writings of St Hildegard of Bingen (1099–1179). It has been used for centuries as a healing herb for injuries, falls and accidents and trauma of all kinds.

Herbal and homeopathic remedy Arnica is a wonderful medicine. It increases resistance to infections including listeria and salmonella and speeds healing after surgery, dental extractions and injuries. It can be taken internally but only in homeopathic doses or using 1 drop of the tincture stirred into a glass of water. It is highly recommended for mental and physical shock, bruises, sprains, pain and swelling, and fractures. Arnica rapidly helps to reduce pain and swelling and causes bruising to disappear, and it reduces the risk of complications following such trauma. Not only can it be taken immediately after recent injuries, but also for incidents several years previously which cause persistent symptoms.

Homeopathic arnica can be taken after unaccustomed exertion to prevent aching and malaise the next day. Arnica can also be taken for the after-effects of concussion, stroke, and loss of or altered consciousness after serious infection.

Externally, arnica tincture can be used in a lotion or a cream to speed healing of wounds, bruises, sprains and swellings, especially in children. Applied over any *unbroken* skin it will ease pain, relieve rheumatic joints and painful, swollen feet.

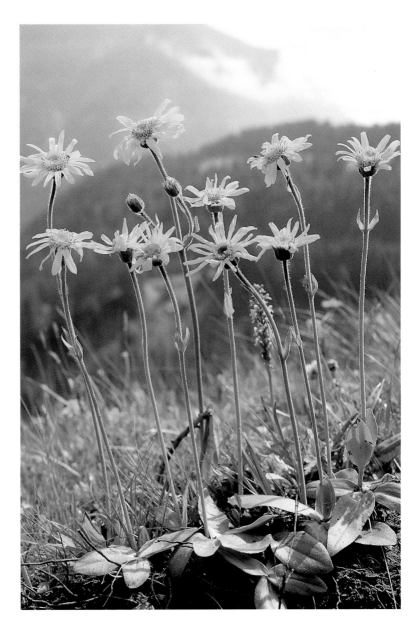

The flower essence Arnica is used to restore a break in the life force after an accident, injury or shock, and to re-establish the connection to the self after trauma. It can be taken as a short-term first aid remedy to speed healing after many different kinds of trauma or injury, and also can be put to good effect where previous accident, injury or deep-seated shock become locked into the body, preventing proper recovery.

Arnica the flower essence can be particularly useful for people who do not respond to other treatment that appears obvious, as the origin of their symptoms lies in past shock or trauma, either emotional or physical.

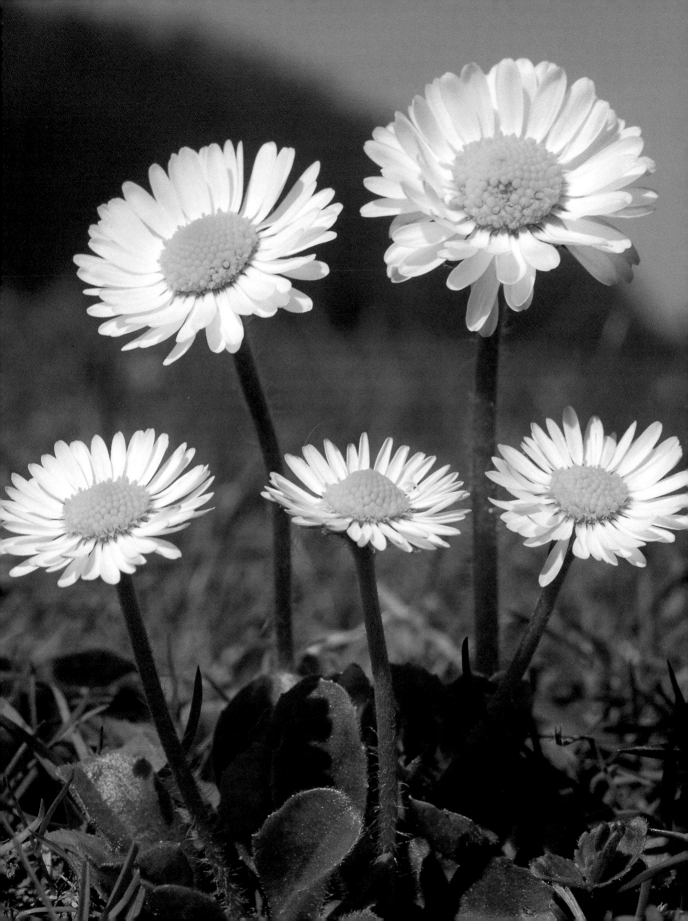

Daisy

The flower of innocence

Of alle the flowers in the med
Then love I most those flowers, white and rede
such as men callen daysies in our town.
  GEOFFREY CHAUCER (1340–1400)

The common daisy, known throughout the world for its cheerful face that flowers from early spring to late autumn, has always been a favourite of children. The country names bairnwort, and baby's pet, reflect children's delight in plucking flowers for posies and daisy chains. Pulling flower petals off one by one, older girls would be told whether 'he loves me, he loves me not'. If they slept with daisy roots under the pillow, they would dream of their love.

In medieval times knights would wear the daisy as a symbol of fidelity, and a token of their lady's love. The name comes from day's eye, because the flower opens in the morning when the sun rises and closes when the sun sets. Its Latin name may come from the Latin *bellis*, meaning beautiful, so *Bellis perennis* can be translated as perennial beauty, as the daisy flowers for so long. Or *bellis* may come from *bellum*, Latin for war, because it grew in fields of battle and can staunch bleeding and reduce bruising and shock. One of the daisy's old names is bruisewort.

The cheerful little daisy is a symbol of innocence, because of its association with children, and of survival. Daisies adapt to almost any landscape and soil type, and will survive being trodden underfoot and all the indignities of the hoe and the lawnmower.

Herbal remedy

The daisy was famous among the Romans as a wound herb and Pliny said it was used to resolve scrofulous tumours. It was used on battlefields to staunch bleeding of wounds and prevent swelling of bruises and sprains. The leaves and flowers were given internally and the bruised herb applied locally. Culpeper said that the daisy was ruled by Venus and was 'used in wound-drinks and are accounted good to dissolve congealed and coagulated blood, to help pleurisy and peripneumonia'. Gerard said, 'daisies do mitigate all kinds of pain, especially in the joints, and gout proceeding from a hot humour.'

Daisy is not commonly used by modern herbalists, although it has useful diuretic properties, aiding the elimination of toxins, thus providing a ready remedy to detoxify the body, useful when treating arthritis, gout, and skin problems such as acne and boils. Its astringent properties are useful in curbing diarrhoea and bleeding and can be used for heavy periods. In fact the daisy used to be a popular remedy for women's problems, given for swellings in the breasts, and swelling and heat in the reproductive system.

According to the doctrine of signatures, the daisy resembles an eye and so should be given for problems affecting the eyes. Daisy was used for making eyebaths to treat inflamed or irritated eye conditions including black eyes. The astringent properties of the daisy would be helpful here. They would also benefit inflammatory skin conditions when daisy tea is used as a lotion and it can be used to apply to varicose veins and haemorrhoids. Daisy will staunch bleeding from cuts and wounds and taken internally and used locally it should be thought of wherever there is shock or bruising from a knock or a fall. It helps us to survive the knocks of life, like the daisy constantly trodden on yet which comes up smiling.

Homeopathic remedy: BELLIS PERENNIS

Bellis perennis is known as the poor man's arnica for it is given for lumps and bumps from knocks or falls, for bruises, wounds and swellings, and the shock that can cause them. Like the herb, Bellis is prescribed for skin problems such as acne and boils, gout, rheumatic pain, varicose veins, women's problems including engorgement of the uterus and breasts. It is prescribed when these complaints follow getting chilled when overheated, or follow injury, accidents or surgery, childbirth or over-exertion.

The flower essence

Daisy is a good remedy for both children and adults. It promotes clarity of mind, and the ability to absorb information and organize oneself in relation to it. Daisy enhances concentration and helps to bring together information from different sources into a focused whole. It is particularly useful for those who suffer from the recurrent problems related, for example, to money, relationships, or learning skills, without understanding why. It is also a good remedy for people involved in planning and organization.

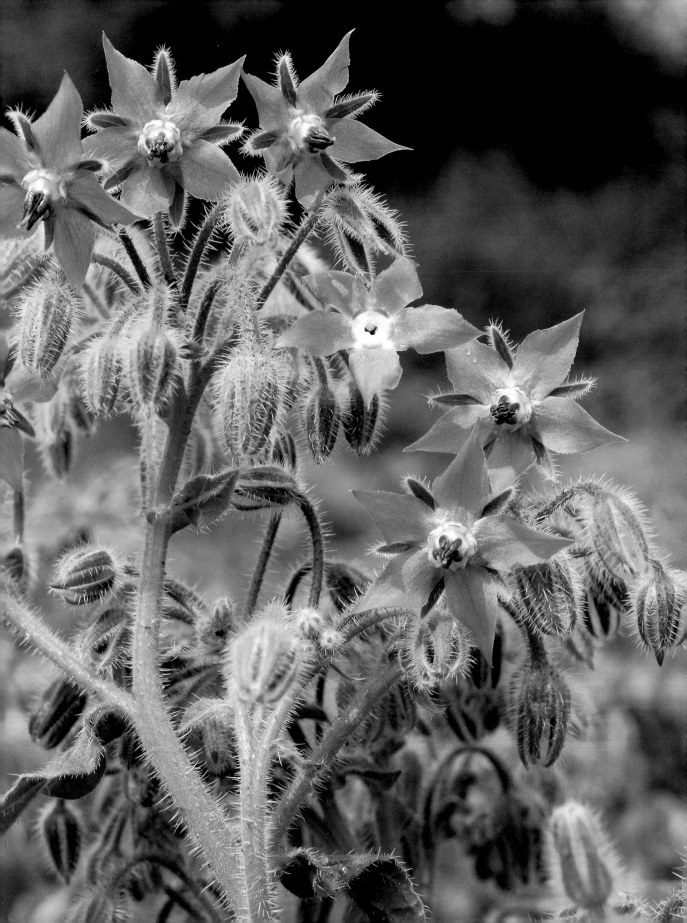

Borage

The flower of courage

Borage ego gaudia semper ago.
[I borage, bring always courage.]
ANON

A native of the Mediterranean countries, borage was taken to Britain by the Romans. It has been highly valued since the time of the Ancient Greeks as a herb to bring courage and dispel melancholy. It was used to promote bravery on the jousting field. The herbalist Gerard writing in 1597 said that a syrup of borage flowers 'comforteth the heart, purgeth melancholy and quieteth the phrenticke and lunatick person'. He also said that Pliny considered 'it maketh a man merry and joyful'. The word borage is said to be a corruption of *cor-ago*; *cor* means heart, *ago* means I bring, as borage has an old reputation as a cordial, a tonic to the heart and lifter of the spirits. It has been used to strengthen weak heart conditions, calm palpitations, and to revitalize the system during convalescence and exhaustion.

The bright blue borage flowers were used by the Ancient Greeks and Romans in their wine cups. The fresh plant has a cool cucumber-like taste, and when added to cider or wine with lemon, sugar and water it was known as a cool tankard. The young leaves are high in potassium and calcium and make a cleansing and nutritious addition to salads. The flowers can brighten any salad, pudding or cake and were crystallized to preserve them for such purposes. Borage is valuable as a companion plant to tomatoes and strawberries and attracts bees.

Herbal remedy

Borage has a relaxing effect generally and is said to dispel grief and sadness. Modern research shows that borage stimulates the adrenal glands, the organs of courage, increasing the secretion of adrenaline, the 'fight or flight' hormone which primes the body for action in dangerous or stressful times. This can prove valuable in countering the effects of steroids and helpful when weaning off steroid therapy to encourage the adrenal glands to produce their own steroid hormones.

The hormonal properties of borage are also present in the seeds which contain gamma linoleic acid. The oil pressed from the seeds can be used for menstrual problems, allergies such as eczema and hay fever, and arthritis. The leaves and seeds have been made into a decoction for increasing milk supply in nursing mothers.

Borage also has an old reputation as a cooling, cleansing herb, used for detoxifying the system and for any condition associated with heat and congestion. It increases sweat production and hastens excretion of toxins via the skin and the urinary system. Borage tea can be taken to clear boils and skin rashes, for arthritis and rheumatism, during infections and to bring down a fever. It is also good for clearing children's eruptive diseases, and for feverish colds, coughs and flu. It has a decongestant and expectorant action in the respiratory system.

The mucilage in borage has a soothing action to relieve any sore, irritated condition of the throat and chest, and to soothe the cough reflex during a dry hacking cough or whooping cough. It has the same action in the digestive and urinary systems. The asparagin in borage lends diuretic, antiseptic action so that it can be used for fluid retention and urinary infections and other irritated or inflamed conditions of the kidneys or bladder.

Externally, a poultice of the leaves and flowers will soothe sore irritated skin conditions. An infusion relieves itching or inflamed skin and sores, ulcers and wounds, and sore inflamed eyes as an eyebath. The fresh juice from the leaves can be applied to burns and to draw out poisons from insect bites, stings and boils. A poultice wrapped around inflamed joints will relieve arthritis and gout. The tea or tincture makes a good gargle or mouthwash.

The flower essence

As a flower essence borage is again the remedy for courage and optimism. Like the cordial herb, it is excellent as a heart remedy to relieve the heavy hearted, ease the broken hearted, and brighten the disheartened. It is particularly helpful for those suffering grief, loss, sadness or discouragement. It lifts the spirits, helping you to rise above the pain you feel and preventing depression.

Borage enhances our resilience, gives renewed buoyancy in adversity, and in this way is useful when feeling low after illness or as old age approaches.

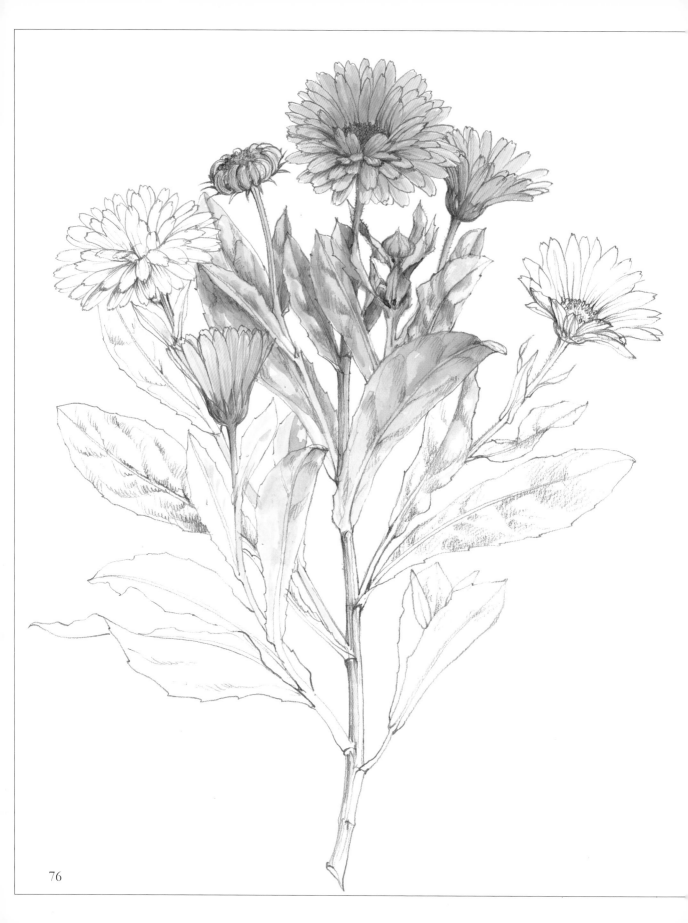

Marigold, Calendula

The flower of the sun

The marigold goes to bed with the Sun
And with him rises, weeping.
WILLIAM SHAKESPEARE (1564–1616)

The common marigold, also known as calendula, with its cheerful orange flower is a familiar sight in cottage gardens and has been popular at least since the days of the Romans. They used the flowers as a tea to relieve fevers and the juice of the crushed flowers to apply to warts. The flowers were used as a cosmetic, a dye and to colour a variety of foods including soups and conserves.

Marigold or calendula flowers, according to Culpeper, are a herb of the sun and under the influence of Leo. They have always been associated with the sun's journey across the sky because they open when the sun rises and close as it sets. Shakespeare, as the lines above suggest, was aware of marigold's association with pain and grief. Some say this is because the flower daily mourns the departure of the sun when its petals are forced to close. Others say that it derives from South American and Mexican lore. After the Spanish conquistadores murdered many Aztecs in their search for gold, the little red flecks which appear on some marigolds were said to symbolize their blood. Another story from Greek mythology tells of Caltha, a girl who fell in love with Apollo the sun god, but was melted by the power of his rays. In her place grew a solitary marigold. The sad association of marigold with grief and pain is said to be dispelled if marigolds are mixed with roses – the two flowers together symbolize the sweet sorrows of love.

Marigold's healing properties were well known to the old herbalists throughout the centuries. It was considered a magic plant: apparently if you wore marigolds you could see who had robbed you. It was also used to protect against evil influences and disease including the plague. Despite its being a symbol of grief, Culpeper and Gerard refer to marigold as a 'comforter of the heart and spirits'. In the Middle Ages St Hildegard and Albert the Great used it for intestinal troubles, liver obstructions, insect and snake bites. In the 16th and 17th centuries marigold tea was used for eye complaints, headaches, jaundice and toothache.

The English name marigold refers to its old use in church festivals in the Middle Ages, being one of the flowers dedicated to the Virgin Mary. It was strewn before cottage doors and made into garlands on May day festivals. The name calendula comes from the Latin *calends*, meaning the first day of every month, because in its warm native climate in Egypt and the Mediterranean, marigold is in bloom on the first day of the month throughout the year. Interestingly, in some traditions marigold is a symbol of endurance.

Herbal remedy

Marigold flowers have antiseptic and astringent properties provided by the volatile oils, tannins and a yellow resin called calendulin. They stimulate the immune system and enhance the body's fight against infection. Research has shown marigold to be effective in controlling flu and herpes viruses, to reduce lymphatic congestion and infections, and swollen lymph glands. It is antibacterial, it can check amoebal infections and worms in the bowel and is one of the best plants for treating fungal infections such as thrush. It has been used for pelvic and bowel infections, including enteritis and dysentery and for viral hepatitis.

In hot infusion marigold stimulates the circulation and promotes perspiration, and thereby helps the body to throw off toxins and bring out eruptions such as measles and chickenpox. It improves poor circulation and varicose veins, and is a good remedy for treating fevers and infections, such as colds and flu, particularly in children.

Marigold has an affinity for the female reproductive system. It regulates menstruation, reduces tension in the uterine muscles and relieves menstrual cramps. It has an oestrogenic effect which helps relieve menopausal symptoms and reduces breast congestion which cause tenderness and mastitis. Its astringent properties help reduce excessive bleeding and uterine congestion. Marigold has a reputation for treating tumours and cysts of the female reproductive system, such as fibroids and ovarian cysts, as well as cysts in the breast and digestive tract. During childbirth it promotes contractions and delivery of the placenta. For this reason it should not be used during pregnancy.

In the digestive tract marigold makes a wonderful healing remedy for gastritis and peptic ulcers, for inflammation and irritation of the lining of the stomach and bowels. It dries catarrh in the stomach, checks diarrhoea and stops bleeding. The bitters stimulate the actions of the liver and gall-bladder, relieving congestion and preventing gallstones. They enhance the secretion of bile and digestive enzymes, improving digestion and absorption. They also stimulate bowel function and relieve 'liverish' symptoms such as headaches, nausea, lethargy and irritability. By enhancing the function of the liver, the great detoxifying organ in the body, marigold helps to cleanse the body of toxins. It also has a diuretic action and increases the elimination of toxins through the urine. Marigold has been used to relieve rheumatism, arthritis and gout – aided by its small salicylic content which adds to its anti-inflammatory action.

Externally, marigold has pride of place as a first aid remedy to staunch bleeding of cuts and abrasions, as an antiseptic healer for sores and ulcers, and to prevent putrefaction of cuts and wounds. Used in tincture, infusion or simply by crushing a flower, it rapidly promotes tissue repair and minimizes scar formation, resolves inflammation, swelling and exudate due to injuries, and reduces venous congestion. Compresses applied to bruises, sprains and strains will reduce swelling and pain. A crushed flower can be rubbed on to insect bites, wasp or bee stings.

An infusion can be used as a mouthwash for inflamed gums, a douche for vaginal infections, or an eyewash for sore, inflamed eye conditions.

Homeopathic remedy: CALENDULA

Calendula is used for injuries where the pain is out of all proportion to the injury. As a tincture, it is taken internally for its remarkable ability to speed healing. It is particularly useful for wounds which may suppurate, and to prevent cuts, injuries and inflammatory problems becoming infected. It can be used after operations and tooth extractions, for skin conditions, particularly erysipelas, and for catarrhal conditions and deafness.

As in herbal medicine, calendula has an affinity for the female reproductive system. It can be taken for heavy or irregular periods, chronic cervicitis, uterine pain with a feeling of stretching and dragging in the groin, an enlarged uterus and vaginal warts.

The flower essence

To the Aztecs marigold represented the cycles of life. As it followed the sun's journey across the sky so also it developed from seed to leaves and stem, then it grew buds and flowers that opened with the sun, and once again produced seed, the womb of the flower. Such is the flow of life eternal. As a flower essence marigold is related to the Word, the source of all creation, the womb of all life. 'In the beginning was the word, and the word was with God ...', as the apostle John wrote. There is a connection between the Word and marigold's affinity with the womb in both herbal medicine and homeopathy. Marigold's use extends into the creative force of the written or spoken word and can be used to enhance communication through this medium. It is particularly recommended for people who lack warmth and receptivity in their communication with others, who tend to use sharp and cutting words, where the spoken word may lead to argument or misunderstanding. Calendula helps such people to listen compassionately to others, to understand their message clearly, and to express warmth and caring in return. This can be applied well to those in healing, teaching or counselling professions and to help authors to be aware of the power of the written word. Calendula helps to balance the feminine aspect of receptivity with the masculine aspect of dynamic activity.

Cayenne

The flower of fire

The greedy merchants, led by lucre, run
To the parched Indies and the rising Sun;
From thence hot pepper and rich drugs they
bear,
Bartering for spices their Italian ware.
    JOHN DRYDEN (1631–1700)

The name cayenne or capsicum comes from a Greek word meaning to bite because of the hot pungent taste and properties of cayenne pepper. It is indigenous to Zanzibar, Mexico and South America and now grows in most tropical and subtropical countries. It was apparently discovered by Christopher Columbus when he was searching for a new source of pepper although it is also said to have arrived in the West from India, as the poem suggests, in 1548.

Apart from being vital in the kitchen for peppering up curries, pickles and relishes, cayenne is invaluable as a medicine. In the past it has been used very successfully as a substitute for alcohol to wean 'hard drinkers' off their tipple. Cayenne tincture was mixed with that of orange peel and some water and gradually reduced in dose as the craving for alcohol diminished. It was also invaluable for delirium tremens as it reduced the tremor and agitation in a few hours and induced a long, calm sleep. Earlier this century capsicum mixed with salt was famous for curing severe influenza with a putrid sore throat.

Herbal remedy

Cayenne is a powerful stimulant and owes its pungency to the alkaloid capsaicin. It is a major stimulant to the heart and circulation, excellent for warming those prone to feeling cold and with poor circulation, and for warding off winter blues, lethargy and chills. Taken hot at the onset of a cold or fever, it causes sweating and enhances the body's fight against infection. It has bactericidal properties and is also rich in vitamin C. It has been used as a strengthening tonic and to ward off senility – probably as it encourages circulation to the brain as well as elsewhere in the body.

Cayenne makes an excellent remedy for the lungs. Its pungency that causes eyes to water also increases the secretion of fluid in the bronchial tubes which thins phlegm in the chest and eases its expulsion. It also acts as an expectorant (through reflex action from its stimulating effect in the stomach). As a decongestant in the head and sinuses, it relieves stuffiness and catarrh, and helps to keep the airways clear, thus preventing as well as treating coughs, colds and bronchitis. Recent research in Sweden has indicated that cayenne blocks irritation and bronchoconstriction caused by cigarette smoke and other airborne irritants.

In the past, cayenne has been used as a remedy for tiredness, lethargy, nervous debility and depression. The burning sensation on the tongue that it causes sends messages to the brain to secrete endorphins – natural opiates – which block pain and induce a feeling of wellbeing, sometimes even euphoria. A couple of drops of tincture can be applied to a sore tooth as an instant remedy for toothache. Research has suggested recently that it may ease the pain of shingles and migraine.

In the digestive tract cayenne stimulates digestive fire and enhances the appetite, promotes the secretion of digestive juices and improves digestion and absorption. It can be added to cooking to relieve sluggish digestion, causing wind, nausea, and indigestion, and symptoms caused by 'cold' such as diarrhoea, abdominal pain and dysentery.

In South America cayenne has long been eaten to kill intestinal parasites. By warming the digestive tract, the health of the whole person is enhanced: toxins are cleared from the gut, stagnant food wastes are removed and the work of the immune system reinforced. However, if you are prone to overheating or acidity of the stomach, cayenne may aggravate your symptoms, and you should therefore exclude it from your diet.

Recent research has indicated that cayenne reduces the tendency to blood clots and lowers harmful cholesterol by reducing the liver's production of cholesterol and triglycerides.

In the reproductive system, the warming effects relieve spasm and pain caused by poor circulation and bring on delayed or suppressed periods. It has been used for infertility and as an aphrodisiac, and it is thought to have rejuvenating powers and to delay the ageing process.

Externally, cayenne is a powerful local stimulant and counter-irritant. It is used in ointment, liniments and plasters as a counter-irritant to treat arthritis, muscular pains, neuralgia, bruises and lumbago, and to paint on unbroken chilblains. It helps bring out inflammation and by numbing the skin, relieves pain. Cayenne powder can be placed in woollen socks to warm the feet on cold winter's days. Use 10–20 drops of cayenne tincture in water to make a good gargle for sore throats and a remedy for colds.

Homeopathic remedy: CAPSICUM

Capsicum is for weak, debilitated people, lacking vital heat and reactive energy. It acts on the mucous membranes and the bones, and is indicated particularly where there is a tendency to suppuration every time there is an inflammatory process: swollen tonsils become infected, eruptions on the skin become ulcerated, congestion in the middle ear turns to infection.

Physically, the burning effects experienced by eating too much hot pepper are the indications for its homeopathic use – symptoms are characterized by heat and burning, as well as constriction. These may be a red, hot face, hot eruptions on the skin, burning and stinging in the ears, hot feeling in the throat, burning on the tip of the tongue and in the stomach, burning with frequency of urination and heat, and soreness of haemorrhoids and with a bowel movement.

Like the herbal remedy, homeopathic capsicum is prescribed for alcoholics withdrawing from alcohol and for delirium tremens. It helps the enfeebled digestion of alcoholics, and their 'peppery' disposition. It is also given for bursting headaches,

swelling and pain in and behind the ears, sore throats of smokers and drinkers, herpes on the lips, sore mouths, flatulence, menopausal problems including heavy bleeding with nausea, constriction in the chest with a dry hacking cough and foetid breath, pain in the legs, sciatica aggravated by coughing, and for fever with coldness and shivering, particularly after drinking and in humour.

The symptom picture is characterized then with burning symptoms but a feeling of chilliness. The person has a great sensitivity to cold and damp, especially draughts. It is useful for older people whose vital energy is depleted, especially by mental exertion. They have a great craving for stimulants such as coffee, and a great thirst, and have a peculiar tendency to shiver after drinking.

The flower essence

This wonderful warming plant again enhances fire and energy, and stimulates movement and change in one's life. The quality of fire is not only warming but also transforming, mobile and creative. It is the fire in the stomach and intestines that transforms food into energy, the light in the eyes, and the spark in the mind. As a flower remedy cayenne is recommended for those who feel stuck in their lives, sluggish, stagnant, and uncreative, not really challenging themselves, caught up in old routines and resistant to change.

Cayenne the flower essence stimulates creative energy and then transforms energy into action. It helps one move decisively into a new phase of life by mobilizing the will and stimulating new motivation. It provides that vital catalytic spark to overcome blocks to transformation.

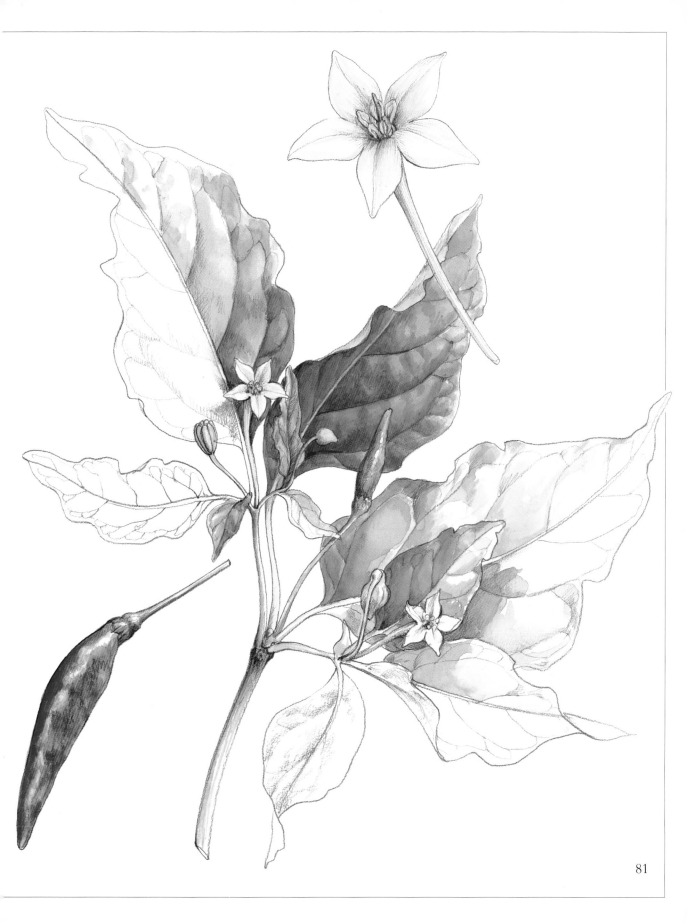

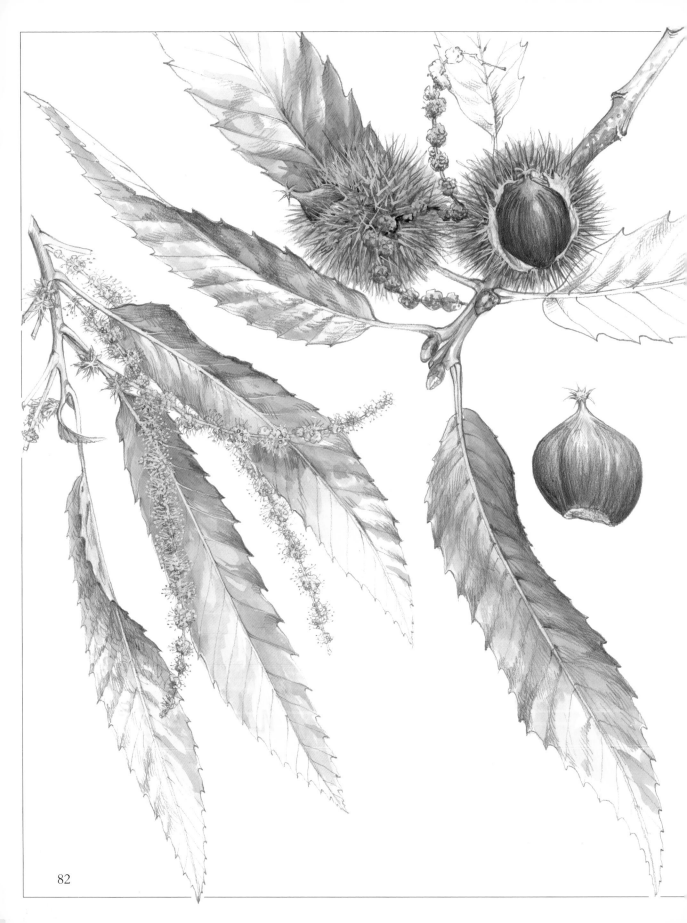

Sweet chestnut

The flower of virtue

The chestnut casts his flambeaux and the flowers
stream from the hawthorn on the wind away,
The doors clap to, the pane is blind with showers
Pass me the can, lad; there's an end of May.
  A E HOUSMAN (1859–1936)

The handsome chestnut tree flourishes all over Europe, but is apparently native to Sardis in Asia Minor, from where it gets its name Sardian nut. It was introduced to Britain by the Romans. Evelyn loved chestnut trees and was said to be responsible for planting many stately avenues of them. He described the chestnuts as 'delicacies for princes and a lusty and masculine food for rusticks, and able to make a woman well-complexioned'.

Sweet chestnuts were known to the Ancient Greeks as *Dios balanos* (Zeus' acorns) and dedicated to Zeus. The name Castanea comes from a town called Castanis on Thessaly, an area where chestnut trees were grown in abundance. In Christianity the sweet chestnut tree is a symbol of virtue, chastity and victory over temptation because of the prickly case that encloses the nut.

Chestnuts contain more starch and less oil than other nuts and make a good flour much like a grain flour which can be made into bread. Roast chestnuts and chestnut stuffing are old winter favourites which are highly nutritious, rich in minerals including calcium, magnesium, phosphorus and iron, and easily digestible. Chestnuts used to be fed to loved ones as an enchanting love spell. *Marrones* are a large sort of sweet chestnut grown in France, Italy and Switzerland, famous for the delicious sweet preserves called *marrons glacés*.

Herbal remedy

The leaves of the sweet chestnut have an anti-spasmodic action used for relaxing spasm particularly in the chest which causes paroxysmal coughing in whooping cough and other irritating convulsive coughs. They also act as a febrifuge, useful for bringing down fevers and were used in the past to treat 'ague' (malaria). The leaves act to soothe and astringe the mucous membranes throughout the body, and have been used in remedies for catarrh, diarrhoea and bleeding. In Culpeper's day, chestnut leaves were used to stop bleeding and coughing up blood and to alleviate heavy menstrual bleeding.

The nuts are strengthening and act as a tonic to the nervous system. They are good to eat in the winter, especially by people who feel cold and weak, and who are involved in physical work.

Homeopathic remedy: CASTANEA VESCA

Castanea vesca is prepared from the leaves and is used for whooping cough, in the early stages when the cough is dry, violent and spasmodic. It is also given for diarrhoea accompanied by severe abdominal pain and rumbling which is relieved by a bowel movement.

The flower essence

Sweet chestnut is the remedy for those who feel so stressed, even tortured, that they have reached the limits of their endurance and feel in a state of utter despair. The mind and the body are completely exhausted from uncomplainingly fighting difficulties, either mental or physical, until a sense of hopelessness and complete darkness sets in. In this 'dark night of the soul' sufferers may come face to face with themselves and this may prove the catalyst for entering a new stage in life.

The intensity of suffering may push us on to the threshold of inner transformation, and to another level of consciousness. Sweet chestnut helps during such crises in our lives; it enhances the process of transformation that is possible in such a state of despair and helps to prevent us from simply going to pieces and deriving little or no benefit from the experience.

Greater celandine

The flower of vision

Greater celandine is a member of the poppy family and shows many of the poppy's actions in healing. It is indigenous to Europe and is remarkably resilient, flourishing where other plants would not survive. It can be found in waste places, growing against walls and fences, and in small cracks in walls and pavements. When cut or bruised it exudes a bright yellow-orange juice that tastes bitter and acrid, much like the juice of a poppy.

The name Chelidonium comes from the Greek word *chelidon*, meaning swallow, because of an old belief that the swallow carried the plant to its nest to open the eyes of its young. It is also thought that the name derives from the simple fact that greater celandine comes into flower when the swallows arrive and fades when they leave. To the alchemists greater celandine was very special and they used it in their search for the philosopher's stone, calling it *coelidonum*, meaning gift of heaven.

Herbal remedy

Greater celandine has been used in healing since the days of the Ancient Greeks and Romans. As the story of the swallow indicates, the plant has a special affinity for the eye, and was given to remedy a whole range of eye problems that caused problems with vision. Francis Bacon said, 'saladyne hath a yellow milk which hathe also much acrimonie for it cleanseth the eyse and is good for cataract', while Gerard stated, 'the juice of the herbe is good to sharpen the sight, for it cleanseth and consumeth away slimie things that cleave about the ball of the eye and hinder the sight'. It is still used by medical herbalists for infections and inflammation of the eye.

According to the doctrine of signatures, the bright orange-yellow juice indicated the plant's use in liver and gall-bladder problems. It was recommended for obstructions of the liver and gall-bladder, jaundice, infections, gallstones, and pain in the liver area. The plant tastes very bitter and by stimulating the bitter receptors in the mouth, greater celandine stimulates the flow of digestive juices and bile.

Paracelsus was aware of the plant's healing properties. He classified it as a 'blood' herb for circulatory problems and as a 'yellow' herb for liver ailments and jaundice. By cleansing the liver and stimulating

the kidneys, greater celandine acts as an alterative, aiding the detoxifying action of the body. As a diuretic it aids elimination of toxins via the urine, and relieves fluid retention. It can be given for rheumatism and gout, as well as allergies and toxic conditions which give rise to skin problems.

Like the poppy, greater celandine has narcotic properties and is only ever used in small doses by qualified medical herbalists. As a sedative it aids sleep, reduces tension and anxiety and relieves pain. It has an antispasmodic effect particularly in the respiratory system.

Externally, the plant is perfectly safe for home use and makes a wonderfully effective remedy for warts and verrucae when the fresh juice is applied directly.

Homeopathic remedy: CHELIDONIUM

Chelidonium reflects much of its action when used as a herb. It is predominantly a liver remedy, indicated by a continual bruised pain or ache under the right shoulder blade, with a variety of symptoms indicative of liver or gall-bladder problems.

Like the opium poppy, chelidonium is given for debility and drowsiness, which tends to occur after eating and on waking, and is given for paralysis. It also acts on the respiratory system and is indicated by dry, racking coughs which are worse at night, with little expectoration and no pain. Chelidonium is also given for rheumatism or arthritis, where oedema, heat, tenderness and stiffness are leading indications.

The flower essence

As the herb was used historically to sharpen the sight, the flower essence is recommended to sharpen the mind and enhance the giving and receiving of information. It is the remedy of communication, and has an affinity for the throat area, and the thyroid gland. It makes a good remedy for singers, teachers and lecturers as it helps articulation. It is useful for people who have difficulty taking in information, such as those who are stubborn and opinionated, or who do not listen, or who cannot concentrate for long. It is said to increase the possibility of telepathic communication, and enhance the understanding of information given in dreams. Thus it affects not only the sight and the mind, but also inner vision.

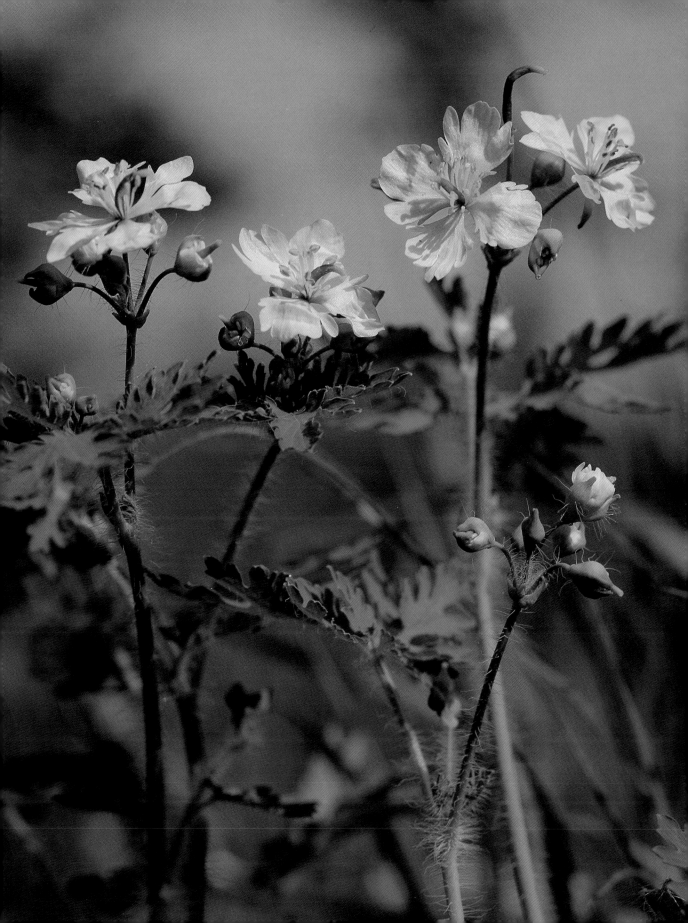

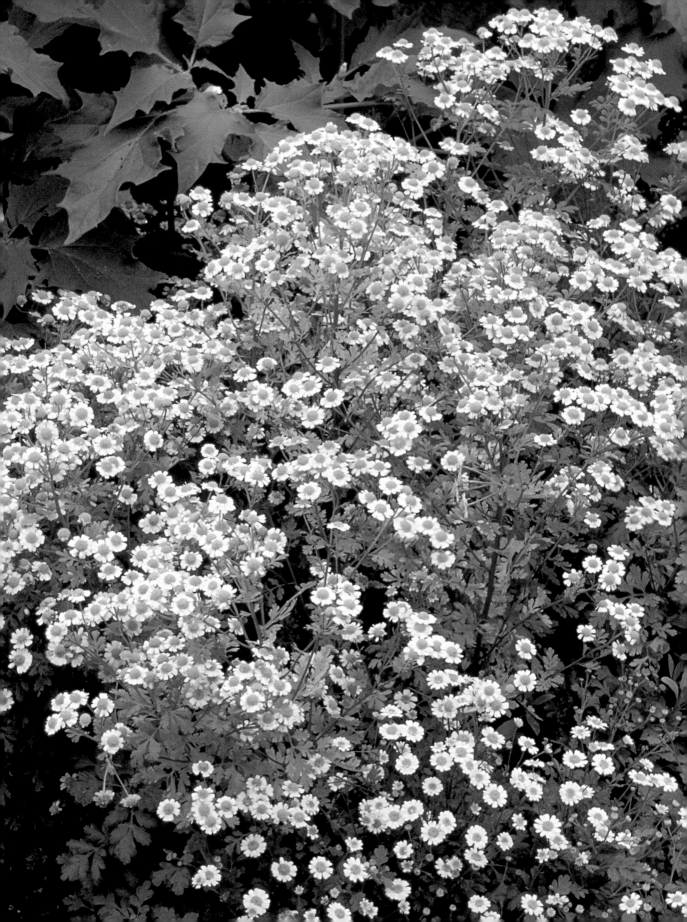

Feverfew

The flower of relief

Feverfew is a pretty member of the daisy family, Compositae. Though now in the genus Tanacetum, it was previously in another Compositae genus, Chrysanthemum, (the others are Matricaria and Pyrethrum). Matricaria was so called because of the plant's beneficial relationship to the *matrix*, the Latin word for womb, and feverfew has been used for centuries for a wide range of women's problems. The name pyrethrum comes for the Greek *pyro* meaning fire, as the roots of feverfew have a hot taste.

Culpeper said that feverfew is ruled by Venus and 'hath commended it to succour our sisters to be a general strengthener of their wombs and to remedy such infirmities as a careless midwife hath there caused; if they will be pleased to make use of her herb boiled in white wine and drink the decoction, it cleanseth the womb, expels the afterbirth and doth a woman all the good she can desire of a herb'.

Feverfew has other names which indicate its usefulness for women. Parthenium comes from the Latin meaning virgin, and it was called maydeweed as it was considered valuable for treating the kind of emotions and 'hysterical distempers' that young women were said to be prone to. The name bachelor's buttons comes from the tradition of young men who wished to gain the love of a lady by carrying the flowers in their pockets. Feverfew also derives its name from its ability to bring down fevers.

Feverfew grows in any soil and seeds itself easily.

Herbal remedy

Feverfew was highly valued in the days of Culpeper and Gerard for relieving ague, or malaria, as well as colds and catarrh. It was frequently used for menstrual problems and other women's complaints. It was also considered valuable for a variety of nervous problems including hysteria, and it is interesting that this emotion was commonly ascribed to women and relates to the womb, (indicated by words such as hysterectomy for surgical removal of the womb). It was used specifically for highly nervous people who were oversensitive to pain, and prone to sudden fits of irritability or anger. It was prescribed for convulsions and for soothing fretful children.

More recently, feverfew has gained fame as an excellent remedy for headaches and migraine. Research and clinical trials have shown that intractable migraines in 70 per cent of sufferers improved when taking feverfew, while one in three had no further attacks. The leaves can be eaten fresh every day between two pieces of bread as a sandwich (taken alone they may cause mouth ulcers in some sensitive people).

Feverfew has a bitter taste, and has a beneficial action on the liver and digestion, enhancing the appetite and digestion, allaying nausea and vomiting and helping to clear heat and toxins from the system. It will help relieve the pain and inflammation of arthritis and reduce symptoms associated with a sluggish liver. It acts as a tonic to the nervous system, relaxing tension and lifting depression and promoting sleep. It has also been used to relieve nerve pain, as in trigeminal neuralgia and sciatica.

Feverfew when taken in hot infusion will, as its name suggests, increase perspiration and reduce fevers. It will also act as a decongestant, clearing phlegm, chronic catarrh and sinusitis. It has also been used for asthma, and other allergies such as hay fever – research suggests that it inhibits release of substances which trigger allergies and migraines.

Externally, a tincture of the fresh plant can be dabbed on to insect stings and bites to relieve pain and swelling, and a dilute tincture used as a skin lotion is said to repel insects, as well as remove pimples, boils and haemorrhoids.

Homeopathic remedy: PYRETHRUM PARTHENIUM

Pyrethrum parthenium is prescribed for a range of nervous symptoms like those indicating the use of feverfew the herb, including convulsions, twitching, restlessness, and delirium.

The flower essence

The flower essence feverfew is taken for headaches and migraines, particularly those experienced in a cyclical pattern by women, according to their cycle of hormonal changes.

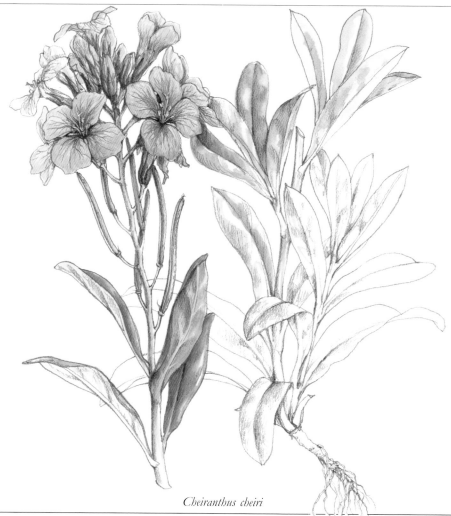

Cheiranthus cheiri

Wallflower
The flower of fidelity

The perennial wallflower comes from the eastern Mediterranean and grows wild on old walls and rocks. The wildflower is yellow, but cultivated for its rustic beauty and sweet smell the flowers range from orange to red and purple.

The name Cheiranthus comes from the Greek words meaning hand and flowers, as bouquets of wallflowers were carried by the Ancient Greeks during festivals and feasts. In the language of flowers, the wallflower is linked more to affairs of the heart. It means 'fidelity in adversity' or 'always true'. A medieval knight who wore a sprig of wallflower was avowing constancy to his lady.

Herbal remedy The wallflower has been used since antiquity, but is not recommended for home use. Culpeper said it was ruled by the moon, which relates to its use in regulating the female menstrual cycle. Rudolph Steiner said it was considered a female remedy, promoting the menses and childbirth. It has been used as a popular remedy for liver and heart problems, and for kidney stones and gravel. Steiner commented that cardiac glycosides, which wallflower seeds contain, are found in plants which fight to establish their own rhythm between inhibiting and accelerating tendencies. Certainly the wallflower blossoms in harsh conditions, which perhaps connects to the old meaning of 'fidelity in adversity'.

Homeopathic remedy Cheiranthus is specifically used for problems when cutting wisdom teeth, such as nasal congestion, and deafness with an ear discharge.

The flower essence Wallflower is used to increase confidence, and to enhance the ability to recognize beauty in the essential self. It is particularly useful for those who compare themselves with others, whether in looks, achievements, accomplishments, career, finance or possessions, and feel under pressure to be different or to achieve more because of lack of self-worth.

88

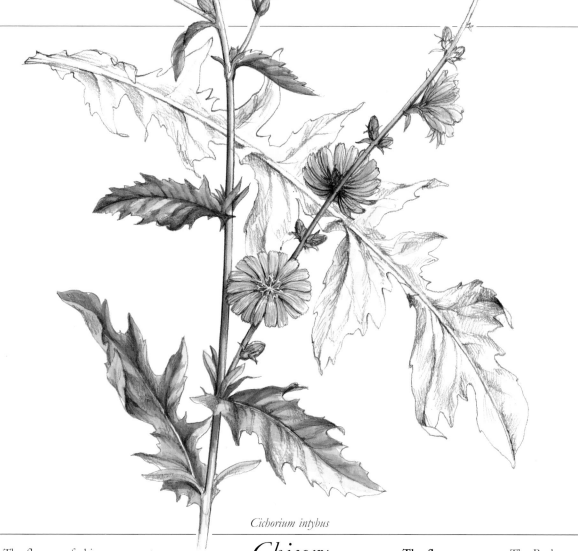

Cichorium intybus

Chicory
The flower of assimilation

The flowers of chicory open at 7 o'clock in the morning and close precisely at midday and so were used by country folk as a guide to the time. Chicory root is best known as a substitute for or addition to coffee; it helps counteract the stimulating effect of caffeine. The Ancient Egyptians and Greeks called it 'liver's friend' as it makes a good medicine for the liver and gall-bladder. The young leaves were cooked or eaten as salad, and considered a health food by the Greeks. The seeds have been used in love potions.

Herbal remedy Chicory has a bitter root and leaves which increase the appetite and promote digestion and absorption, enhancing liver and gall-bladder function. As a diuretic chicory treats fluid retention and also helps eliminate toxins via the kidneys; by increasing excretion of uric acid it makes a good remedy for rheumatism and gout. It is also helpful to diabetics as it reduces blood sugar. Research shows it has antibacterial effects and may be useful for heart problems.

Homeopathic remedy Cichorium is used for sluggish digestion, and heaviness in the stomach with a general disinclination to physical or mental exertion. It is prescribed for over-relaxed bowels, leading to constipation and headaches.

The flower essence The Bach Flower Remedy chicory is for people who are possessive, domineering, excessively interfering and manipulative. Very demanding, they require a lot of support from those around them, needing love, sympathy and a great deal of attention. If this is not available they may lapse into self-pity and use emotional blackmail or illness to obtain the attention they need. Behind this overbearing personality is an insecure person who fears being alone, or losing friends, family or possessions. Easily feeling slighted or hurt, they are over-concerned with what other people owe them. Chicory helps to create a more secure feeling in yourself, so that you are more able to give love unselfishly.

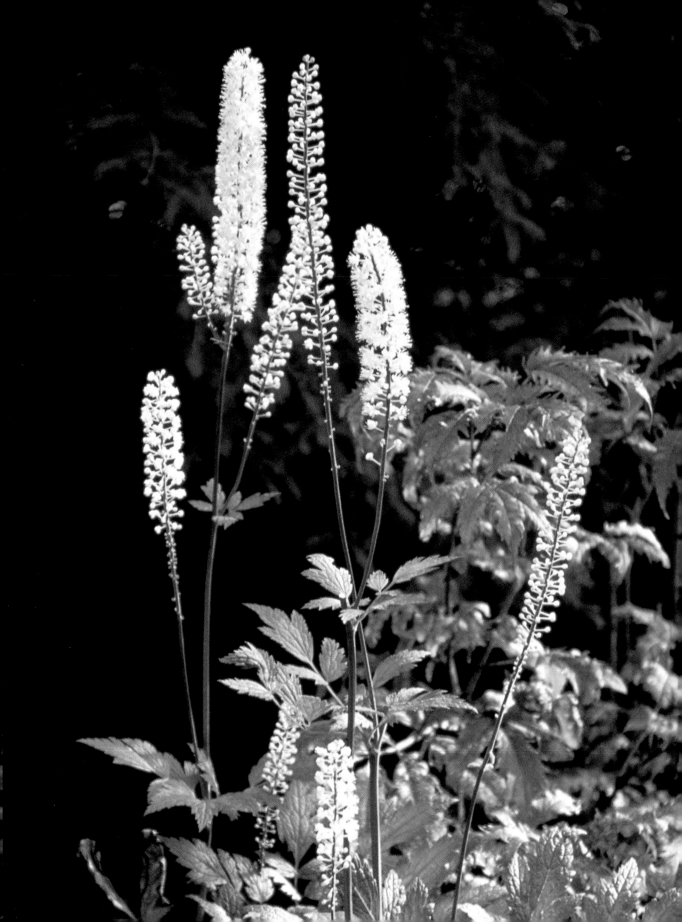

Black cohosh

The flower of medicine women

Black cohosh, brother to the blue
Has uses two
The leaping nerve is wooed to rest
The weary muscle, having work to do,
Gives of its best.
 MRS LEYEL

Black cohosh is a beautiful plant growing 4–8 feet (1–2 metres) high with small white feathery flowers in graceful slender spikes. It is a hardy perennial, native to the shady woods of North America and Canada. The name Cimicifuga derives from the Latin *cimex*, a bug, and *fugo,* to drive away, as its rank smell was known to repel insects; this explains its names bugwort and bugbane. From Siberia and India to Europe, bugbanes like black cohosh have been used for centuries to drive away insects.

Black cohosh was a popular medicine among the indigenous tribes of America who called it squaw root because of its great ability to treat uterine disorders and to aid childbirth. In 1831 a certain Dr Young introduced black cohosh to the American medical world where it was used for a wide variety of ailments including heart problems, epilepsy, bronchitis, whooping cough (it was considered one of the best remedies for this), rheumatism, neuralgia, hysteria, menstrual problems, scarlet fever, measles and smallpox. It became a leading remedy in America for acute rheumatism, arthritis and neuralgia. In both America and China black cohosh was considered a powerful remedy to antidote the poison of rattlesnakes, to ward off old age and as a general preventative against disease. It was also famous as a nerve tonic, to relieve depression with fear and dread of impending evil. Tea made from the roots was sprinkled in a room to stop evil spirits from entering.

Herbal remedy

The root of black cohosh is specific for nerve and muscle pain. It was widely used by the native Americans for treating neuralgia. The anemonin in the plant depresses the central nervous system, making it an excellent pain reliever for a range of problems including rheumatoid and osteoarthritis, headaches, ovarian and uterine pain, contractions during childbirth and breast pain. The salicylates with their anti-inflammatory action are helpful in pain relief. It is a good remedy for tinnitus and vertigo.

Black cohosh has an antispasmodic action, easing cramping and muscle tension and can be taken to relieve asthma, whooping cough, menstrual cramps and painful contractions in childbirth. Taken several weeks before the birth, it prepares the uterus for childbirth. It normalizes the function of uterine muscles, helping them to work as effectively as possible to enable a safe and easy delivery. Black cohosh also relaxes and dilates the muscles in the blood vessels, helping to lower raised blood pressure. While acting as a sedative to the nerves and a relaxant to the muscles, black cohosh also normalizes heart function. It strengthens a slow and irregular pulse.

Black cohosh has a generally very beneficial effect on the female reproductive system. It can be used to treat menstrual pain and irregularities, heavy bleeding and breast pain and swelling. It strengthens the uterine muscles and with its oestrogenic properties helps to relieve problems associated with the menopause such as depression, hot flushes and low libido.

Homeopathic remedy: CIMICIFUGA

Cimicifuga is useful particularly for women who are prone to bouts of depression, as if a black cloud has descended on them with a sense of impending evil. This is likely to occur during pregnancy or after childbirth and may be accompanied by a great fear of losing her senses or of dying. The bout of depression is followed by excitable, even manic behaviour.

Cimicifuga, like the herbal remedy, is recommended to relieve muscle and nerve pain. It is also a good remedy for female problems such as ovarian pain, irregular periods, heavy bleeding, pains after childbirth and breast pain.

The flower essence

Black cohosh is for women, particularly those prone to dark, morbid thoughts and who tend to become caught up in destructive relationships in which they feel powerless. This negativity may express itself in physical illness, particularly in the reproductive system. Black cohosh increases your positivity and energy to transform negative, threatening circumstances into ones that are more life-enhancing and fulfilling.

Caution The fresh root is poisonous; always used dried root

Blessed thistle

The flower of independence

The haughty thistle o'er all danger towers
In enemy place the very wasp of flowers.
    JOHN CLARE (1793–1864)

Blessed or holy thistle derives its name from its reputation as a heal-all, as described by Mattiolus: 'It helpeth inwardly and outwardly; strengthens all the principle members of the body, the brain, heart, stomach, liver, lungs and kidneys; it is a preservative against all diseases; it expelleth the venom of infection; it consumes and wastes away all bad humours, therefore give God thanks for his goodness, Who hath given this herb and others for the benefit of our health.'

Blessed thistle was even said to cure the plague. As it was used to protect against physical illness, so also it was valued as a herb to protect from evil spirits and negative influences. It was made into incense and ritual cups for use at religious ceremonies to invoke the god Pan.

Culpeper said, 'Mars rules this thistle. It is cordial and sudorific, good for all sorts of malignant and pestilential fevers'. He also said it was under the sign of Aries. Holy thistle was a symbol of independence, retaliation and austerity. Certainly the prickly, hairy thistle is good at protecting itself.

The fresh green leaves used to be eaten with bread and butter for breakfast, like watercress. They are an indication of good soil and are found growing in uncultivated land. In a compost heap thistles and nettles together impart the heat required to break down the waste material.

Herbal remedy

Holy thistle is an excellent tonic, useful after illness or when feeling tired and run down. The bitters enhance the appetite and aid digestion, while stimulating the liver and the flow of bile. It is a good remedy for anorexia, indigestion, wind, colic and any condition associated with a sluggish liver such as skin problems, headaches, lethargy and irritability. Its astringent action is useful for treating diarrhoea.

The bitters also have an antimicrobial action, useful for enhancing the function of the immune system. Blessed thistle has also been shown to act as an antineoplastic, useful in cancer treatment. It has diuretic properties and when taken in hot infusion is a useful diaphoretic for fevers and an expectorant for chest problems. Blessed thistle also has a reputation as a fine tonic to the nervous system. It has been used for headaches, migraines, dizziness and poor memory. According to Gerard, 'Blessed thistle taken in meat or drinke is good for the swimming and giddiness of the head, it strengthens memories and is a singular remedie against deafness'.

Blessed thistle has been taken to relieve both nerve pain and backache. It is also beneficial to the circulation and helpful for varicose veins.

A very useful herb for women, blessed thistle can be taken to relieve painful periods, and for menstrual headaches. As an emmenagogue it will help bring on suppressed periods (and so should be avoided during pregnancy). It is excellent for increasing milk production in nursing mothers and can be helpful during problems with the menopause, such as heavy bleeding.

Externally, blessed thistle can be used to staunch bleeding of cuts and speed healing of wounds. It also acts as an antiseptic.

Homeopathic remedy: CARDUUS BENEDICTUS

Carduus benedictus has a strong action on the eyes and is prescribed for twitching or flickering eyes, visual disturbances and pain in the eyes with a feeling of the eyes being too big. Symptoms characterized by burning respond well to this remedy – bitter burning in the stomach, burning in the hands after sweating, and burning in the arms after exercising them.

The flower essence

This proud thistle with its threatening points is excellent at defending itself, a symbol of independence and valued for its reputation to protect against negative influences. Similarly, the flower remedy is recommended for defending your beliefs and upholding your integrity. The thistle flower remedy enhances self-respect and dignity, and the ability to trust your own inner judgement and guidance. It helps you to recognize your inner strength, reducing the need for defensive speech or actions.

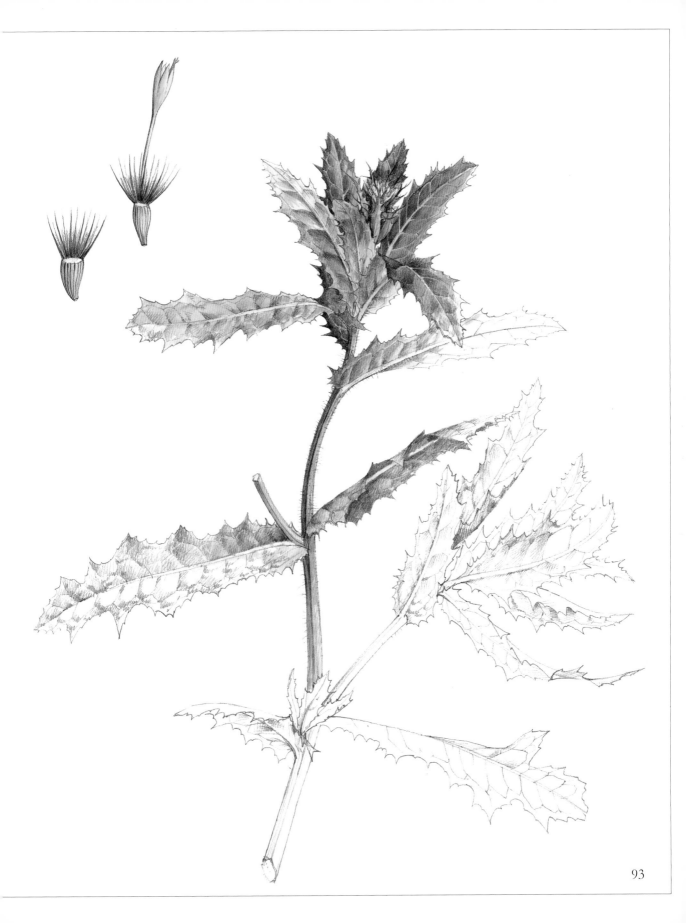

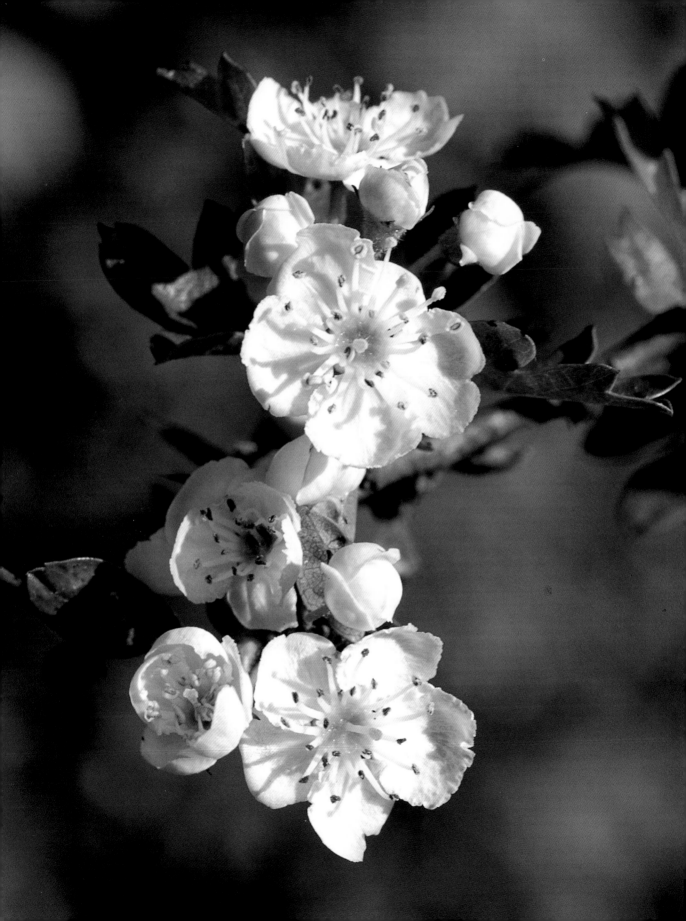

Crataegus oxyacantha or *monogyna*

Hawthorn

The flower of the heart

This attractive member of the rose family has sweet-scented snow white blossoms covering hedgerows in spring as a herald to summer, and bright red berries in autumn. Almost all parts of the plant have been used in healing since the Middle Ages.

Hawthorn has long been considered a sacred and protecting plant. Sprigs of hawthorn were attached to the cradle of a newborn baby to afford protection against illness and evil influences. It was said to give psychic protection, to lift the spirits and banish melancholy if worn or carried, but said to be unlucky to bring indoors. Spirits and faeries had their meeting place under the hawthorn tree.

Hawthorn has traditionally been connected with May Day customs in the Northern hemisphere where it blooms in May. The ancient spring festival of May Day was named after the Greek goddess Maia. The girl crowned Queen of the May represents the goddess. The maypole ceremony is symbolic of renewed life, fertility and spring. The maypole represented an *axis mundi* around which the universe revolves; the tree stripped of its changing foliage symbolizes the changeless centre. The pole is phallic, the ribboned discus at the top representing the feminine principle and the union of the two represents fertility. It was customary to erect hawthorn trees outside your sweetheart's house and to decorate porches with hawthorn on May Day in many parts of Europe.

Hawthorn has been associated with fertility and affairs of the heart since the days of the Ancient Greeks and Romans. At Greek wedding feasts the guests used to carry sprigs of hawthorn to bring happiness and prosperity to the newly married couple. In Rome, the bridegroom would wave a sprig of hawthorn as he led his bride to the nuptial chamber, which was lit with hawthorn torches.

The Christian church re-dedicated the hawthorn, like other sacred trees, to the Virgin Mary. Hawthorn was reputedly used for Christ's crown of thorns and . it was one of these thorns, piercing the robin's breast, that gave the bird his red breast. It was believed for centuries that lightning would never strike a hawthorn tree – lightning was the work of the devil and could not strike a plant that had touched the brow of Christ.

Herbal remedy

Hawthorn is veritably the best remedy for the heart and circulation. The flowers, leaves and berries all act as a wonderful heart tonic and have a vasodilatory effect, opening the arteries and thus improving blood supply to all body tissues. It makes an excellent remedy for high blood pressure, particularly that associated with hardening of the arteries.

Hawthorn can be used to improve poor circulation associated with ageing arteries. It acts to open the coronary arteries, improving blood flow through the heart and softening deposits, allieviating hardening of the arteries which causes angina. It is ideal for all heart conditions, including arrhythmias, palpitations, breathlessness, degenerative heart disease and heart failure.

The berries have an astringent effect and are used for diarrhoea. In addition the leaves, flowers and berries have a relaxant effect in the digestive tract. In the nervous system they relieve stress and anxiety, calming agitation and restlessness, and inducing sleep in insomniacs. They also have a diuretic effect.

Externally, a decoction of the flowers and berries can be used as a lotion for a blotchy complexion and acne rosacea. A decoction of the berries makes an astringent gargle for sore throats and a douche for vaginal discharges.

Homeopathic remedy: CRATAEGUS

Crataegus is also a wonderful heart tonic. It is used for chronic heart disease with extreme weakness, for heart failure that threatens from the slightest exertion, for pain in the heart area, high blood pressure and arteriosclerosis of the elderly. The berries are used in a mother tincture as a heart remedy.

The flower essence

On an emotional level hawthorn is said to work on the heart chakra, opening the heart and enhancing the expression of love. It can be used where there are problems both giving and receiving love. It is a remedy recommended to heal broken hearts, disappointment, anger or bitterness after a failed love affair. It eases emotional extremes which would contribute to physical illness such as heart disease.

Lady's slipper

The flower of serenity

The cyprepedium with her changeful lives
As she were doubtful which array to choose.
    MRS LEYEL

There are 50 species of Cypripedium, one of the
most beautiful of the wild orchids, which in the past
could be found in Europe, Asia and North America.
Lady's slipper is now an endangered plant having
been far too popular and overpicked for enhancing
bouquets. It grows naturally in woods and damp,
shady places, and was once common enough to be
sold to travellers by the roadside in the north of
England. The name Cypripedium comes from the
Greek words *kypris*, one of the names of the goddess
Venus, and *podion* meaning a little foot or slipper.
It came to be called Venus' or Aphrodite's slipper
and lady's slipper because the shape of the flower
resembles a shoe.

Lady's slipper was a popular herb amongst the
native peoples of North America. There is an old
Blackfoot legend that tells of a little Indian princess
who, while out playing, encountered a rabbit which
had injured its foot, so that it could not get home to
its family. The princess took off her moccasins and
gave them to the rabbit. Returning home she began
to feel the effect of the sharp stones that had hurt
the rabbit's feet, and her feet too became sore and
bleeding. Becoming exhausted from the pain she sat
down to rest and fell asleep. A bird flying by spotted
her sorry state and implored the Great Spirit in the
sky to help her. When the princess awoke she found
hanging on stems by her side the most beautiful pair
of lady's slipper moccasins she had ever seen. Her
feet fitted perfectly into them and she joyfully made
her way home. The native American name for lady's
slipper is, not surprisingly, moccasin flower. It is said
that the red-purple spot and scarlet lines inside the
flower are the marks left from the little princess's
feet. In the language of flowers lady's slipper means
capricious beauty.

Herbal remedy

Lady's slipper, known to generations of native
Americans, and adopted by herbalists, is used for
nervous problems and to allay pain. It acts as a tonic
to the nervous system, supporting it through times of
stress and overwork. Lady's slipper makes a good
remedy for nervous exhaustion, for depletion after
illness, for anxiety, tension, restlessness, over-excitement and insomnia, for palpitations, neuralgia and
depression. It is useful for restless children who will
not sleep. In the past it was used for epilepsy and
convulsions. It can be given for all kinds of stress-
related problems such as tension headaches, stomach
aches, colic and muscular pains.

Lady's slipper has antispasmodic properties,
relaxing smooth muscle throughout the body and
relieving muscle pain such as cramps and period
pains. It is an excellent remedy for use during childbirth, when a woman feels tired or anxious. Lady's
slipper combined with raspberry leaves and ginger
will help to relax a rigid cervix and ease the birth.
As a diaphoretic lady's slipper can be used for fevers
accompanied by great restlessness and anxiety.
Since lady's slipper is an endangered species it must
only be used when it is obtained from a cultivated
crop and not picked as a wild flower.

Homeopathic remedy: CYPRIPEDIUM

Cyprepedium is prepared from the fresh root of
lady's slipper and is an excellent remedy for the
nervous system. It is prescribed for people who are
agitated, restless, irascible, and who sleep badly and
fitfully. The limbs may twitch and the mind may be
full of ideas just when one is trying to sleep. It is
good for children who wake in the night and want to
play with no desire to go back to sleep. It is also
recommended for sexual and nervous debility and
depression, and is good for women, for stress and
anxiety around a period, and for menstrual pain.

The flower essence

Lady's slipper is for those people who are unable to
draw upon their inner wisdom and strength to guide
them and provide them with energy for the demands
of daily life. They may suffer from nervous exhaustion and sexual debility. Lady's slipper acts as a tonic
to the nervous system, enabling you to connect with
inner resources of strength and calm and to apply
these inherent gifts to daily life.

NB This is an endangered species. Never pick wild plants. The fresh plant can cause dermatitis

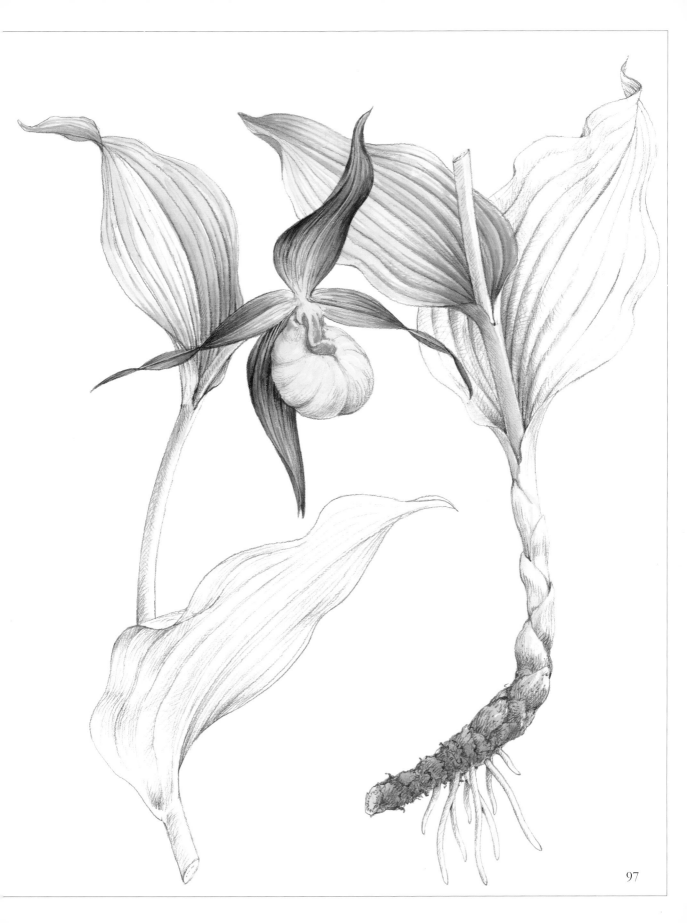

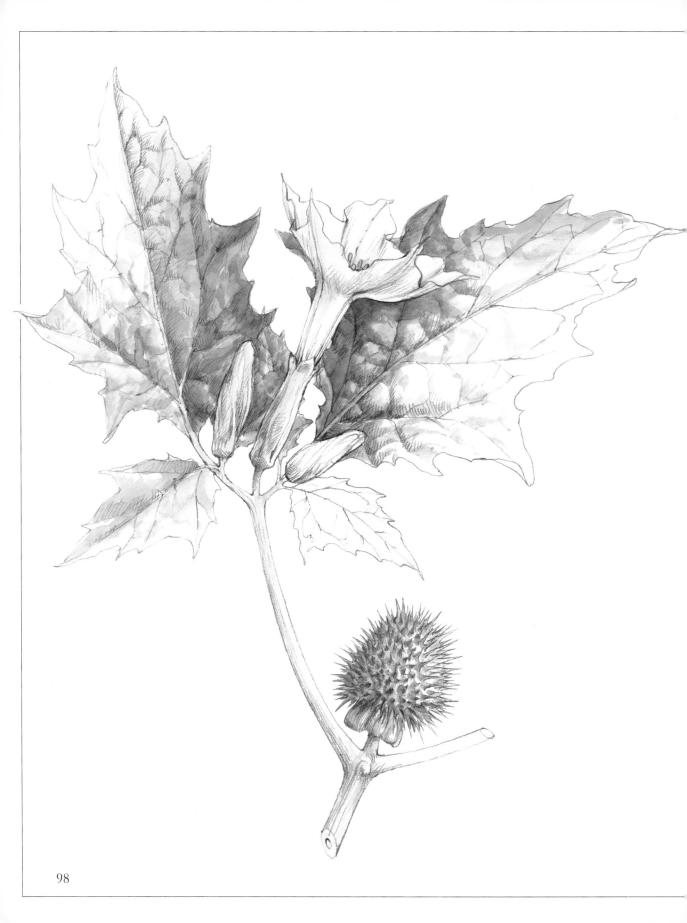

Thorn apple

The flower of initiation

This exotic-looking plant, also called Jimson weed, with its gaudy trumpet-shaped flowers and overpowering narcotic smell, is a member of the nightshade family and shares many of the virtues and dangers of belladonna. The genus Datura consists of at least 15 species distributed throughout the warmer parts of the world, which vary in habit from herbs to shrubs and even trees. Datura is easily grown from seed, sown in early summer in open, sunny positions or raised under glass earlier and transplanted. In temperate climates it is an annual.

Most daturas contain similar alkaloids which all have narcotic properties. These have led to their wide use as medicines and as mind-altering substances for thousands of years in both the Old and New Worlds. Avicenna, the 11th century Arab physician, wrote of datura's value as a medicine and the intoxicating effect of small amounts of the seed. The name datura in fact derives from early Arabic names *datora* and *tatorah*, which both originate from earlier Sanskrit names, *dhustura* and *unmata*.

Datura metel is a native of India, where concoctions of powdered datura seed in water were made into intoxicating drinks and used by unfaithful wives to drug their husbands conveniently for hours, and were popular amongst thieves and criminals to stupefy their victims. Datura was also used for drugging young girls and exploiting them as prostitutes, and 'dancing girls' would use such concoctions to excite or stupefy their clients while they took advantage of them, knowing that the poor victim would have no recollection of what had happened. So datura came to have an evil reputation in India and was known as drunkard, madman, deceiver and fool maker.

In China, however, datura was sacred and said to receive droplets of water when the Buddha spoke, and to have descended to the earth from heaven at the time of the Buddha. In India datura was used medicinally to treat a variety of illnesses including heart disease, hysteria, epilepsy, pneumonia and mumps. In China, where it was called *man-t'o-lo*, it was employed for treating swollen feet, prolapse, colds, cholera, skin problems and nervous and mental imbalances. When mixed equally with cannabis, pulverized and steeped in wine, it was used as an anaesthetic for operations and cauterizations.

The thorny seed capsules of datura (giving the name thorn apple) contain black seeds which can remain dormant for many years and probably travelled over Asia and Europe with gypsies or buried in the earth ballast of trading ships. In Ancient Greece, the priests of Apollo used datura to achieve altered prophetic states. Seed remains found in the Temple of the Sun in Sagomozo in Colombia show that *Datura sanguinea* was similarly used in rites to produce a sedated state in which the prophet could communicate with the spirit world and see the souls of the departed. Temple priests of the Peruvian Incas used *Datura fatuosa* to sedate their patients when performing surgery. In the Choco and Darien areas of South and Central America extracts of datura seed were given to children to make them wander around in a semi-conscious state until they fell down in a coma. Where they fell was thought to indicate the site of an ancient grave containing treasure, preferably gold.

In both North and South America datura has played a dominant role in coming-of-age rituals and to sustain people through grief following the death of a native tribe member, as well as to simulate death and resurrection in rituals of the shaman. In the trance state produced by datura it was believed there could be communion between man and god – Zuni priests chewed the root to commune with the gods who brought rain. It was given once in a lifetime to boys at puberty, during which time their prophetic dreams and other-worldly experiences would prepare them for manhood. Symbolically, they would undergo a ritual of dying as a child and being reborn a man, and after several days in an altered state they were supposed to have forgotten their childhood.

Herbal remedy

In North America datura was available over the counter of most drugstores until 1968 when it was placed on 'prescription only' lists because of its growing use as an hallucinogen. It is used predominantly for its antispasmodic action in the treatment of asthma and for Parkinson's disease because it is an antagonist to acetyl-choline. Atropine has the power to paralyse the vagus nerve endings, and so relieves spasm in the bronchial tubes. Under medical supervision, it can be taken internally, used as an inhalant or smoked.

In India Ayurvedic physicians use datura in medicines for patients suffering from cerebral or mental disorders, for bronchial asthma, coughing fits in whooping cough and for spasms of the bladder. The seeds are used to dampen sexual desire. Datura is also used in India for hydrophobia (rabies) and its efficacy in the treatment of this is leading to further studies in the West.

Gerard introduced datura into England and boiled it with hog's grease to make a salve for 'all inflammations whatsoever, all manner of burnings or scaldings, as well of fire, water, boiling lead, gun powder, as that which comes by lightning'.

Today datura is still used in ointments, liniments and plasters for the relief of neuralgia, rheumatic pain and haemorrhoids. Its pain-killing and sedative action can be put to good use when taken internally, and when applied to bruises, sprains and strains.

Homeopathic remedy: DATURA

Datura exerts its main action on the mind and the musculature, relaxing spasm, much like the herbal remedy. It makes a good remedy for suppressed secretions and excretions, such as suppressed urination. Interestingly, it is also used for hydrophobia with acute fear of the sight of water, or anything glistening which can spark off spasms, causing, for example, inability to swallow or to urinate, convulsions and asthma.

A datura person can change rapidly from being happy to sad; they fear being alone and in the dark. They may suffer from terrifying delirium or hallucinations, as in the delirium tremens of alcoholics. They may have religious mania or even be violent or lewd. In great panics, such as that set off by visions

of dogs or the sight of water, they have a great desire to escape.

Physical symptoms that datura people may suffer include boring head pain preceded by visual disturbances; loss of vision, staring eyes, dilated pupils, and small objects looking large; and the face may be hot and red as blood rushes to the head. There may be an expression of terror or great pallor; the throat and mouth are dry, accompanied by violent thirst but an aversion to water and inability to swallow. There may be vomiting of mucus or green bile sparked off by bright light; convulsions, trembling, hot flushes, red rashes, violent pain in the left hip and violent fevers with rashes, accompanied by delirium and convulsions.

Datura people are worse in a dark room, when alone, looking at bright shining objects (such as the sun), after sleep and swallowing. They are better with company, warmth, motion, touch and pressure.

The flower essence

Datura meteloides is used for those who feel confused, disorientated, unearthed, detached from reality or in a dream-like state. They may suffer from delusions, altered perceptions, and have a great fear of losing touch with reality, of losing control, of insanity, of losing their identity. They may feel very lonely and separated from others by their separate reality. They may feel like an alien. Datura is also for those experiencing the break-up of a regular pattern in their life, such as a relationship or a career; it is for shattered dreams and for disillusionment. It helps to ease confusion and fear often experienced during changes in one's life or changes in perception, and lends courage to let go of the familiar and secure. It helps to open the 'doors of perception' and allow a new, expanded experience of reality.

NB Datura is highly poisonous, particularly the seeds, and must only be used in therapeutic doses under the supervision of a practitioner. Overdose can cause dizziness, double vision, thirst, inability to pass water, palpitations, restlessness, confusion and hallucinations. Avoid in pregnancy, prostatic disease, tachycardia, glaucoma and when taking antidepressants. In case of overdose, induce vomiting

Eucalyptus

The flower of purification

The eucalyptus is an attractive evergreen tree with bluish-green leathery leaves which are full of glands containing a fragrant volatile oil. It is indigenous to Australia and Tasmania where it can attain a height of 375 feet (112 metres), ranking one of the largest trees in the world. There are hundreds of species, but the one used medicinally has the highest proportion of eucalyptol (cineole) in its essential oil.

The eucalyptus is also known as the fever tree. It exhales an aromatic odour which exerts an antiseptic effect in the area in which it grows. It was planted in low-lying marshes or swamps because it absorbs great quantities of water. Such places were breeding grounds for diseases such as malaria, and the eucalyptus was deliberately planted to purify these areas. It was first introduced into Europe in 1856 for such purposes by Baron Ferdinand von Muller, a German botanist and explorer, and director of the botanical gardens in Melbourne. He was keen to spread the knowledge of eucalyptus' powerful antiseptic properties all over the world and was instrumental in its cultivation in North and South Africa, California, and non-tropical parts of South America. He was the first to suggest that the oil may be of use as a disinfectant in fever districts.

Herbal remedy

Eucalyptus is a traditional Aboriginal remedy for fevers and infections as it is a highly antiseptic febrifuge. The volatile oils in the leaves stimulate the circulation, enhancing blood flow to the skin and causing sweating. This process clears toxins from the blood, lowers fever and pushes out eruptions, speeding resolution of eruptive fevers such as chickenpox and measles. It was an old folk remedy for typhoid and scarlet fever, remittent fevers, malaria and cholera. It also makes an excellent decongestant and expectorant. It is used for colds, flu, croup, coughs, asthma and chest infections such as whooping cough, pneumonia and bronchitis, for catarrh, sinusitis and ear infections. It is best taken at the onset of symptoms such as sore throat, aches and pains, feverishness and malaise.

Russian research on eucalyptus species has shown some to be effective antiviral remedies while other are antimalarial or highly antibacterial.

In Chinese medicine decoctions of the leaves are used for pulmonary tuberculosis. The dried leaves also used to be smoked for asthma. They are burnt in South American countries to purify the atmosphere. A decoction of the leaves in hot water can be used for fumigation, to cleanse the air of infection in the sick room, or during a flu epidemic. A decoction kept simmering in a pot all day will continually disinfect the air and prevent the spread of contagious diseases.

In China eucalyptus leaves are taken in decoction to treat aching joints. The herbal oil is applied externally as a rubbing oil for painful inflamed joints in arthritis and gout, to relieve neuralgia, and when applied to the temples for headaches and migraines.

In our grandmothers' day eucalyptus was made into wine and used as an aperitif and digestive. Its antiseptic properties are exerted throughout the digestive tract and when taken in decoction eucalyptus leaves were used for bacillary dysentery, typhoid, diarrhoea and vomiting. The gum and tannins in the leaves have an astringent action, also useful in resolving diarrhoea, dysentery and to check bleeding. The volatile oils from the leaves are excreted via the urinary system so that a decoction will relieve infections such as cystitis and pyelonephritis. Recent research suggests that eucalyptus may lower blood sugar.

Externally, eucalyptus can be used as an antiseptic and to speed healing, applied in compresses to wounds, burns, ulcers, boils and abscesses. It will stop bleeding of cuts and abrasions and promote tissue repair. A fluid extract diluted in a little water was a folk remedy for nosebleeds. In traditional Aboriginal medicine eucalyptus leaves were used in poultices for wounds and inflammation. A decoction of the leaves can be used as a gargle for sore throats and as a mouthwash for infected gums, thrush and mouth ulcers. It also makes an effective douche for vaginal discharges and infections such as thrush, and a wash for haemorrhoids.

Aromatherapy oil

The oil obtained by steam distillation of eucalyptus leaves is an excellent natural antiseptic. Dr Jean Valnet (the well-known French doctor who has written extensively about aromatherapy) reports that

101

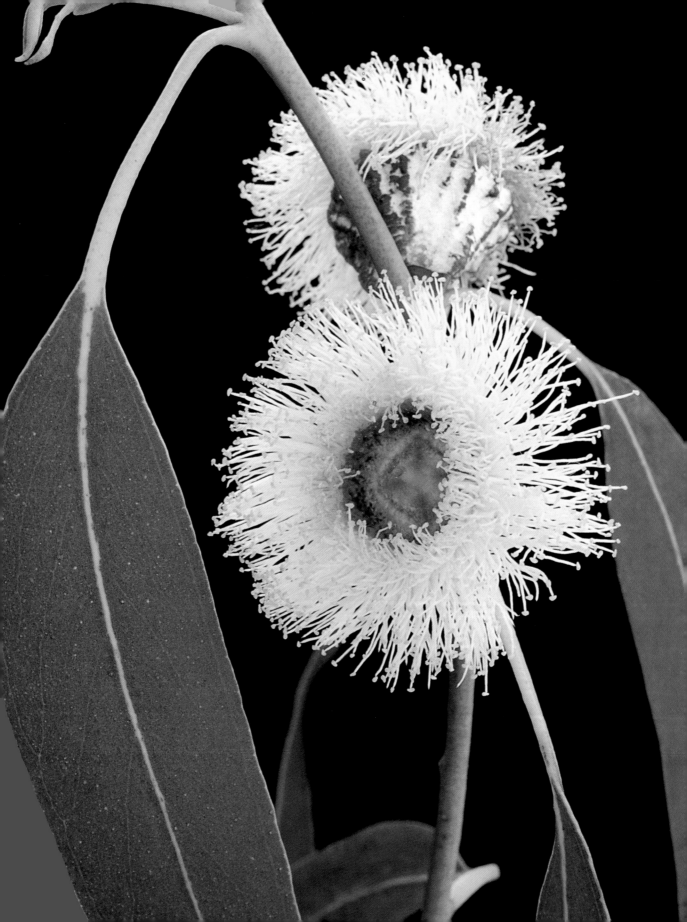

2 percent dilution spray will kill 70 percent of airborne staphylococci and still recommends it for treatment of cholera, malaria, typhoid, as well as scarlatina, measles and flu.

Externally, the dilute oil is useful for cold sores, shingles, chickenpox and other skin infections, as well as inflammatory complaints such as boils, chilblains, and varicose ulcers. It also makes a good insect repellent.

Since the actions of the herbal remedy are mostly attributed to the high volatile oil content, the use of eucalyptus oil in aromatherapy very much resembles its herbal action. It increases circulation, promotes sweating and thereby relieves fevers. Used as an inhalant it is an exceptional decongestant, clearing the airways of phlegm – useful in colds, flu, sinus congestion, headaches, chest infections and asthma.

Applied locally, eucalyptus oil increases circulation and has anaesthetic properties. It is good for aching muscles, sprains, arthritic and rheumatic pain, especially when combined with rosemary, lavender or marjoram oil. It promotes urination and relieves urinary infections such as cystitis. It enhances the digestion and relieves diarrhoea and is useful to diabetics as it can lower blood sugar levels. Its stimulating properties aid concentration, invigorating and refreshing both mind and body.

Homeopathic remedy: EUCALYPTUS

Eucalyptus is similarly prescribed for acute infections, including malaria, typhoid and influenza. It is used both preventatively and curatively. Eucalyptus will relieve fevers particularly if they are intermittent, eruptive infections such as measles and scarlet fever, as well as catarrhal conditions throughout the body and congestive headaches. It is indicated for asthma with thick phlegm, bronchitis, whooping cough, emphysema, and for sore throats and enlarged, ulcerated tonsils.

The remedy can also be given for gastric and intestinal conditions, particularly where there is sluggish digestion giving rise to dyspepsia, offensive wind and an empty feeling in the stomach. Gastric pain is relieved by eating. It is excellent for acute diarrhoea, and dysentery with colic, blood and mucus discharge in the stools, with a feeling of heat in the rectum.

In the urinary system, symptoms indicating eucalyptus include blood in the urine, spasmodic stricture of the urethra, pain on urination and when urine has the odour of violets. It is given for acute nephritis as a complication of flu.

The homeopathic remedy is also prescribed for stiff and painful joints, pain in the limbs on walking, stiff weary feelings, gout and pricking sensations in the muscles followed by painful aching. Herpes and varicose ulcers also respond well to it. Eucalyptus is given for those feeling tired and sluggish, in mind and body, often a consequence of chronic catarrh in the head. Such people have a desire for exercise, and their symptoms tend to be worse at night.

The flower essence

Eucalyptus is said to have a liberating effect, helping one to accept life as it is.

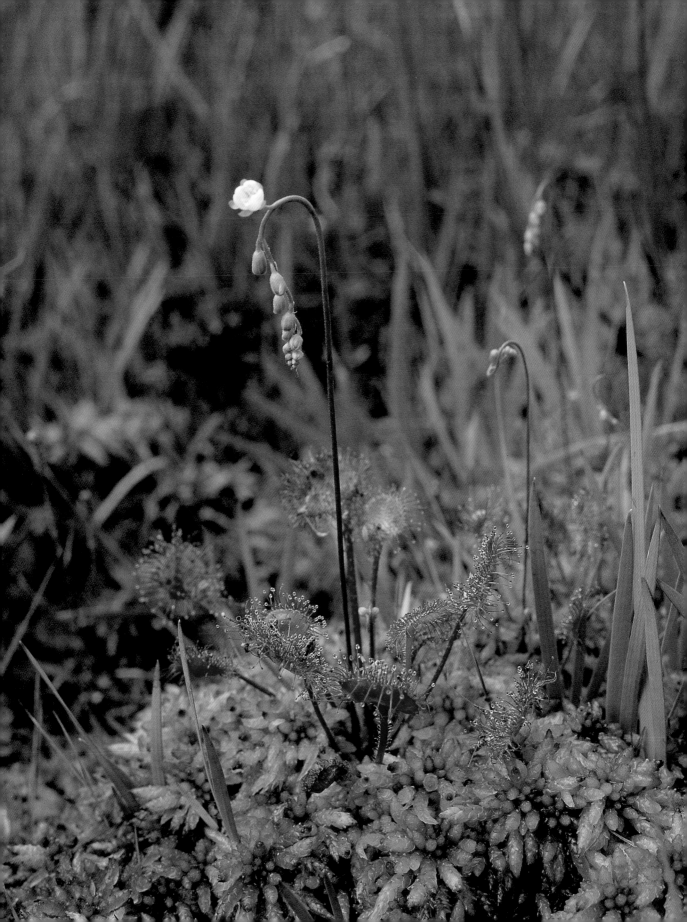

Sundew

The flower of dewdrops

Queen of the marsh imperial Drosera treads,
Rush-fringed banks, and moss embroidered
beds;
Redundant folds of glossy silk surround
Her slender waist, and trail upon the ground.
    ERASMUS DARWIN (1731–1802)

Sundew is a carnivorous plant, one of 90 species of Drosera, which is found growing in the damp marshy edges of ponds and rivers in North and South America, Europe and Asia. Having once grown plentifully it is now increasingly hard to find. Its leaves which are nearly round (hence the name rotundifolia), form a flat rosette around the stem of the white flower, and have long red hairs like tentacles. These hairs have small secreting glands at their tips which exude a sticky substance that entangles unwary insects settling on the plant. The leaves contain digestive juices similar to pepsin which then dissolve and absorb the plant's victims. The glands secrete more sticky exudate in the sunshine, and when the sun shines on the leaves they look as if they are glistening with dewdrops – hence the names sundew and dew plant. Its name Drosera comes from the Latin *drosos*, meaning dew.

Herbal remedy

Sundew has an affinity for the throat and the lungs and has a long history of use as a remedy for coughs, bronchitis and asthma. Its antispasmodic effect relaxes spasm in the bronchial tubes and makes it an excellent remedy for the spasmodic coughs of whooping cough and croup. Its demulcent effect soothes irritated conditions of the mucous membranes throughout the respiratory system. This is helpful in sore throats, laryngitis and harsh, dry irritating coughs as in early bronchitis and tuberculo-

sis. Sundew was used frequently in the past for treating TB and pneumonia.

The relaxant and soothing effects of sundew extend to the digestive system, where it can be used for irritated stomachs and bowels, for colic, nausea and indigestion.

Sundew was used in the days of Culpeper who said, 'The sun rules it and it is under the sign of Cancer. The leaves, bruised and applied to the skin, erode it and bring out such inflammations as are not easily removed. The juice destroys warts and corns, if a little be frequently put upon them.'

Homeopathic remedy: DROSERA

Drosera is prepared from the entire fresh plant gathered when it is flowering. It is used almost specifically for whooping cough and other dry, hacking coughs where the cough is deep, barking, dry and comes in violent fits. It can be suffocative, irritating and accompanied by pain in the chest so that the patient wants to hold the chest during coughing fits. The face may go blue with coughing as breathing can be difficult and there is often retching after coughing and nosebleeds. Coughing can be set off by lying down or after drinking. Drosera is also given for sore throats, hoarseness and laryngitis. In babies, it is used for tummy pains with wind and rumbling.

The flower essence

The Australian sundew, *Drosera spathulata,* is used for people who are vague, uncentred, indecisive and who tend to daydream, especially when there is work to be done.

Sundew helps to keep one focused and in the present; it increases motivation and attention to detail, and reduces the need in such people to escape from the realities of daily life.

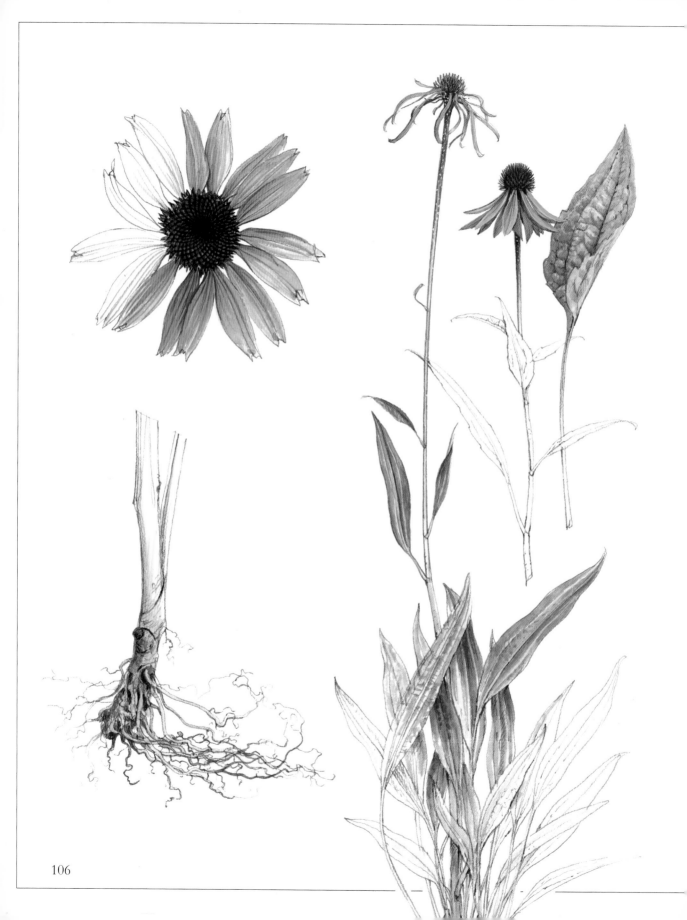

Purple coneflower

The flower of wholeness

The Echinaceas are beautiful plants with pink to purple daisy-like flowers. Their petals fall to reveal black spiny seed heads – the name Echinacea comes from the Greek *echinos,* meaning hedgehog. Three of the nine species of Echinacea that are native to North America have medicinal benefits. These are *E. purpurea*, the common purple coneflower; *E. angustifolia*, the narrow-leafed purple coneflower; and *E. pallida*, the pale purple coneflower. The name coneflower comes from its conical flower heads. Local American names include snakeroot, comb flower, black sampson, Kansas snakeroot, scurvy root, Indian head, black Susan and hedgehog.

Purple coneflower was one of the most important medicinal plants known to the native Americans. They applied it externally to wounds, burns, insect bites and swollen lymph glands and took it internally for headaches, stomach aches, coughs and colds, measles and gonorrhoea. They chewed the root to relieve toothache and neck pain, and commonly used it as an antidote for rattlesnake bites. The root was the part most commonly used, although tribes such as the Comanche, Cheyenne and the Sioux used the juice and a paste of the macerated fresh aerial parts of the plant. The root made a local anaesthetic to deaden sensation and relieve pain. You can feel this on your tongue when taking a few drops of the tincture. The Cheyenne chewed the root to stimulate the flow of saliva, which was particularly useful as a thirst-quencher for those undergoing the ritual Sun Dance. They also drank the tea to relieve rheumatism, arthritis, measles and mumps.

Herbal remedy

Scientific information on the medicinal benefits of Echinaceas comes from two fronts. From 1895 to 1930 American doctors proved the effects of *E. angustifolia* in a wide range of complaints including boils and abscesses, blood poisoning, post-partum infection, malaria, typhus and TB. German studies over the last 50 years using *E. purpurea* have proved the remedy to be extremely valuable in septic conditions, rheumatoid arthritis, antibiotic resistance, whooping cough in children, flu, catarrh, chronic respiratory tract infections, gynaecological infections,

pelvic inflammatory disease, urinary infections and a variety of skin problems.

Purple coneflower has an antibiotic and antifungal effect, an interferon-like antiviral action and an anti-allergenic action. This means that it can be taken at the first signs of sore throats, colds, chest infections, tonsillitis, glandular fever as well as for candida and postviral fatigue syndrome (ME). Taken in hot infusion, it stimulates the circulation and stimulates sweating, helping to bring down fevers. As a blood cleanser it will help to clear the skin of infections, and will help to relieve allergies such as urticaria and eczema. It is particularly useful for people whose deficient immune system makes them prone to one infection after another. The anti-inflammatory effect helps relieve arthritis and gout, skin conditions and pelvic inflammatory disease.

Externally, this is a good anti-inflammatory and antiseptic remedy for skin problems, wounds, ulcers, burns, stings and bites. It makes a good gargle and mouthwash for sore throats and infected gums and a douche for a wide range of vaginal infections.

Homeopathic remedy: E. ANGUSTIFOLIA

Echinacea angustifolia is used much like the herbal remedy. It is specific for blood poisoning, poisoned wounds, gangrene, boils and carbuncles, septicaemia, diphtheria and the effects of vaccination. It is prescribed for catarrh, abdominal pain and griping, loose yellow stools, diarrhoea, offensive wind and nausea.

An Echinacea person may feel cross and irritable, and does not wish to be contradicted. So nervous they cannot study or concentrate, their head feels dull, and their senses numbed. They may also be depressed and out of sorts, particularly in the afternoon. They generally feel worse after eating, and after physical and mental exertion and better for rest.

The flower essence

Echinacea is used specifically for those who feel shattered by severe trauma in their lives. They may feel profoundly alienated, unable to contact that inner place of strength and calm. Echinacea helps to bring about a sense of wholeness, and greater resilience when under enormous stress.

Yerba santa

The flower of emotional release

Yerba santa or holy herb was regarded as a panacea by the indigenous peoples of American living in the dry, rocky, mountainous regions of what are now the western United States, notably California and Northern Mexico where it grows. The Spanish settlers who observed the natives' respect and use of this plant gave it the name holy herb.

Yerba santa is an aromatic evergreen shrub, with woolly leaves which exude a glutinous resin. The funnel-shaped clusters of lavender-to-white flowers are loved by bees; the honey produced from nectar from yerba santa has a slightly spicy flavour, because of the pungent taste of the plant.

The native Americans boiled the fresh or dried leaves of yerba santa to make medicines to treat colds, coughs, catarrh, sore throats, stomach aches, vomiting and diarrhoea. They chewed or smoked the leaves for asthma and applied them externally for rheumatism, aching limbs, sores and swellings. Settlers in the 19th century considered it a good blood purifier and used it for rheumatism, tuberculosis and fevers.

Herbal remedy

The leaves of yerba santa have a warming, pungent taste and make a good drying remedy for clearing chronic phlegm, for colds, hay fever and sinusitis. They act as a stimulating expectorant for shifting phlegm from the chest in coughs, bronchitis, asthma and a variety of chest infections. The relaxing effect of this plant helps to reduce spasm in the bronchi associated with asthma and wheezing during chest infections. It is also helpful in croup, laryngitis and harsh, irritating coughs.

The bitter taste of the leaves stimulates the flow of saliva in the mouth and of digestive juices, enhancing appetite, digestion and absorption, and helping to resolve digestive problems.

Yerba santa acts as a urinary antiseptic because of the presence of phenols, resin and essential oils, and so it makes a useful remedy for bladder and kidney infections. As a diuretic it aids elimination of toxins from the body via the urinary system, and so acts to cleanse the system. For this reason it is considered good for rheumatism and arthritis. Its stimulating effect upon the circulation brings out sweating and so it can be used to treat fevers.

Externally, yerba santa makes a useful antiseptic for cuts, wounds and insect bites. It has been used to soothe rashes such as those caused by poison oak or poison ivy and to reduce swelling and inflammation in bruises and sprains. It can be applied to heal haemorrhoids and used as gargle and mouthwash for mouth and throat infections.

Homeopathic remedy: ERIODYCTION

Eriodyction is prepared from the whole plant of yerba santa, and like the herbal remedy, has a particular affinity for problems in the chest. It is prescribed for asthma with copious mucus, bronchitis and TB with night sweats. It is also used for the symptoms of hay fever and cold, such as sneezing and runny nose, fevers, sore throat and sharp pain in the right lung. It can be given for nausea which is aggravated by running and changing positions.

The flower essence

Yerba santa is used for unresolved grief and sadness buried in the heart and causing depression and a melancholy that pervades life. Breathing problems such as in asthma, TB or pneumonia may be caused by congestion in the chest, and aggravated by a need to smoke. Yerba santa promotes the release of unresolved emotions and restores life and joy to the heart, enabling the free flow of natural feelings again and the ability to breath without constriction.

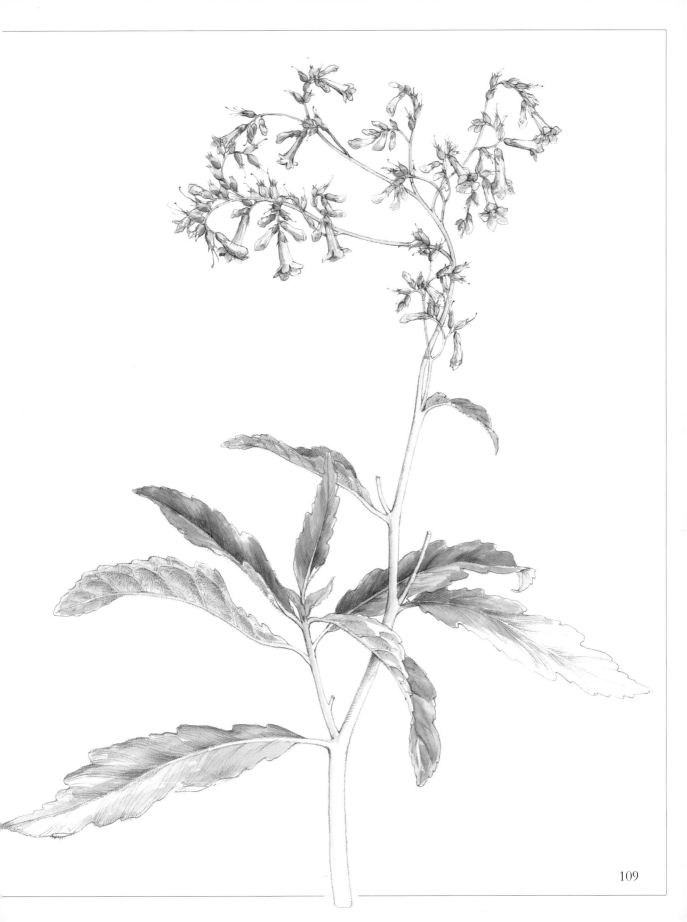

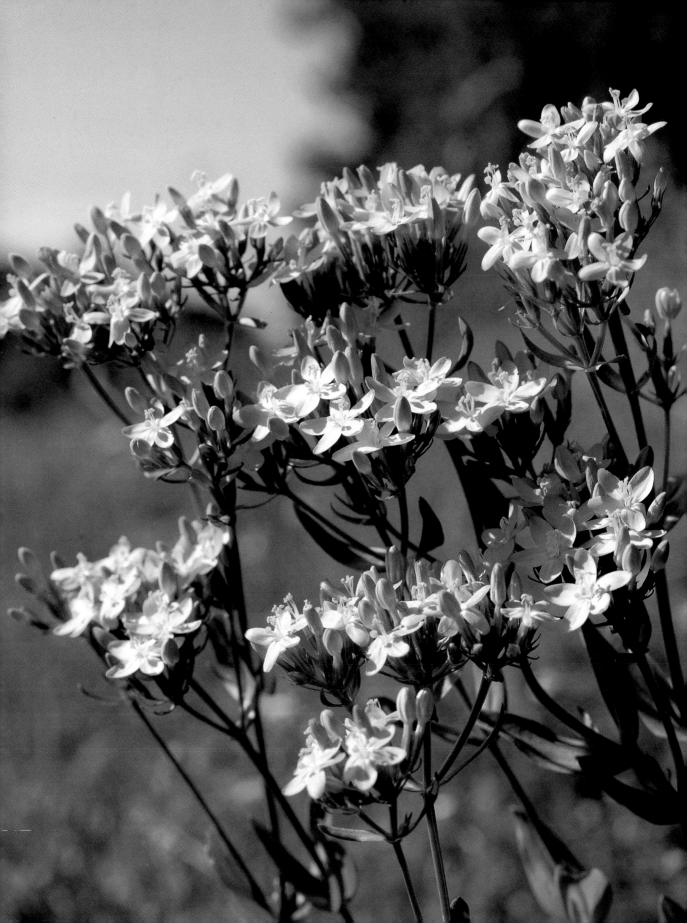

Centaury

The flower of Chiron

This small annual with its pink or white flowers grows wild on chalk downs, sandy pastures and hedgerows throughout Europe. It is said to dislike being cultivated. It derives its name from the centaur physician of Greek mythology, Chiron, from whom humankind is said to have obtained knowledge of medicinal plants. Chiron taught Asclepius, the god of medicine, and the warrior Achilles. Dioscorides, the Greek physician, used the 'great Kentaurion' for treating injuries. Its name Erythraea comes from the Greek *erythros*, meaning red, alluding to the pinky-red colour of the flower, or maybe the efficacy of the remedy in the treatment of skin rashes.

For 2000 years, centaury has been revered by many cultures. The Romans believed it had magical powers to drive away snakes, so did the Gauls of the Dark Ages, who used it to antidote snakebite. In the south of England it was known as 'herb of the sun', and the Saxons also used it for snakebite and intermittent fevers – hence its common name of feverwort. Another name for centaury was the 'universal purifier', since it drove poisons and infections out of the body, as well as negative influences from the psyche. Medieval witches took it to increase their psychic powers and to take them into trance-like states. It was also considered to protect against evil. In Ireland it was known as a herb of good luck.

The flowers of centaury open early, but only in fine weather, and close at 12 noon. A single cloud obscuring the sun is enough to keep the flowers tightly closed. Culpeper said, 'they are under the dominion of the sun as appears in that their flowers open and shut as the sun either shews or hides his face. This herb is so safe that you cannot fail in the using of it, only give it inwardly for inward diseases. Use it outwardly for outward diseases. 'Tis very wholesome, but not very toothsome'.

Herbal remedy

The ancients also called centaury *fel terrae*, gall of the earth, because of its very bitter taste. It is used in vermouth and other bitter aperitifs and liqueurs. Its bitterness, like that of its relative gentian, accounts for much of its medicinal value. It acts as a digestive tonic and liver remedy, increasing the flow of digestive juices and bile from the liver and gall-bladder. It can be used for weak digestion, poor appetite, heartburn, nausea, intestinal parasites, jaundice, gallstones and liver problems. Centaury acts as a blood purifier, cleansing toxins from the system and increasing the efficiency of the bowels. It will effectively reduce fevers when taken hot and has been used as a substitute for quinine. One of its bitter glycosides, gentiopicrin, reputedly has antimalarial properties. It helps to combat both bacterial and viral infections and treats postviral syndrome (ME). As a blood cleanser and anti-inflammatory, centaury treats rheumatism and gout, and skin problems such as eczema and boils. Centaury also has an affinity for the nervous system, lifting the spirits and calming the nerves. Generally it has a strengthening effect, useful when recovering from illness of stress, and as a blood tonic in anaemia.

Externally, centaury makes an anti-inflammatory antiseptic for cuts and grazes, boils and other skin conditions and is used to heal ulcers.

The flower essence

Centaury is a wonderful remedy for people who are very sensitive to others and to their environment. They are easily hurt and upset and can become ill as a result of disharmony and negative influences. Centaury people are good-natured and kind but stronger personalities will readily take advantage of them. As children they are obedient and good, responding well to praise and discipline. They may spend too much of their time helping others, sacrificing their own lives in their service. They can be 'doormats', and martyrs, and neglect their own mission in life in their desire to please.

Centaury helps you to develop your will, and recognize your own individuality and personality and to see it as valuable. It turns submissiveness into an ability to relate to others on an equal footing, to say 'No' when necessary and to use service to others as part of your own transformation.

California poppy
The flower of gold

Pleasures are like poppies spread,
You seize the flower the bloom is shed.
ROBERT BURNS (1759–96)

The poppy symbolizes the ephemeral pleasures of life – here one minute, gone the next. The California poppy with its vibrant yellow-orange flower is the state flower of California, and native to the west of North America. It was first introduced to Europe as an ornamental and medicinal plant in the last century and rapidly gained a reputation as a non-addictive alternative to the opium poppy. It was used for colicky pains and toothache by the native Americans and early settlers.

According to the doctrine of signatures, California poppy resembles a cup of gold, and the saying 'all that glisters is not gold' may be very appropriate to many in the state of California attracted to mind-altering drugs and glamorous spiritual practices.

Herbal remedy
California poppy is a cousin to the opium poppy but far less powerful, making it a safe remedy to calm excitability, restlessness, anxiety, tension and insomnia. It acts as a gentle sedative and is suitable for calming children. Its antispasmodic action relaxes muscles throughout the body, useful for treating colic in the stomach and gall-bladder, as well as for soothing tense, aching muscles and relieving tension headaches.

As an anodyne, California poppy can be used internally and applied externally to allay pain. It can be taken to relieve headaches, migraine, neuralgia, back pain, arthritic pain, sciatica and the pain of shingles.

Externally, it can be applied to areas of local pain such as toothache. Through its calming action in the nervous system California poppy also influences the heart and circulation. It slows down a rapid heartbeat and relieves palpitations, and helps to lower high blood pressure.

Generally, California poppy can be thought of as a gentle balancer to the emotions and a calming remedy in times of stress. It is well worth using when trying to withdraw from addiction, be it to alcohol, drugs, orthodox drugs or tobacco.

Homeopathic remedy: ESCHSCHOLZIA
Eschscholzia is used in tincture form for insomnia, slowness of the circulation and general weakness.

The flower essence
California poppy is for those who seek spiritual highs from external sources, who are attracted to the glamour and brightness of psychedelic drugs, charismatic teachers or occult rituals. Their spiritual life lacks discipline and solidity and they may be susceptible to techniques or influences which open the psyche too quickly, causing inner disharmony. California poppy helps to develop a more solid inner life, awakening the light within and enhancing self-reliance.

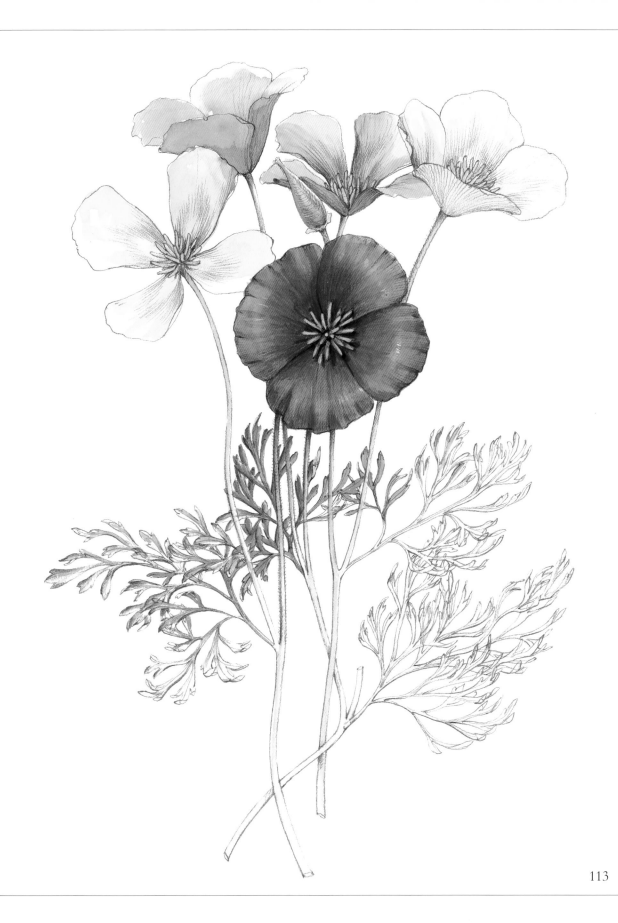

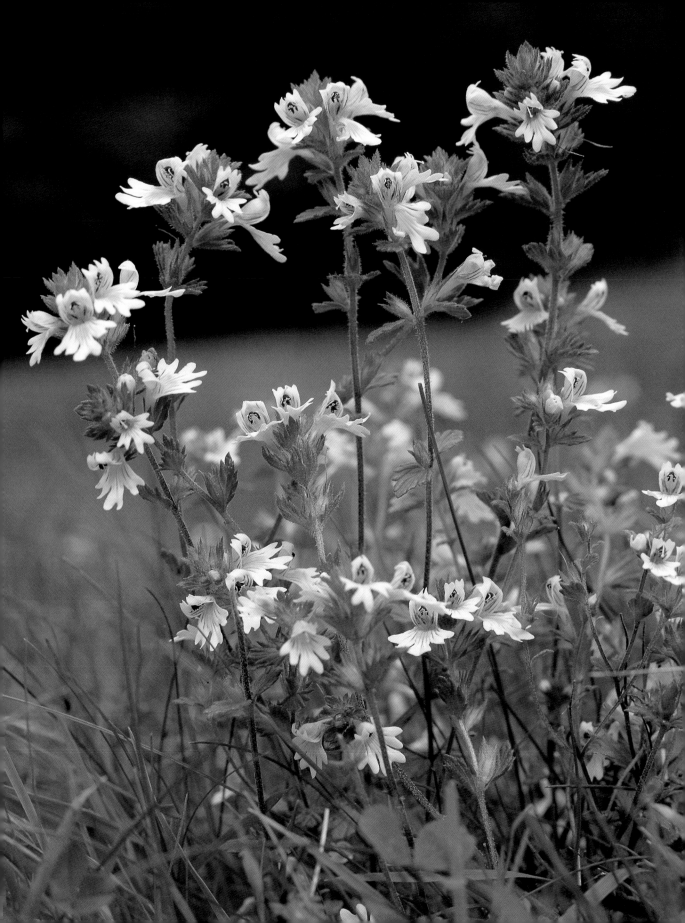

Eyebright

The flower of insight

...To nobler sights
Michael from Adam's eyes the film removed
Then purged with Euphrasine and Rue
His visual orbs for he had much to see.
  JOHN MILTON (1608–74)

Eyebright is a delicate little flower that grows in dry sunny pastures, commons and hillsides and is loved by bees. It is an annual plant which is partially parasitic, taking nourishment from roots of grasses. It is a member of the foxglove family and comes originally from Europe and Asia, although it grows throughout the United States.

Eyebright has been famous for centuries for its ability to preserve and restore eyesight. Its Latin name comes originally from the Greek word for linnet as the Ancient Greeks said that the healing power of eyebright was first discovered by a linnet who used it for her young in the nest. The linnet then gave her knowledge of eyebright to humankind and tells of her gratitude continuously in song. The Greek name for eyebright, *Euphrosyne*, was also the name of one of the Muses who represented joy and gladness. This plant clears the sight, it 'gladdens the eye' or lifts the spirits of the one whose sight is improved. Eyebright was said to be a visionary herb, increasing insight and enhancing inner vision, the ability to see things as they truly are. It was prescribed for troubles of the mind and according to Culpeper, 'it also helpeth a weak brain or memory'.

The doctrine of signatures interpreted the dark spot in the middle of the flower as bearing a resemblance to the human eye, and the purple and yellow spots and stripes inside the flower indicated a variety of inflammatory eye problems. Culpeper said, 'if eyebright were as much used as it is neglected, it would have spoilt the trade of the spectacle makers'.

Herbal remedy

Although modern herbalists may be more moderate in their claims about the power of eyebright than the ancients, it is still an excellent remedy for a variety of eye problems. Its astringent properties are good for relieving inflammatory eye infections such as styes, conjunctivitis, blepharitis, watery eye conditions, and catarrh. It is particularly good for sore, itching eyes

accompanied by a discharge, often seen in hayfever or measles, and for catarrhal conditions affecting the nose, throat, sinuses, ears, upper chest and causing sinusitis, headaches, and coughs. It will also help those with oversensitive eyes, which tend to run in cold and wind, or are irritated by smoky or stuffy atmospheres. It can be used either locally in lotions for the eyes or taken internally: 30 drops of the tincture in a glassful of rosewater makes an excellent eyewash. Eyebright can also be used in gargles for sore and catarrhal throats, and in mouthwashes for mouth ulcers.

The bitters in eyebright stimulate the digestion and enhance the flow of bile from the liver, making this a good tonic and a cleansing remedy. Several plants that improve the function of the liver are also recommended for the eyes, such as greater celandine, marigold, chamomile and centaury. According to Culpeper, all these herbs, including eyebright, are under the dominion of the sun which governs circulation, vital energy and eyesight. By detoxifying the system via its action on the liver, eyebright helps to clear the eyes and by improving circulation to the eyes, it improves feeble eyesight in the elderly and tired, strained eyes from overwork. By clearing mucus from the system, eyebright will keep the mucosa of the eye clear and healthy.

Homeopathic remedy: EUPHRASIA

Euphrasia is an excellent medicine for the eye. Like the herbal remedy it is prescribed for watery, burning eyes, discharges from the eyes, sensitive eyes aggravated by both light and windy weather, for swollen, inflamed eyelids and eyes as in blepharitis and conjunctivitis. It is good for catarrh, sore throats, colds, catarrhal throats, hay fever and coughs, and for eye and catarrhal problems accompanying measles.

The flower essence

Eyebright is again the flower of sight, insight, inner vision and perception. It is given to those whose brain feels weak and tired and whose memory is poor. Eyebright increases your sensitivity and perception of others and their conditions, which makes it helpful for those in the caring professions. It helps you to get things in a clearer perspective.

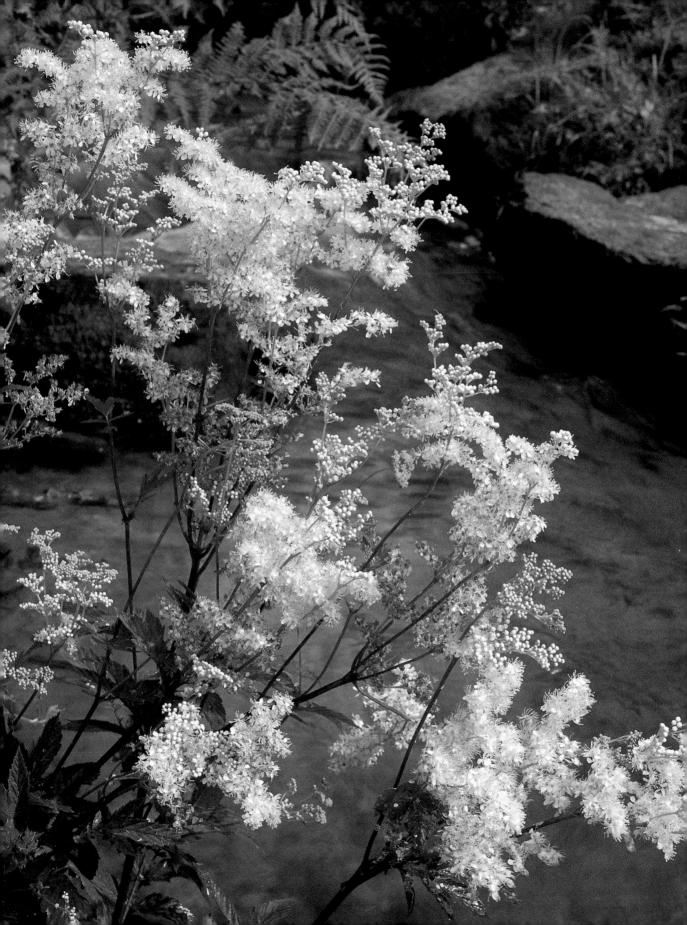

Meadowsweet

The flower of summer meadows

The meadowsweet taunts high its showy wreath
And sweet the quaking grasses hide beneath.
  JOHN CLARE (1793–1864)

The elegant meadowsweet flower with its sweet almond scent lives in damp fields and by rivers and streams. The plant well deserves its country name of queen or lady of the meadow. It was also know as bridewort, as its feathery white plumes and attractive red-stalked leaves were strewn in churches at weddings and made into garlands and posies for brides and bridesmaids. In Anglo-Saxon times it was used for sweetening mead and it was a favourite strewing herb in Tudor times. Gerard said that when strewed the smell of meadowsweet 'makes the heart merrie and joyful and delighteth the senses'. Along with vervain and watermint it was one of the most sacred herbs to the Druids. When gathered on St John's Day it was said to reveal a thief. In Iceland, where it also grows, not only is it believed to do this but also to indicate the sex of the robber by sinking in water for a man and floating for a woman!

Herbal remedy

The medicinal virtues of meadowsweet are very similar to those of aspirin. When crushed, meadowsweet flowers give off the characteristic smell of the salicylic aldehyde, which when oxidized yields salicylic acid, from which acetyl-salicylic acid or aspirin can be derived. The name aspirin comes from the old Latin name for meadowsweet, *Spiraea ulmaria*. Unlike aspirin, meadowsweet contains tannins and mucilage which protect the stomach lining and have an anti-inflammatory action.

Meadowsweet is one of the best antacid remedies for acid indigestion, heartburn, gastritis, peptic ulcers and hiatus hernia. It relieves wind and flatulence, and can be used in any inflammatory condition of the stomach or bowels. The astringent tannins protect and heal the bowel's mucous membranes and make it an excellent remedy for enteritis and diarrhoea, especially for children and the elderly. Its mild antiseptic action is helpful where there is infection, and its relaxant properties soothe griping and colic.

For aches and pains, rheumatism, arthritis and gout, meadowsweet offers welcome relief. The salicylates and gaultherine contained in the flowers have a powerfully anti-inflammatory action for hot, swollen joints and the diuretic properties of the plant help eliminate toxic wastes and uric acid from the system. Meadowsweet's analgesic properties soothe arthritic pain, headaches and neuralgia, and its relaxant properties release spasm and induce restful sleep.

Its cleansing diuretic effect has given meadowsweet a reputation for clearing the skin and resolving rashes. Given its mild antiseptic action it makes a good remedy for cystitis and urethritis, fluid retention and kidney problems. The salicylate salts soften deposits such as kidney stones and gravel as well as atherosclerosis in the arteries. Meadowsweet is a cooling diaphoretic, bringing blood to the surface of the body and causing sweating, making it useful for colds and flu and all eruptive infections.

Externally, the flowers which are rich in vitamin C, iron, magnesium and silica, speed healing of connective tissue and help to resolve inflammation. This may explain the folk use of meadowsweet of applying it to cuts and wounds, ulcers and skin irritations. The astringent tannins also promote healing and staunch bleeding. A decoction of the flowers can be used in a compress to promote tissue repair and for painful arthritic joints. It can also be used as a mouthwash for mouth ulcers and bleeding gums.

Homeopathic remedy: *SPIRAEA ULMARIA*

Spiraea is indicated by symptoms of heat which can be general as well as local. There may be heat in the cheeks with fever, vertigo, or headache, or a feeling of blood rushing to the face. It is also given for cramp and heaviness in the limbs with sleepiness and a feeling of dullness or heaviness in the head.

The flower essence

People who feel anxious and tense, and as a result suffer from tightness and tension in the head and neck muscles, benefit from the flower essence. It helps you relax and drift peacefully, as on a lazy summer's day on the banks where the plant grows.

Gentian

The flower of bitterness

See how the giant spires of yellow bloom
of the sun-loving gentian, in the heat
are shining on those naked slopes like flame.
    MRS LEYEL

Gentian is a large perennial herb indigenous to central and southern Europe and Asia Minor. It is a
highly ornamental plant with yellow star-shaped flowers. Yellow gentian will grow in most deep, loamy
soils in full sun and is easily grown from seed.

According to Dioscorides, gentians were named
after Gentius, King of Illyria, an ancient country
located on the Adriatic Sea. Gentius lived in the 2nd
century BC and was the first, apparently, to discover
the medicinal properties of gentian against the
plague. As a medicine gentian has been used at least
since the time of the Ancient Egyptians and was
employed by Pythagoras in 6th century BC as an
antidote to poisons. In the Middle Ages, gentian was
valued as a panacea for all ills. Before the days of
quinine it was taken for malaria.

Culpeper said that gentian was ruled by Mars, and
claimed, 'it resists putrefactions and poisons; a more
sure remedy cannot be found to prevent the
pestilence than it is'.

Herbal remedy

Gentian root contains one of the most bitter substances in the plant world, the glycoside amarogentin.
The bitter receptors in the mouth, on contact with
gentian, stimulate the flow of digestive juices and
enzymes throughout the digestive tract. The appetite,
digestion and absorption are enhanced, and elimination of wastes improved. Gentian increases the flow
of bile from the liver and promotes the movement
of food and wastes through the digestive system.

Gentian can be given for a wide range of digestive
problems, and for problems associated with inflammation. Its excellent effect on the digestion gives
gentian pride of place as a strengthening tonic, useful
in cases of general debility, weakness following illness
and lethargy from poor absorption and weak digestion. Gentian has traditionally been added to
alcoholic drinks and to this day several bitter aperitifs
include extract of gentian. Gentian was also traditionally taken as a spring bitter tonic to purify the blood.

It is a useful herb for clearing worms and infections
from the system. One constituent of gentian,
gentiopicrin, is highly poisonous to plasmodium,
accounting for its wide use as a malaria remedy.

Gentian with its detoxifying action has also been
used to treat rheumatism, arthritis and gout. It acts
as a febrifuge, bringing down fevers, and has cooling
properties. Gentian has a stimulating effect on the
female reproductive system, bringing on periods and
regulating menstruation. It was a considered a valuable remedy for 'female weakness' and hysteria, and
was given as a tonic to the nervous system.

Homeopathic remedy: GENTIANA

Gentiana is also given as a general tonic and as a
remedy for digestive problems. It helps nausea,
acidity and colic. A Gentian person tends to feel
dejected and morose.

Like the herbal remedy, gentiana is used for
rheumatic pains, headache and vertigo. Gentiana is
also prescribed for fevers, with febrile shuddering
like electric shocks, followed by lassitude, depression
and tension in the limbs.

The flower essence

The Bach Flower Remedy uses *Gentiana amarella*, a
variety of gentian with small lavender-to-crimson
flowers. It benefits those easily discouraged and
prone to despondency and depression. A gentian person at worst is the eternal pessimist, often bitter, and
almost gaining satisfaction from seeing things go
badly for them. They worry constantly and analyse
everything that could be of some benefit to them so
that they become sceptical of its ability to help them.
The 'doubting Thomas' in them prevents their
believing in anything they cannot grasp with their
constantly active minds, so that they cut themselves
off from their higher self, and the source of light and
clarity in their lives.

Gentian helps people to have more faith in themselves and others, and more confidence and trust in
their innate healing abilities and those of others.
With gentian they should be able to cope better with
setbacks and difficulties and be less prone to despondency and despair, realizing that conflict and
challenge are an integral part of human life.

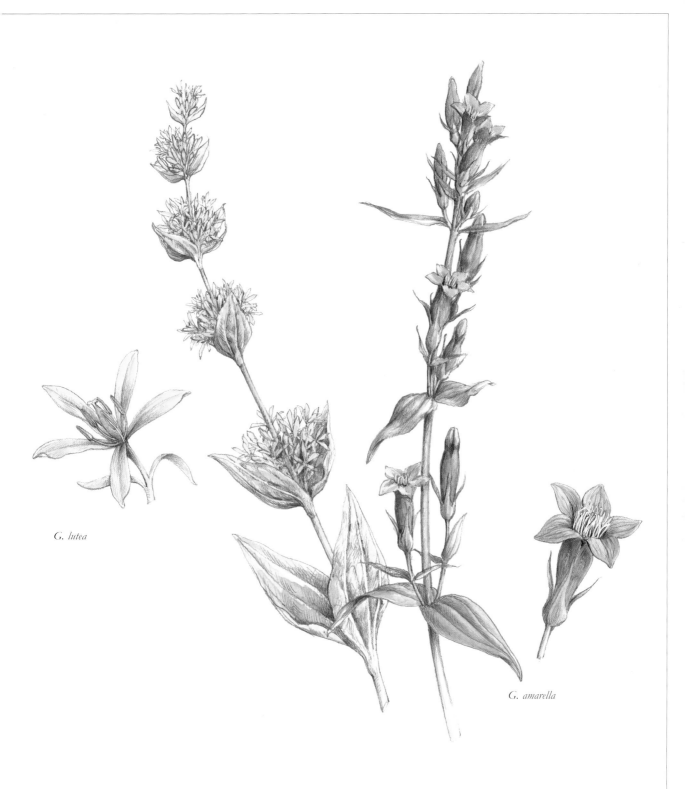

G. lutea

G. amarella

119

Cranesbill

The flower of constancy

...how gay
with his red stalks upon this summer's day!
And, as his tufts of leaves he spreads, content
with a hard bed and scanty nourishment
mixed with the green, some shine not lacking
power
To rival summer's brightest scarlet flower.
  WILLIAM WORDSWORTH (1770–1850)

There are many different varieties of wild geranium. American cranesbill is an attractive hardy perennial with rose-purple flowers and mottled leaves, found growing wild in woodlands throughout North America. In England and Europe the best known wild geranium is herb Robert, also known as stinking cranesbill because of its unpleasant smell, to be found growing in woods and open ground, even in cracks in walls and steps.

The name cranesbill was inspired by the beak-shaped fruit of the plant which resembles the bill of a crane. It also derives from the Greek word *geranos* meaning crane. For relatives of American cranesbill and herb Robert in the geranium family, the French botanist, L'Herifer, coined the names Erodium from *ero dios* meaning heron and Pelargonium from *pelargos* meaning stork. Our non-hardy garden geranium came from the South African species of Pelargonium and was introduced into Europe in the 17th century. They became increasingly popular because of the brightness of their flowers and varieties of colour so that by Victorian times they were found in almost every summer garden. They were also greatly appreciated for the beautiful scents from their leaves which varies from one species to another, from almond to lemon, nutmeg and rose.

According to an old Arab legend, geraniums are descended from the mallow. Once the prophet Mohammed washed his shirt in a stream and hung it out on a mallow plant to dry in the sun. The humble mallow blushed at so great an honour and turned a deep shade of pink and was thus transformed into the magnificent geranium.

Herb Robert was named after a Frenchman, the Abbé Robert, who founded the Cistercian order in the 11th century; perhaps this is why in the language of flowers, geranium means steadfast piety. In the language of love it means constancy and availability. However, to dream of geraniums was taken to mean a change of interests. In medieval times geranium was used as a protective herb to ward off evil influences and ill-health. According to Culpeper, it was under the dominion of Venus, and in his time it was a symbol of love and the desire to please. The flowers were used in love potions, and also as a cordial to lift the spirits and comfort the heart.

Herbal remedy

The wild geraniums, American cranesbill and herb Robert, are both powerful astringents due to the high percentage of tannins they contain. This makes them very useful for diarrhoea and dysentery, any kind of internal bleeding and heavy periods, and externally to heal cuts and wounds, ulcers and sores. American cranesbill was well known among the native Americans and early settlers for its healing properties. The Blackfoot Indians kept the powdered root in their pouches as a first aid remedy for stopping bleeding from cuts and wounds; the Meskwakis of the mid-west used the root to heal sore gums, pyorrhoea, for toothache and piles; the Cherokees made a mouthwash from a decoction of the root and used it for thrush in children while the Iroquois treated sore throats, mouth ulcers and infections, sores on the skin with cranesbill and used it for babies' navels when they did not heal. The early settlers boiled the root in milk and made a popular remedy for children's bowel problems including diarrhoea and dysentery since cranesbill tasted pleasant and had a gentle action with no adverse effects.

Both herb Robert and American cranesbill can be taken to astringe flaccid muscles, causing problems such as stress incontinence, prolapse and constipation, and also to dry up excess secretions as in catarrh and vaginal discharge. When used as a wash on the skin they can be used not only for cuts and grazes, sores and ulcers but also burns, greasy skin and blocked pores that cause pimples. They have also been used as a wash for the nipples when they become sore and tender (not on the whole breast as this may dry up breastmilk).

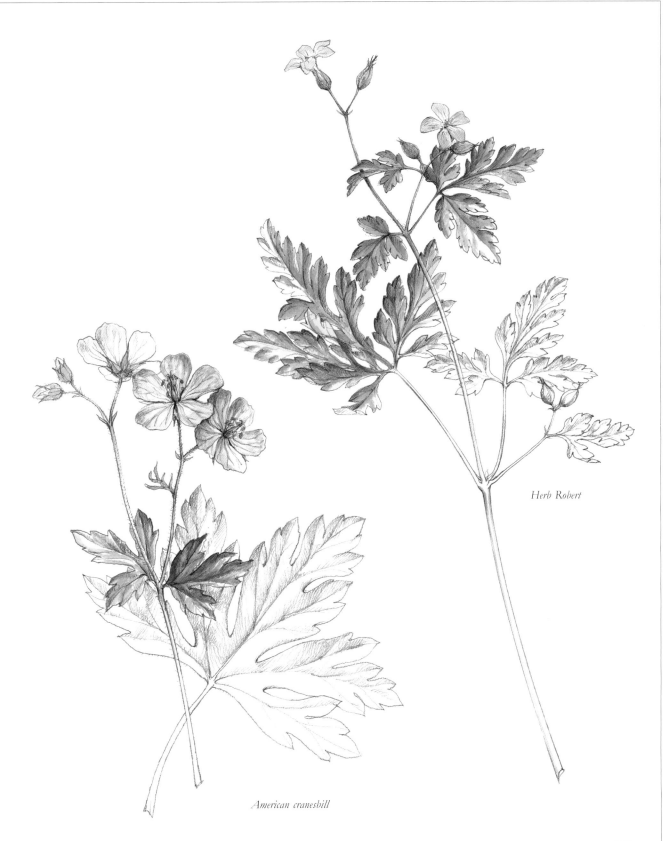

Herb Robert

American cranesbill

121

Homeopathic remedy: G. MACULATUM

Geranium maculatum root is also used for diarrhoea, dysentery, heavy periods, haemorrhages, ulcers, sore nipples, vaginal discharges and sore throats. Other symptoms indicating its homeopathic use are giddiness with double vision, relieved by closing the eyes and lying down, dilated pupils, difficulty walking with the eyes open, though better with them closed, dryness of the mouth, burning at the tip of the tongue, pain on left side of forehead, and a constant desire to empty the bowels but inability to do so. There may be symptoms indicating stomach ulcers including vomiting of blood.

Aromatherapy oil

Rose geranium, *Pelargonium graveolens*, is a relative of the cranesbills, and is used for its rosy sweet smell. It has a beneficial effect on the nervous system, and has astringent properties. Rose geranium is ideal for stress-related disorders such as headaches, stomach aches, menstrual cramps and debility. It helps to relieve tension and anxiety, and lifts the spirits, dispelling melancholy and depression. Its balancing effect on the emotions reduces mood swings and can be put to good effect when treating PMS and menopausal problems. Its hormone-regulating properties are very helpful in this respect.

As an astringent rose geranium will tone up lax muscles, relieve diarrhoea and heavy periods, stop bleeding from grazes and cuts, and is good used as a skin toner for excess sebum production, spots, greasy skin and acne. It can also be used in washes for piles, varicose veins, chilblains, burns and cellulite, and skin complaints such as eczema. Its antiseptic properties help prevent infections from cuts and can be used when treating boils, abscesses and head lice. It also makes a good insect repellent and deodorant. Used on the breasts, geranium reduces swelling and engorgement, and makes a good remedy to prevent and treat mastitis.

The flower essence

Geranium is for those who feel down and depressed, lacking colour in their life. Geranium helps to lift the spirits and to bring joy and happiness to your daily activities. It is also helpful for those who need strength and motivation to bring plans and projects into action. It helps to get things started in a well ordered way by providing the energy and clarity that is needed.

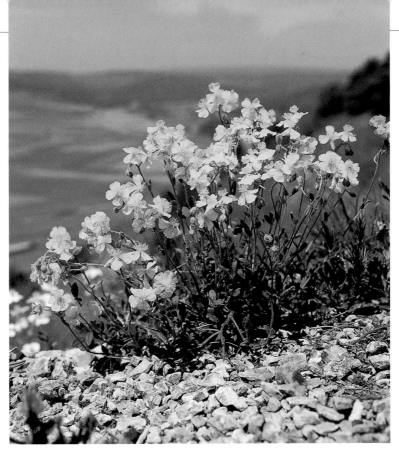

Helianthemum nummularium, H. canadense

Rock rose
The flower of heroes

The name Helianthemum derives from the Greek *helios* (sun) and *anthemon* (flower), since the flowers only come out when the sun shines. The American or Canadian rock rose, *H. canadense*, grows in dry, sandy soils and is an old remedy for scrofulous symptoms, gangrene and skin problems. The English or European rock rose, *H. nummularium*, grows wild on chalky, sandy or gravelly soil in hilly pastures.

Herbal remedy As an astringent, *H. canadense* can be used to treat diarrhoea and dysentery, when taken in small amounts (large amounts may prove emetic). As a gargle, rock rose will help to relieve sore mouths and throats and mouth ulcers. It can be used as an eyewash for inflammatory eye problems and as a skin lotion for skin problems, such as acne, eczema, varicose veins and ulcers, insect bites and stings.

Rock rose is not commonly used today, but in the past it was used often in the treatment of secondary syphilis, and scrofula. It was also prescribed for swollen glands and sore throats in scarlatina. Its old name was scrofula plant.

Homeopathic remedy Cistus or Helianthemum canadense is prepared from a tincture of the whole plant and is used for diarrhoea and dysentery, for shingles and its accompanying painful blisters on the skin and pain along the nerve pathway. It is also used for swollen glands and scrofulous conditions, as well as itching of the skin and sore throats including those associated with scarlet fever. A sensitivity to cold air runs through the symptom picture which is suggested by the peculiar habit of the plant forming ice crystals around its root in winter. A Cistus or Helianthemum person tends to be anxious and trembles when ill with a fever. Their symptoms are aggravated by all kinds of mental excitement.

The flower essence Rock rose (*H. nummularium*) is a remedy of emergency, where there is terror, panic or extreme fright, which spreads from the person affected to those around them. It may be the terror of a child after a nightmare, or of someone involved in or witnessing an accident. It is one of the components of Dr Bach's Rescue Remedy, and can be used for acute fear or terror in any situation when feeling unable to cope. Rock rose frees one from the almost paralysed state of panic, and can help to turn fear for oneself into courage, even to the point of forgetting oneself in times of emergency for the sake of others. It is the remedy of heroes, where people can grow beyond their natural capabilities.

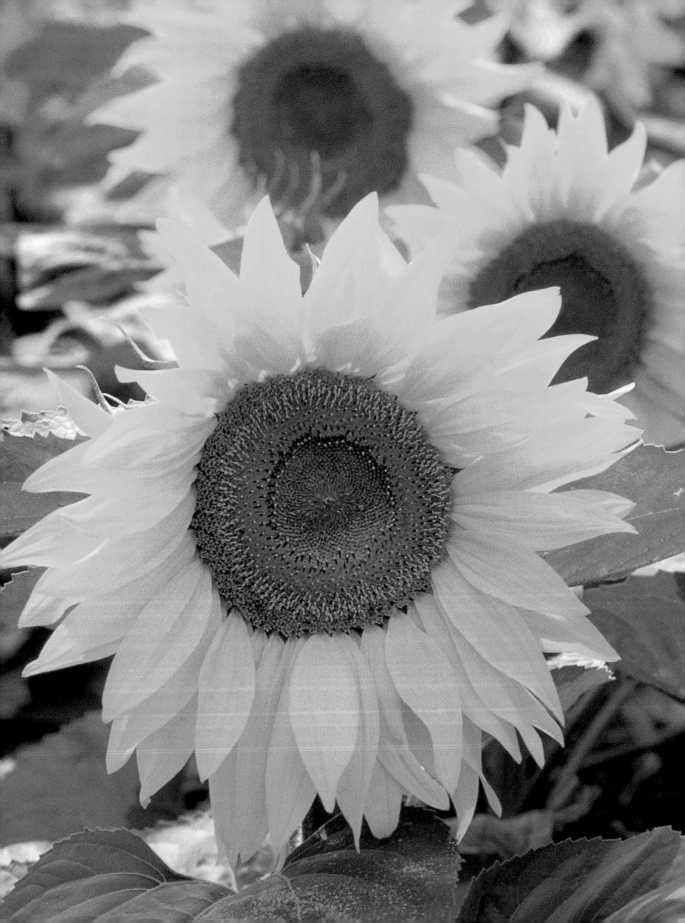

Sunflower

The flower of the Incas

The heart that has truly lov'd never forgets
But as truly loves on to the close,
As the sunflower turns on her God when he
sets,
the same look which she turn'd when he rose.
  THOMAS MOORE (1779–1852)

The magnificent sunflower is a native of Mexico and Peru and was brought to Europe in the 16th century because of its extraordinary economic value. Every part of the plant has something to offer: the leaves and stalks make fodder, cloth and paper, and a tobacco substitute; the flowers contain a useful yellow dye; the seeds are highly nutritious and can be made into bread, or roasted to make a drink; and the seed oil is excellent for salads and cooking, being high in polyunsaturated fats. It is made into margarine, paint and soap. The pith of the stalk is one of the lightest natural substances and was used to make lifebelts.

The name Helianthus comes from the Greek *helios* meaning sun, and *anthos* meaning flower, because the flowers always turn towards the direction of the sun. In Italian it is called *girasole*, and in French *tourne sol*. The marigold does the same, hence the name marigold of Peru. It may also be called sunflower because its golden-rayed flowers resemble the sun.

The sunflower was worshiped as a symbol of the sun and an emblem of the sun god Atahualpa by the Incas of Peru and later by the native people of the Americas. It was carved in the sculptures of their temples and woven in gold into the fabrics of their clothing; the priestesses wore crowns made of gold carved into the shape of sunflowers. The early Spanish invaders found beautiful carvings of the sunflower in gold and said their workmanship far outvalued the gold they comprised.

The legendary origin of the sunflower is described in the Greek myth in which Clytie, a beautiful water nymph, fell in love with the sun god Apollo. However, Apollo loved another, Caliope, and so Clytie pined away and died of a broken heart. Where she died her limbs dissolved into the earth and took root; her body was transformed into a slender stem and her lovely face into the sunflower.

Herbal remedy

As the sunflower was dispersed around the world as a crop it began to acquire a reputation as a good folk remedy for sore throats, colds, coughs, bronchitis, asthma, whooping cough and tuberculosis.

The seeds were used for intermittent fevers and 'ague' and were considered better than quinine for the treatment of malaria. The 19th century settlers in America planted sunflowers near their homes as a protection against the disease. They are very useful for drying damp soils as they have a remarkable ability to absorb water. They can therefore reduce disease that abounds in damp areas, including malaria carried by mosquitoes. They were also popular in Russia, Turkey and Persia for this reason.

Sunflower seeds have been the subject of much investigation and found to be highly nutritious, rich in minerals including phosphorus, calcium, iron, fluorine, iodine, potassium, magnesium and sodium. They are also high in protein, and vitamins B and D. Inulin contained in the oil has been found effective in the treatment of asthma.

Sunflower seeds also have diuretic properties, and since they aid the elimination of toxins, have been used in treatment of gout and rheumatism. The oil has also been used externally as a rub for arthritis and rheumatism.

The flower essence

In the language of flowers the sunflower, perhaps because of the lofty heights to which it can grow, symbolizes haughtiness. As a flower remedy sunflower can be used for people who have a tendency to be egotistical, arrogant, haughty or vain.

Sunflower can also be used for those who suffer from low self-esteem, or lack of self-confidence, perhaps because of conflicts with their parents, particularly fathers or father-figures, during childhood. As a symbol of the sun with its light, warmth and power, sunflower relates to the light in our lives that emanates from the inner self.

Sunflower was used in the past to increase happiness in one's life, to attract joy to replace sorrow, and today it is still used as a flower remedy to enhance our ability to shine like the sun.

Witchhazel

The flower of divination

Witch hazel is an attractive deciduous shrub native to the eastern part of North America. It is often grown in gardens for its bright yellow flowers which appear in the depth of winter to enliven an otherwise bare garden. It enjoys part sun and part shade. The name Hamamelis comes from the Greek, indicating its resemblance to an apple tree. One of its common names, snapping hazel, refers to the violent ejection of its seeds when ripe.

The bark, twigs and leaves have similar actions. It was used dried as snuff to stop nosebleeds. The native Americans used witch hazel mixed with flax seed for inflamed swellings and painful tumours. The branches made good divining rods for detecting underground water and metals. Because hazel was used in divining rods in Britain, it became known as 'witch' hazel in the New World.

Herbal remedy

Extracts of witch hazel were much used in the days of our grandmothers as a general household remedy for scalds and burns, swelling and inflammation of the skin and to stop bleeding. Its main action is astringent because of the high levels of tannins that occur in the plant. This makes it an excellent remedy for bleeding, both internally and externally, and it has been used to stop bleeding from the lungs, stomach, uterus and bowels. Witch hazel makes an excellent remedy for diarrhoea, dysentery, mucous colitis, and respiratory catarrh. It used to be prescribed for uterine prolapse and a debilitated state after miscarriage or childbirth, to tone up the uterine muscles. It can be used to good effect for excessive menstruation, and uterine blood stagnation with feeling of fullness, heaviness and discomfort around a period.

Externally, either as a decoction, tincture or in distilled form, witch hazel can be applied to cuts and wounds, used as a mouthwash for bleeding gums, and as a lotion or in an ointment for bleeding piles. The tannins not only stop bleeding, but also speed healing, reduce pain, inflammation and swelling, and provide a protective coating on wounds to inhibit the development of infection. They also check mucous discharges throughout the body and have a tonic, contracting action on the muscles and blood vessels giving witch hazel a wonderfully wide variety of therapeutic uses. As a lotion or ointment it will relieve the pain and swelling of varicose veins and phlebitis, the itching of haemorrhoids, and speed the healing of varicose ulcers. A poultice or compress will relieve burns, swollen inflammatory skin problems, swollen engorged breasts, bed sores, bruises, sprains and strains.

As a lotion it can be applied to soothe the pain, irritation and swelling of insect and mosquito bites and stings, to relieve tender aching muscles, as a toning skin lotion to tighten the tissues and reduce broken capillaries. Mixed with rosewater it makes a refreshing eyebath, and eye pads soaked in witch hazel will relieve sore, tired or inflamed eyes, including conjunctivitis.

As a lotion, decoction or tincture it can also be used as a douche for vaginal discharge and irritation; or as a gargle for sore throats and infections, such as tonsillitis and laryngitis, and a mouthwash for an inflamed mouth and mouth ulcers.

Homeopathic remedy: HAMAMELIS

As a homeopathic remedy hamamelis similarly acts on the nervous circulation and the mucous membranes. The deep red colour of the tincture is a signature of its therapeutic action: there is no better remedy for bleeding and blood vessel disorders.

It is prescribed for passive haemorrhage from any part of the body, and for venous congestion, varicose veins and ulcers, and haemorrhoids with a bruised soreness of the affected part. It is very valuable after operations, to speed healing of wounds, and to remedy the weakness associated with loss of blood.

The flower essence

Witch hazel is used for those who put themselves under pressure by trying to live up to the expectations of others.

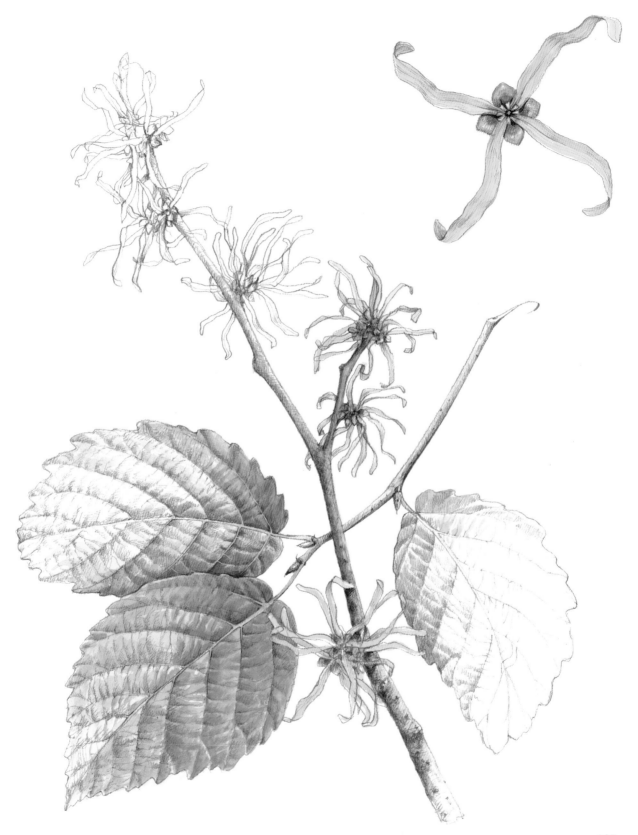

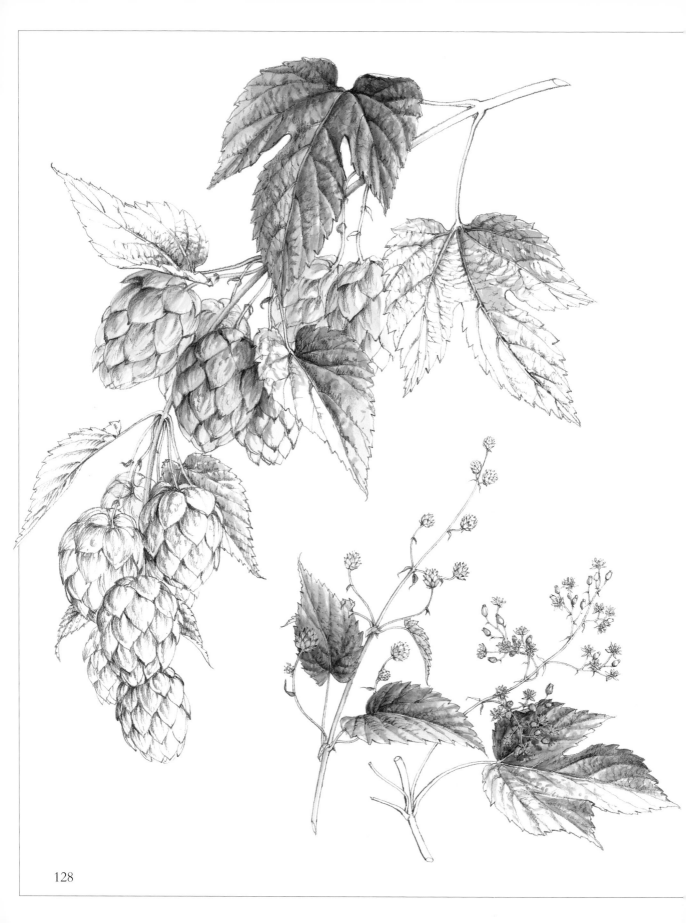

Hops

The flower of restful sleep

Hops are trailing plants that grow wild all over Europe, Central Asia, North America and Australia. They wind clockwise around tree trunks or other supports, clinging to them with tiny barbs. The Romans believed, wrongly, that in this way they sucked life out of the supporting trees and they called hops *lupulus*, meaning little wolf. The name *humulus* probably derives from the fact that hops prefer moist, humus-rich soils. The name hops comes from the Anglo Saxon *hoppan*, meaning to climb.

Hops are most famous for their relationship to beer. They were widely used to flavour beer by the 14th century in most parts of Europe but only used in English breweries since 1524. King Henry VIII of England had forbidden their use as he said they caused melancholy. Small yellow glandules on the fruits of the hops secrete a sticky substance called lupulin which contains several bitter compounds. These help to preserve beer, make it more foamy and give it a bitter taste.

The Jewish captives in Babylon drank barley beer with hops to protect them from leprosy. Pliny says that the Romans grew hops in their gardens and ate the young shoots as a vegetable. Hops have been smoked for their narcotic properties and used in sleep pillows to relieve insomnia. They have been a favourite herb of gypsies who use them to relieve uncontrolled sexual desires and quarrelsome natures.

Culpeper said that hops were ruled by Mars and could be used to cleanse the bloodstream of heat and toxins by stimulating the liver and kidneys.

Herbal remedy

The dried flowers of hops, or strobiles, have a sedative action which explains the use of hops in pillows to this day. Not only do they relieve insomnia, but they also help in cases of tension and anxiety, soothing pain, restlessness and agitation. Hops has an antispasmodic action which reduces tension in muscles throughout the body, including spasm in the gut and other digestive problems such as nervous indigestion and irritable bowel syndrome which could be stress-related. The bitters in hops aid digestion, enhancing the action of the liver and the secretion of bile and digestive juices. There are also tannins which aid healing of irritated and inflammatory conditions and stem diarrhoea, while the antiseptic action of hops relieves infections.

Despite the masculine image of beer-drinking, hops are a good remedy for women. Along with the essential oil, they have an oestrogenic action, making them excellent for any problem around menopause. Hops have also been used to enhance milk supply when breastfeeding and for suppressed and painful periods. They depress men's libido but have the opposite effect on women.

The asparagin in hops is a soothing diuretic, reducing fluid retention and hastening elimination of toxins from the system. This combined with the action on the liver have given hops a reputation for clearing skin problems such as eczema and acne. Its relaxant and antihistamine action is also useful here.

Externally, hops are used in creams to keep the skin soft and supple and delay wrinkling. Their antiseptic action is useful for cuts, wounds and ulcers.

Aromatherapy oil

Hop oil can be added to a night-time bath to ease aching tense muscles and promote a restful sleep. Inhalations or baths will help relieve pain and reduce tension, anxiety, irritability and restlessness. Like the herbal remedy hop oil helps to calm sexual desire in men, and enhance women's libido, while the oestrogenic effects will be helpful through the menopause.

Homeopathic remedy: LUPULUS

Lupulus is used in the advanced stages of sleepiness that the narcotic effects of hops in large amounts produce.

The flower essence

Hops are a good remedy for adolescence when the playful energy of children transforms into sexual energy and greater bodily strength. It eases this transition, and also stimulates physical and spiritual growth. It helps to improve group interaction.

St John's wort

The flower of light

The bright yellow flowers of this wild woodland plant have always been associated with light. Its flower symbolized the sun which casts out all evil, dispelling the forces of darkness. The name Hypericum comes from the Greek *huper eikon*, meaning 'over an apparition' because of its apparent power to protect against evil spirits. Mattiolus said, 'certain writers have said that St John's wort is so detested by evil spirits that they fly off at a whiff of its odour.' In the past people who suffered from mental illness, melancholy and epilepsy had to sniff the juice to drive out their evil spirits. Sprigs of St John's wort were hung at house and church doors on Midsummer's Eve, the pagan summer solstice, and the longest day, to protect them from negative influences, thunder, lightning, fire and witches.

With the coming of Christianity, the herb was dedicated to St John the Baptist, and Midsummer's Day became St John's day. The red pigment that exudes from the flowers represented the blood of St John the Baptist. It was also called heart of Jesus oil. On the night of St John young girls would hang the herb over their doors or sleep with it under their pillows, to foresee their husbands. In several countries the dew that had fallen on the flowers before daybreak on St John's Day was gathered and used to protect the eyes from all harm throughout the coming year. In the language of flowers St John's wort means superstition.

Herbal remedy

St John's wort is a wonderful remedy for the nervous system, relaxing tension and anxiety, and lifting the spirits. Research confirms this remedy as an antidepressant and sedative. The mood-elevating properties take 2–3 months to produce lasting effects, brought about by the plant's ability to enhance the effect of neurotransmitters in the brain.

St John's wort increases sensitivity to sunlight, and can help those not over-sensitive with seasonal affective disorder (SAD) during winter, caused by lack of sunlight. It may well be helpful with jetlag. It is excellent for emotional problems during menopause, and reduces blood pressure, capillary fragility and benefits the uterus. St John's wort can be used for painful, heavy and irregular periods as well as PMS.

It has a diuretic action reducing fluid retention and hastening elimination of toxins via the urine. It relieves bedwetting in children and incontinence by its tonic effect on the urinary system. It is also a useful remedy for gout and arthritis.

St John's wort also has an expectorant action, speeding recovery from coughs and chest infections. Its antibacterial and antiviral action aids the fight against TB and influenza A, and may help treat AIDS, HIV and cancer. Hypericin seems to interfere with the reproduction of retroviruses. In the digestive tract its astringent and antimicrobial action relieves gastro-enteritis, diarrhoea and dysentery.

Both internally and externally, St John's wort is a wonderful remedy for nerve pain and any trauma to the nervous system. It can be used for trigeminal neuralgia and sciatica (fibrositis), back pain, shingles, headaches and rheumatic pain. It is also worth taking after surgery, and laceration of nerve tissue.

Externally, 'heart of Jesus oil' applied to sites of nerve pain such as sciatica and shingles will ease pain and speed healing. It soothes and heals burns, cuts, wounds, sores, and ulcers. It is also useful for sprains, haemorrhoids, varicose veins and ulcers.

Homeopathic remedy: HYPERICUM

Hypericum is called the arnica of the nerves; it is used to treat any trauma or injury to areas of the body that are rich in nerve tissue such as the spine, fingers, eyes, lips, mouth and toes. Often arnica should be given first to prevent swelling and bruising, and then hypericum given for pains that are tearing and sensitive to touch or pressure, and for shock.

The flower essence

St John's wort is again the remedy of light. It is best suited to sensitive people, prone to fears, often of the dark, or of psychic attack, causing restless, disturbed sleep and often nightmares. It is also for those who are oversensitive to sunlight and heat. Such people may be prone to allergies and oversensitive to their environment. St John's wort helps to engender a feeling of being protected from negative influences and to dispel fears by giving a feeling of being strong and full of light. It also allows light to illumine rather than to threaten in one's life.

NB The phototoxins in St John's wort may cause photo-sensitivity in fair-skinned people when taken internally

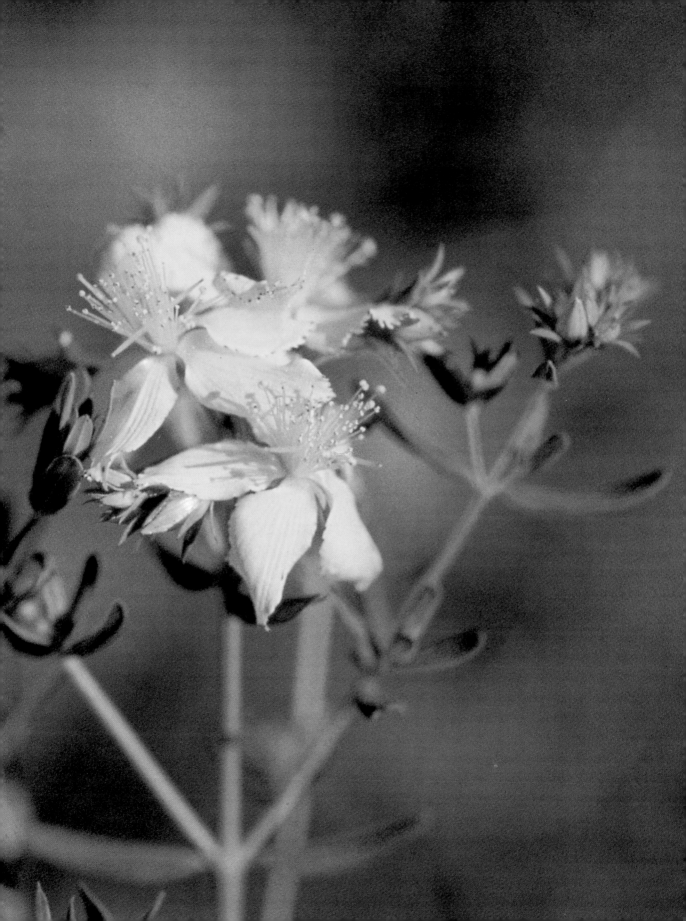

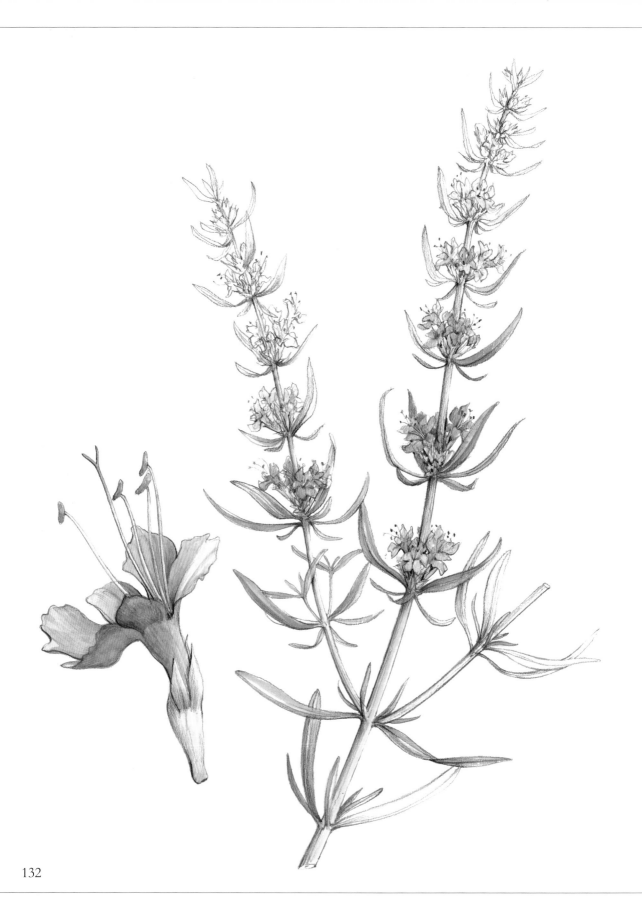

Hyssop

The flower of forgiveness

Purge me with Hyssop and I shall be clean,
wash me and I shall be whiter than snow.
PSALMS

Hyssop is an attractive evergreen member of the
mint family, with a sweet, powerful and long-lasting
scent that has been used often in perfumery, pot-
pourris and herb pillows. The white, pink, blue or
purple flowers are loved by bees and butterflies.
Hyssop was planted in medieval monastery gardens
and by the 17th century it was often featured as an
ornamental flower in English gardens.

The name hyssop derives from the Hebrew word
ezob. To the Hebrews hyssop was a sacred plant,
used for cleansing holy places. Since early times hyssop has been a symbol in many cultures of purity,
cleanliness, baptism and forgiveness of sins. It was
used in the Water of Purification that God
commanded Moses to prepare.

The Greeks valued hyssop in the same way.
Dioscorides referred to it as a 'holy herb' since it was
an ingredient of incense employed in cleansing ceremonies. The Romans valued it to protect them
against sickness, including the plague. Later it was
used to clean churches and houses of the sick including leper houses; it was a strewing herb in the
Middle Ages and made into nosegays and bouquets
to ward off contagion and bad smells.

Hyssop can be grown from seed in the spring or
cuttings taken during the summer. It prefers a sunny
position and well-drained soil.

Herbal remedy

Hyssop is an excellent herb for warding off infection
and enhancing immunity. It has an affinity for the
respiratory tract, and makes a good stimulating
decongestant and expectorant for colds, flu, catarrh,
sinus problems, coughs, bronchitis, asthma and
pleurisy. It is particularly useful for children. The
volatile oils in hyssop are mainly responsible for its
antiseptic and expectorant action; it has been shown
to be effective against the tuberculosis bacillus and to
have antiviral properties – useful in the treatment of
colds, flu and herpes simplex which causes cold
sores. Hyssop can be taken as a gargle for sore

throats and tonsillitis, and as an inhalation for catarrh
and hay fever.

Hyssop is warming and pungent tasting. It stimulates the circulation and causes sweating which helps
to bring down fevers and cleanse the blood. It
warms and invigorates the stomach, increasing the
appetite and enhancing digestion. It can be used for
indigestion and flatulence, all kinds of spasm, and
constipation. Hyssop was used in the past for epilepsy; its tonic properties make it a restorative to the
nervous system, good for debility and convalescence.

Externally, hyssop can be applied to bruises,
sprains, cuts and wounds to relieve swelling and
speed healing. It can also be added to the bath to
relieve rheumatism and arthritis.

Aromatherapy oil

Hyssop oil makes a nerve tonic to relieve anxiety,
tension, exhaustion, depression and to support during
times of stress. In a vaporizer it will help to purify
the atmosphere, particularly useful where there is
infection in the house, and when studying for exams
will help clarify the mind and steady the nerves.

As an inhalant it will help to clear respiratory
infections and catarrh, and enhance immunity, making it useful in asthma, chest infections, bronchitis,
fevers, flu and hay fever.

Hyssop oil, like the herbal remedy, will also aid
digestion and stimulate appetite. Rubbed into painful
swollen joints it will help ease the pain. It has also
been used for scanty periods, vaginal discharges and
as a diuretic for urinary infections and stones.

The flower essence

Hyssop is used again for purifying and cleansing,
emotionally and spiritually, reflecting its use in early
times as a symbol of the forgiveness of sins. It will
help to release tension throughout the system which
has its origin in emotional problems and specifically
feelings of guilt. In this way hyssop will help one to
let go of such feelings and allow self-forgiveness. It
is particularly useful for children who may blame
themselves for strife between their parents, and for
parents who feel guilty because their child-rearing
does not mirror their ideals.

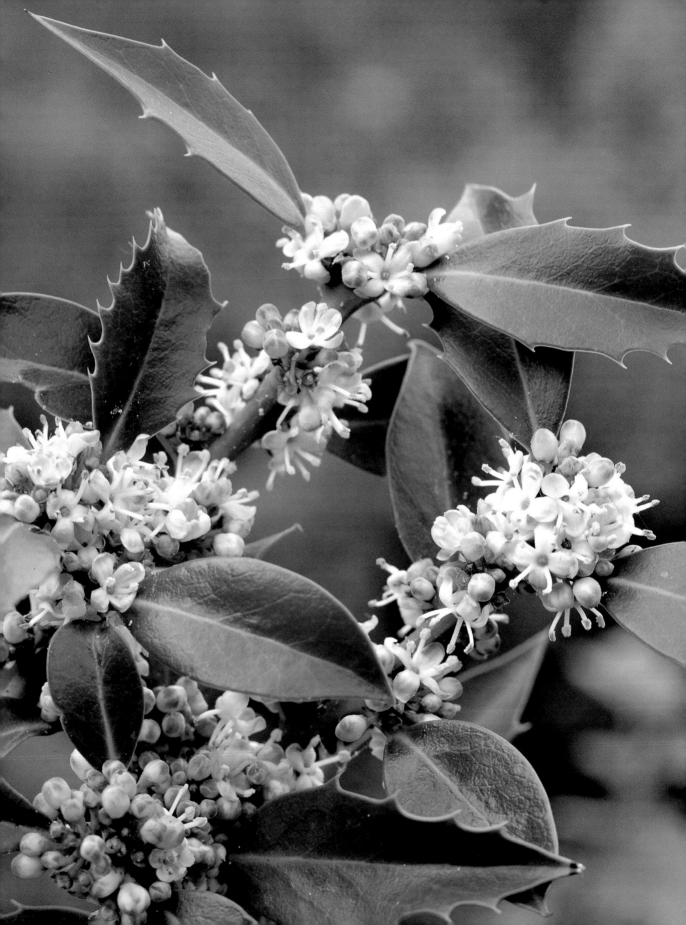

Holly

The flower of goodwill

The Holly and the Ivy
when they are both full grown
of all the trees that are in the wood
The Holly bears the crown.

Holly is a handsome evergreen, native to Central and Southern Europe, and is widely cultivated in Europe and the United States specifically for Christmas decorations. Holly's association with the winter solstice goes back many hundreds of years. In Ancient Roman mythology holly was dedicated to Saturn, and during the Roman festival saturnalia, between 17–23 December, branches of holly were exchanged as a symbol of health and happiness. In pagan mythology the oak king (ruler of the waxing year) slays the holly king (of the waning year) at yule and is himself slain at midsummer by the holly king. In the Christian calender Midsummer's Day is St John's Day, and St John the Baptist came to be equated with the oak king. Yuletide is Christmas, the birth of Christ, so Christ was equated with the holly king and holly became known as a symbol of joy and goodwill.

In other old legends holly first grew in places where Jesus walked when he was alive. The spiny leaves and red berries, the colour of blood, were thought to represent the suffering of Christ and so holly derived the names Christ's thorns and holy tree.

Holly was a tree of good omen; its evergreen leaves symbolizing life amidst the apparent death of winter. In the days of Pliny, holly was considered a tree of protection; if planted near a house or hung over the door, it defended the place and its inhabitants from poison, evil spirits, lightning and witchcraft. It was carried by men for good luck (women carried ivy) and if the wood was thrown at a wild animal it would make the creature lie down quietly. Holly water was sprinkled on newborn babies for protection. Holly was also used by the Druids to decorate their huts in winter, making a suitable dwelling for sylvan spirits. It was one of the seven sacred trees of the Irish chieftains and illegal to fell.

Herbal remedy

The leaves of several species of holly are used in different countries for making tea. The best known is *Ilex paraguayensis* from Brazil, known as yerba maté,

which is drunk throughout South America as a revitalizing tonic (it is high in caffeine). In the German Black Forest holly leaf tea was commonly drunk as a substitute for ordinary tea, and as a tonic.

The astringent properties of the leaves will tone mucous membranes throughout the body and make a good remedy for catarrhal problems. They also act as an expectorant, useful for persistent coughs, and were taken in the past for bronchitis, pleurisy and pneumonia.

As a diuretic, holly helps relieve fluid retention and hastens elimination of toxins from the body. It has long been used for arthritis, gout and rheumatism for this reason. It can also be taken for urinary infections and to prevent urinary stones.

Taken in a hot infusion holly leaves have a diaphoretic effect, bringing blood to the surface of the body and causing sweating. This helps to bring down fevers and to bring out rashes.

Homeopathic remedy: ILEX

The fresh leaves, berries and young shoots are used in homeopathic preparations for catarrhal problems, inflammatory eye symptoms, pain in the spleen, diarrhoea with mucus and intermittent fevers. Symptoms are generally better in winter.

The flower essence

Holly is for people who are full of hatred, jealousy, envy, thoughts of revenge, and resentment. Such feelings arise from a lack of love in their lives or within themselves. They feel insecure, suspicious of others and malicious. Such feelings are often clear to see in a first child, who becomes jealous, moody, aggressive or rebellious when the new baby is born, terrified their parents' love may switch to the new sibling. Holly was said by Dr Bach to open the heart and unite us with divine love.

The holly tree symbolizes the birth of Christ and the love of God, and love is the antithesis of the hatred felt by those needing holly. Holly helps us to release such emotions, and to be able to experience love towards others and within ourselves, so that we can be happy, unthreatened by others and their achievements or attributes and accepting and understanding of the various vexations of life.

NB The berries of the holly tree are mildly poisonous. They cause vomiting and diarrhoea

Blue flag
The flower of the rainbow

O flower de luce, bloom on and let the river
linger to kiss thy feet!
O flower of song, bloom on and make for ever
The world more fair and sweet.
    HENRY LONGFELLOW (1807–1882)

There are few flowers to match the iris in beauty or
popularity. It was aptly named by Linnaeus after Iris,
Juno's messenger who, in Greek mythology, descended from Olympus and appeared to mortals as a rainbow. The Greek *iris* means eye of heaven, used both
of the centre of the eye and the rainbow. Iris's speed
in flight is mirrored in the short flowering time of
the flower, and her rainbow is reflected in the many
different colours of irises. Iris accompanied the souls
of the departed to their eternal resting place along
the path made by the rainbow, and so the iris was
placed on graves to symbolize hope and the eternal
spirit. The custom of decorating graves with white
irises in Eastern Muslim countries, white being their
colour of mourning, has spread all over the world. In
the language of flowers iris means a message.

The iris has also been a symbol of royalty since
the days of Ancient Egyptians. Iris flowers feature in
tomb paintings dating back more than 4000 years in
the Valley of the Kings, and appear as decorations
on the sphinx's brow. The shape of the iris is that of
the sceptre, symbol of power and majesty.

The iris has had close links with the history of
France since around 496AD when Cloris, king of the
Franks, was baptised along with 3000 of his followers and adopted the iris as his emblem. In the 12th
century Louis VII also used the iris as his emblem
during the crusades, and the iris became known as
the *fleur de Louis* which became *fleur de luce* or *lys*, and
the *fleur de lis* remains the royal emblem of France,
the petals representing faith, wisdom and valour.

There are about 250 species of iris found wild
throughout the northern hemisphere, thriving in
damp soil and river and pond margins. *I. versicolor*
comes from North America and was long used in
healing by the natives and early settlers.

Herbal remedy
Blue flag has a particular affinity for the lymphatic
system, enhancing lymphatic circulation and the
action of the immune system. It is therefore highly
valued as a blood purifier and a detoxifying herb,
useful when treating skin disease. Its diuretic properties help elimination of toxins via the urinary system.

Blue flag acts on the liver and gall-bladder,
increasing the flow of bile, a further cleansing action
as the liver is the great detoxifying organ. It benefits
the digestion, stimulating the flow of digestive juices,
relieving wind, flatulence, constipation, heartburn,
indigestion and nausea and can be given for
headaches, skin problems and lethargy associated
with poor digestion.

William Turner, the 16th century English herbalist,
similarly recommended flag iris for 'gnawings in the
belly' and 'for them that have taken a thorowe cold'.
Blue flag can be taken to help clear catarrh, congestion in the chest, throat and nose, and for swollen
glands and sore throats. It has been used to treat
thyroid and pancreatic problems.

Externally, iris root was used in poultices to treat
sores on the limbs; it can also be used for bruises.

Homeopathic remedy: IRIS
The tincture of the fresh root is used mainly for
digestive complaints and skin problems, particularly
those characterized by burning. An Iris person feels
low-spirited and easily discouraged.

The flower essence
Iris versicolor, or *I. douglasiana*, with all its rainbow
colours and its special symbolical ability to carry
messages between the earth and the heavens, is a
remedy of creativity and inspiration for those who
feel that their 'feet of clay' have weighed them down
in the mundane material world. It is for those who
feel uninspired, creatively stifled or blocked and lack
trust in their innate abilities to be creative and happy.
Iris people may feel insecure, tense about the future,
feeling the need to be constantly planning for all
eventualities. They may feel angry and frustrated by
their lack of inspiration or their imperfections. The
flower remedy helps to release such blocks to
creativity and allow one to draw on inspiration from
within and without, to become more fully alive. It
helps to eliminate negative feelings about oneself and
lack of trust in one's inner resources.

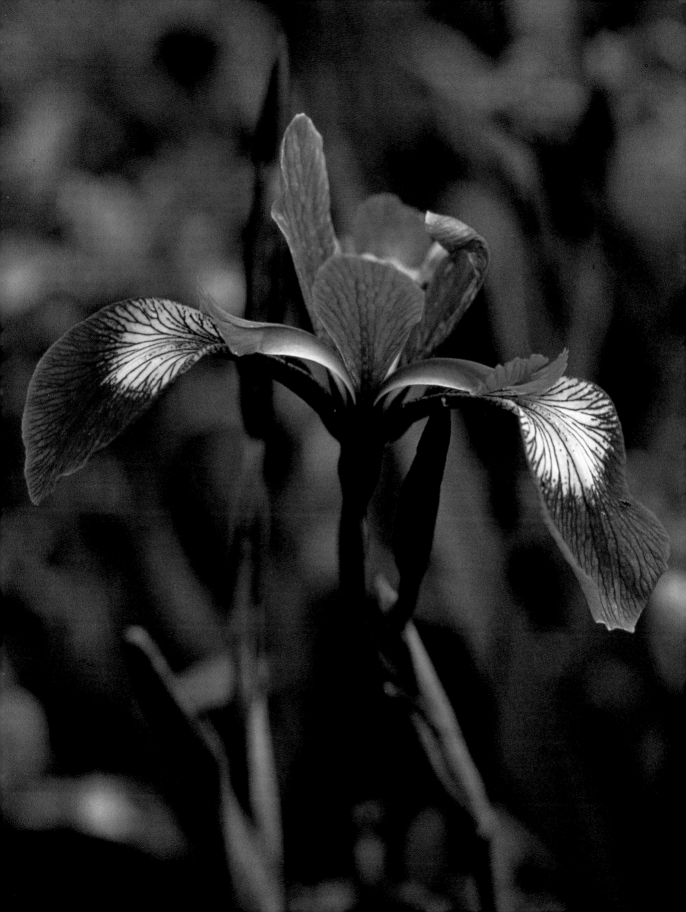

Jasmine
The flower of luxury

Known in India as Queen of the night, the delicate jasmine flower has one of the loveliest and most distinctive perfumes, particularly intoxicating at night. The common white jasmine, *J. officinale*, is a native of Northern India and Persia, while the Spanish jasmine, *J. grandiflorum*, is a native of the Himalayas and has slightly larger, highly perfumed flowers grown for use in perfumery. There are between two and three hundred species of jasmine, mostly native to Asia.

The old name jessamine, and jasmine, come originally from the Persian name *yasmin* and the Chinese *yeh-hsi-ming*. In China jasmine has been a symbol of feminine sweetness and beauty, and Indian jasmine is a sacred flower, known as 'moonlight of the grove' and traditionally woven into bridal wreathes, and worn as scented ornaments by women. The flower oil has been a favourite scent and hair oil of Indian women. Jasmine is held sacred to Vishnu and Indra.

For centuries the luxurious perfume of jasmine has been associated with femininity, love and fertility in the Hindu and Muslim traditions. The oil and the flowers have long been major ingredients in love potions and were historically associated with the moon, the goddess Diana and the maternal, creative aspect of the universe. With the coming of Christianity, jasmine was dedicated to the Virgin Mary and the star-shaped flowers symbolized heavenly felicity. White jasmine flowers were known as 'the star of divine hope' and associated with the Virgin Mary. In the language of flowers white jasmine symbolizes deep affection, happiness and elegance.

Herbal remedy
Jasmine has an affinity for women and the female reproductive system and has been used in healing women for many centuries. In Ayurvedic medicine jasmine is used for calming the nerves and soothing emotional problems, relieving period pains, PMS and tension headaches. Its astringent properties will stem bleeding and so it is used for heavy periods, and locally for vaginal discharges and infections. It helps to regulate menstruation and as an antispasmodic relaxes the uterus and soothes pain during childbirth. It is widely known as an aphrodisiac. Jasmine's antiseptic properties are useful for treating a range of infections including respiratory infections and

problems in the genito-urinary system, including cystitis and salpingitis. According to Culpeper, jessamine is a warm cordial plant which could be used to facilitate childbirth and remove diseases of the uterus, and also to 'dissolve cold swellings and hard tumours'. The astringent properties of the flowers treat inflamed eyes and skin, and as gargles and mouthwashes relieve sore throats and mouth ulcers. Jasmine has a decongestant action in the uterus and the respiratory tract, clearing catarrh and relieving sinisitus and coughs.

Aromatherapy oil
Jasmine has an uplifting, even euphoric effect on the emotions and has an affinity for women. It is often used to treat emotional problems relating to sexuality, such as impotence and frigidity. Its warming sensual fragrance is relaxing and reassuring, useful in a whole range of stress-related problems, including grief, heartbreak, anger and depression. When combined with clary sage or bergamot it helps to relieve postnatal depression. Its aphrodisiac effect can be enhanced by combining it with rose, ylang ylang or clary sage. It is antiseptic, antiviral and antifungal and can be used in treatment of herpes and thrush. It strengthens and relaxes the uterus and is excellent for use during childbirth. During the menopause, it reaffirms a woman's confidence in her femininity and sensuality, and brings a feeling of optimism, warmth and wellbeing.

Homeopathic remedy: J. OFFICINALE
Jasminum officinale is prepared from a tincture of the berries and is prescribed for symptoms of tetanus, including convulsions, vomiting and coma.

The flower essence
Jasmine is recommended for people with problems of excess mucus clogging the nose, throat and chest and causing a feeling of cloudiness and sluggishness. Jasmine clears the passageways and the head and promotes mental clarity. It stimulates the brain, increases perception and allows the mind to grasp deep questions about the essence of all life and our purpose on this planet. It increases awareness of innate femininity and the wisdom that brings.

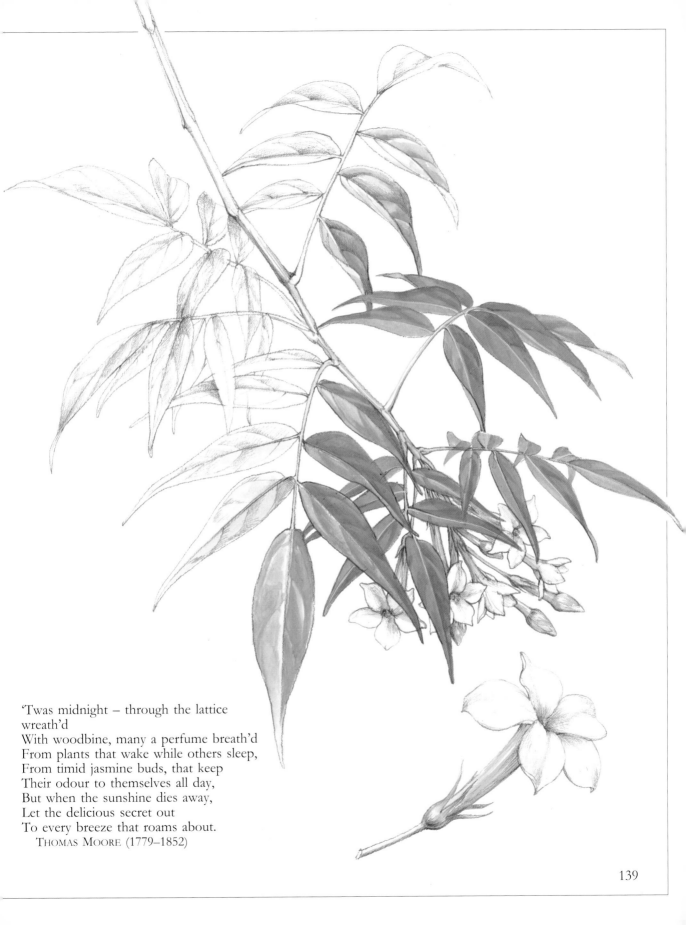

'Twas midnight – through the lattice
wreath'd
With woodbine, many a perfume breath'd
From plants that wake while others sleep,
From timid jasmine buds, that keep
Their odour to themselves all day,
But when the sunshine dies away,
Let the delicious secret out
To every breeze that roams about.

Thomas Moore (1779–1852)

139

Walnut

The flower of royalty

Let the air with Hymen ring:
Hymen! lo! Hymen sing!
Soon the nuts will now be flung:
Soon the wanton verses sung.
GAIUS CATULLUS (87–54? BC)

The handsome walnut tree with its large spreading boughs is probably a native of Iran and grows throughout Asia and Europe. Walnut trees can live for up to 1000 years. Many of the large walnut trees seen in Europe were planted by monks for their nutritious nuts and the medicinal value of their leaves and green outer nutshells. There are about 50 species of walnut, some, such as the black walnut and various kinds of hickory, native to North America.

Juglans regia means royal nut of Jupiter from *glans* (acorn) and *Jovis* (Jupiter), alluding to the ancient days when men lived on acorns and the gods lived on walnuts. The name walnut comes from the German *wallnuss* or *welsche nuss*, meaning foreign nut.

In Ancient Greece the walnut was dedicated to the goddess Artemis, and the tree symbolized wisdom, fertility and longevity, as well as strength in adversity. Nuts were used in love spells and served at Greek and Roman weddings, as the poem suggests. Their purpose was to symbolize the end of the frivolities of youth for the newly-wedded couple. In Romania a woman wishing to remain childless would, on her wedding day, stuff as many roasted walnuts as the number of years she did not want to conceive into her bodice. The walnut tree was also said to symbolize selfishness because nothing can grow underneath it. However, a gift of a bag of walnuts was said to make all your dreams come true. The husks of walnuts when boiled in water made a hair thickener and dye (to cover grey hair).

Herbal remedy

The leaves, best picked before mid-July, have a beneficial effect on mucous membranes throughout the body. In the digestive system they are astringent, combating irritation and inflammation of the gut lining and relieving indigestion, gastro-enteritis, nausea and diarrhoea. In the respiratory system they clear catarrh and catarrhal coughs; they also have a diuretic and depurative action, aiding the elimination of toxins from the body via the urinary system. They help clear skin problems such as acne, and to clear congestion in the lymphatic system and swollen glands. They are reputed to lower blood sugar.

Externally, an infusion or decoction of walnut leaves can be used as a lotion for skin problems such as cold sores and shingles blisters, for chilblains, and for excessive perspiration of the hands and feet. They are a good remedy for piles, varicose veins and ulcers, for styes and sore throats.

The bark of the walnut tree has a blood-cleansing and laxative effect, while a vinegar of pickled young nuts makes an effective gargle for sore throats. Walnut oil is a good source of linolenic acid, which aids the immune system, heart and circulation, helping to protect them from degenerative disease and problems associated with harmful cholesterol.

Homeopathic remedy: JUGLANS REGIA

Juglans regia is a good remedy for acne, cradle cap, boils, itching and inflammation of the scalp, and ulcers. In the digestive tract it relieves wind, bloating and diarrhoea and can relieve catarrh in the throat, chest and ears, in those who are mentally either over-excited as if intoxicated or peevish and discontented.

The flower essence

Walnut is the remedy for times of change in life, when one has to make a big step forward, starting a new life and breaking away from restrictions or past habits, releasing oneself from conventions. Old beliefs, family ties, the force of habit can be hard to shake off and can inhibit transformation and development. Walnut is the link breaker, the remedy to protect us from powerful outside influences such as the opinion of significant others that restrict our freedom and limit our potential for self-fulfillment. It is excellent for those going through periods of biological change such as puberty, pregnancy and menopause and finding them hard to accept. It is just as good for starting a new relationship, a new job, when moving house, retiring, or after divorce or bereavement and yet still linked emotionally to the past. Walnut is the remedy to enhance our inner strength and stability, the springboard to real change and freedom from misgivings from the past.

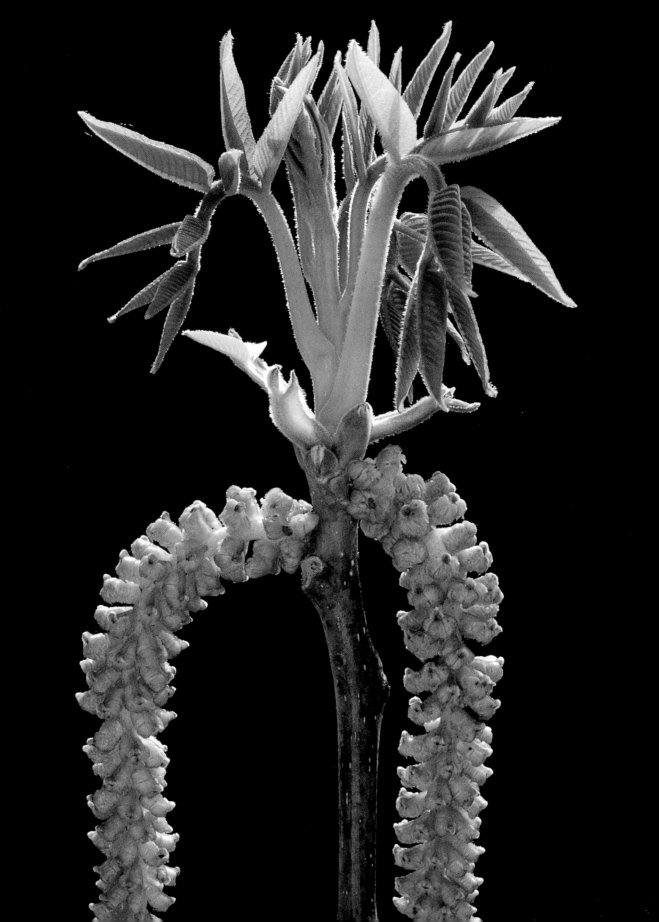

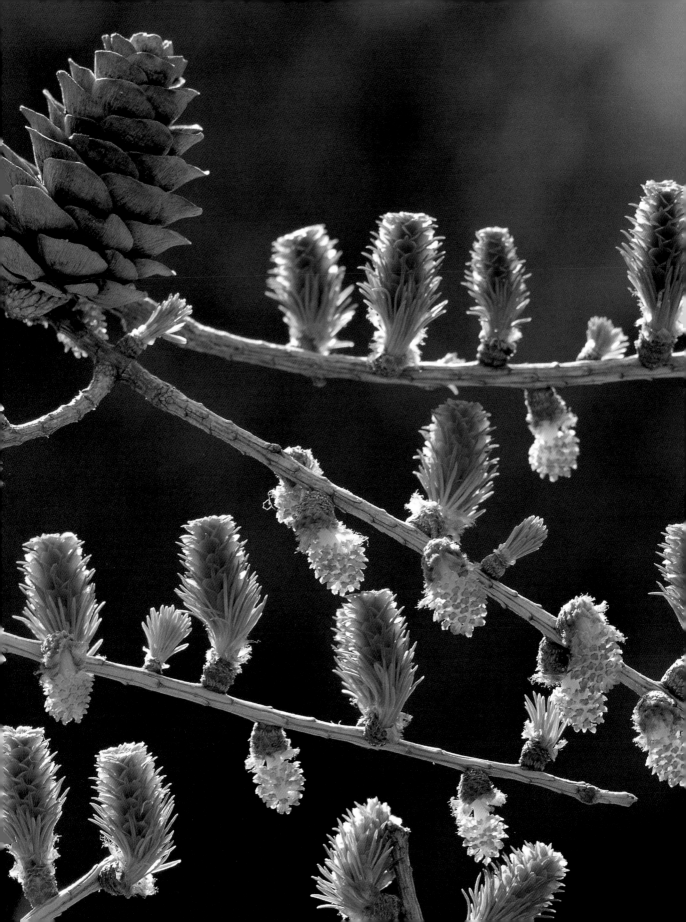

Larch

The flower of durability

When rosy plumelets tuft the larch,
And rarely pipes the mounted thrush;
or underneath the haven bush
flits by the sea-blue bird of March.
ALFRED, LORD TENNYSON (1809–92)

Larch is a conifer which is indigenous to hilly areas throughout Central Europe where it can be found in large forests. It was introduced into England in 1639 for its enormous value in housing and shipbuilding. The wood is stronger and more durable than most other conifers, and is almost indestructible by fire. The Romans used it in building castles, which were often apparently almost impossible to destroy in sieges. Augustus used it for building the Forum in Rome and Tiberius found it very useful for making bridges. Larch is also valuable because it grows so quickly – six times faster than oak; some of the beams of larch found in houses in Venice are over 100 feet (30 metres) long. As a result, larch has been worshipped in many parts of the world as a symbol of immortality and incorruptibility, also of boldness and audacity. It has been used to protect against evil influences, witchcraft and disease.

The larch is not evergreen like other conifers and the appearance of its bright green leaves in spring symbolized renewal of life, regeneration of energy, death and rebirth. Large amounts of its resin, turpentine, are collected from larch trees when they are fully grown and has been used for centuries in medicine and for making varnish, when it is known as Venice turpentine – it used to be exported exclusively from Venice. The resin and sap were regarded as the soul of a tree, a source of fire and regeneration. Resin represents immortality and the undying spirit. Larch is said to be ruled by Mars.

Herbal remedy

Larch is mainly used as a stimulating expectorant for catarrhal coughs and bronchitis. Its astringent properties can be put to good use in treating heavy periods, diarrhoea and bleeding. As a diuretic, larch can be taken to relieve fluid retention and to aid elimination of toxins via the kidneys. This makes it a useful remedy for arthritis and gout. A weak decoction makes a good eyewash for inflammatory eye problems and a lotion for skin problems such as eczema and psoriasis, as well as piles and varicose ulcers. Larch has also been used to lift the spirits and dispel melancholy and despondency.

Externally, the turpentine can be used in compounds to apply to rheumatic joints and gout. The new twigs and bark can be boiled and employed as an antiseptic inhalant for catarrh and respiratory infections. Turpentine was used in the past in massage oils in cases of paralysis and in hospitals to stop the onset of gangrene.

The flower essence

The Bach Flower Remedy larch is again used to dispel melancholy and despondency that arises from a sense of failure and inferiority. A larch person suffers from lack of self-confidence, and an inbuilt, almost unconscious, feeling that they are less able than others. This means that they often do not attempt to do things, convinced as they are of failure. They deprive themselves of opportunities in life and the chance to live life to the full. The more such people think they cannot do things, the more they fail in their self-fulfilling prophesy and hence a vicious circle is created. They feel increasingly useless and impotent.

Larch people are not resentful or jealous of others' abilities, admiring others for their successes in matters a larch person would never even attempt. In fact such people are usually just as capable as others, despite their modesty.

The larch flower remedy can be taken to help dissolve negative ideas of oneself from the past that are inhibiting proper development and fulfilment. It can be used for adults and children alike. It enables one to recognize otherwise hidden abilities and to increase self-confidence and self-esteem, making it particularly useful during periods of challenge such as exams, and for children venturing to do things for themselves, such as homework, without parental assistance. It helps one to persevere despite setbacks and to tackle projects with a more positive or open attitude about the outcome.

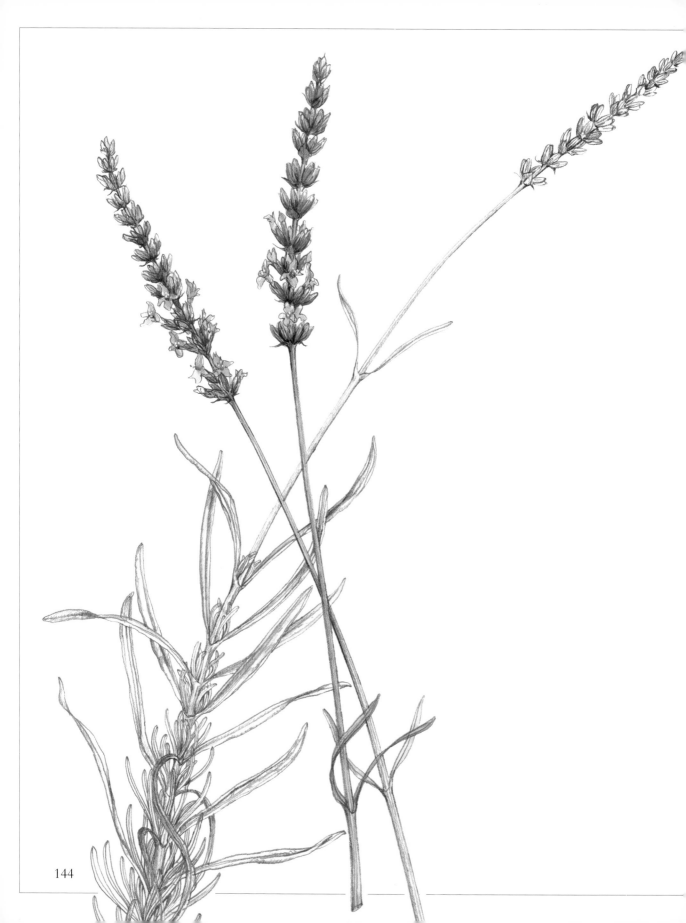

Lavender

The flower of the Virgin Mary

Lavender has been one of the best loved scented herbs for thousands of years. Its fragrance when brushed against lifts the spirits and also attracts bees. It makes delicious honey. Dioscorides considered that its fragrance surpassed all other perfumes, and it was venerated also for its cleansing and purifying qualities. The Romans used lavender to perfume their baths, hence its name which comes from *lavare*, to wash. It was used to sweeten the breath and for perfumes, in preparation for childbirth and to keep away infection. It was dedicated to Hecate, the goddess of witches and sorcerers and was said to avert the evil eye. The Virgin Mary is reputed to have been especially fond of lavender because it protected clothes from insects and also preserved chastity.

During the Middle Ages and Renaissance lavender was the favourite strewing herb for floors of houses and churches to keep off the plague. Housewives placed it in linen cupboards, wardrobes and drawers to scent clothes and repel moths. It was hung in the corners of rooms to keep away flies and mosquitos. The 16th century herbalists recognized its medicinal virtues and recommended it for improving eyesight, relieving headaches and faintness and to comfort the heart. Mattiolus the Italian herbalist said, 'it is much used in maladies and those disorders of the brain due to coldness, such as epilepsy, apoplexy, spasms and paralysis; it comforts the stomach and is a great help in obstructions of the liver and spleen'.

Herbal remedy and Aromatherapy oil

The volatile oils in lavender account for the major part of its medicinal action, so that the uses in herbal medicine and aromatherapy are very similar. Parkinson said lavender is 'of especiall good use for all griefes and pains of the head and brain'. An infusion or tincture of lavender flowers or inhalation of the essential oil has a wonderfully relaxing effect on the mind and body. It makes an excellent remedy for anxiety and nervousness, and physical symptoms such as tension, headaches, migraines, trembling, palpitations and insomnia. A few drops of oil in the bath will soothe a fractious child into restful sleep.

In aromatherapy lavender oil is considered a balancer to the emotions. It lifts the spirits, and has a stimulating edge, acting as a tonic to the nervous system. It restores strength and vitality to those suffering from nervous exhaustion.

Lavender relaxes the digestive tract, soothing away spasm and colic related to tension and anxiety. Its powerful antiseptic volatile oils are active against bacteria including diptheria, typhoid, streptococcus and pneumococcus. As a tea, inhalation or vapour rub on the chest, it relieves colds, coughs, bronchitis, pneumonia, flu, tonsillitis and laryngitis. Its decongesting and expectorant action hastens the expulsion of phlegm from the chest, making it a useful remedy for asthma. The tea or tincture can also be taken for stomach and bowel infections causing vomiting and diarrhoea. When taken as hot tea lavender causes sweating and reduces fevers. It increases elimination of toxins through the skin and the urine.

Externally, the antiseptic oils in lavender make it an extremely useful disinfectant for applying (as a dilute oil, strong infusion or tincture) to cuts and wounds, sores and ulcers. It stimulates tissue repair and minimizes scar formation when the oil is applied neat to burns, and diluted to skin inflammation and infection as in eczema, acne and varicose ulcers. The neat oil repels insects and relieves insect bites and stings. Diluted it soothes the pain and swelling of bruises, sprains, gouty and arthritic joints, and when used as a massage oil or added to the bath, soothes away tension and spasm in the muscles. It can be rubbed on the chest and inhaled for chest infections, coughs, colds and catarrh. The tea or tincture makes a gargle for sore throats, tonsillitis and hoarseness, a mouthwash for mouth ulcers and inflamed gums, and a douche for leucorrhoea (vaginal discharge).

The flower essence

Lavender can be taken to balance the emotions, to relieve anxiety, depression and reduce stress and conflict. It is particularly recommended to those who have used the herb or the oil over a long period and have become used to it. The flower remedy could be added to enhance their effects. It is also valuable for people involved in spiritual practices, for it calms the mind and helps to ease emotional conflicts blocking spiritual growth. Lavender is said to activate the crown chakra; it stimulates awareness and alertness and helps to connect people to their higher self.

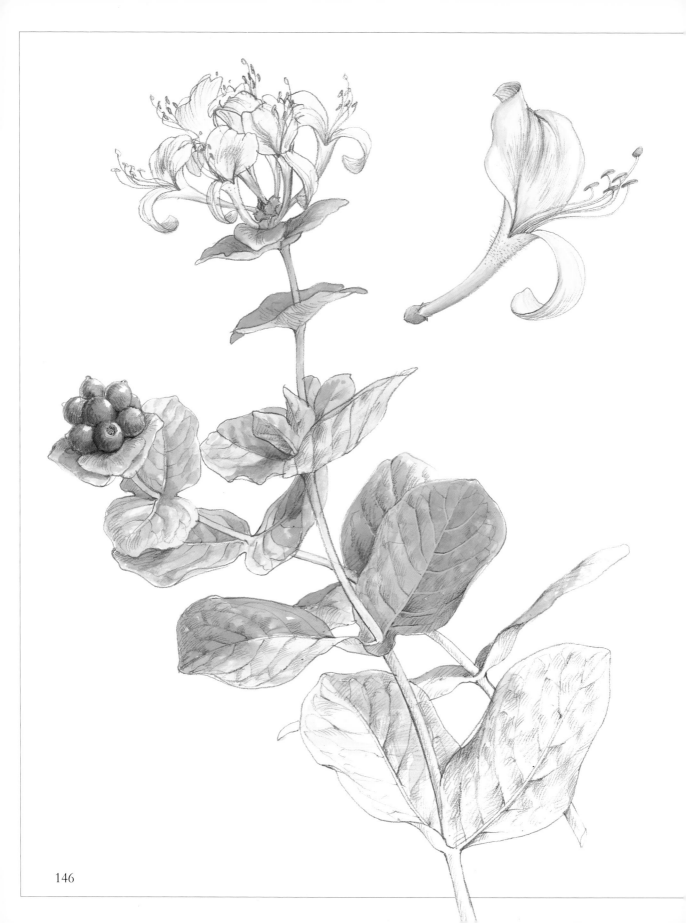

Honeysuckle

The flower of unity

I am drunk with the honey wine
Of the moon-unfolded eglantine
which fairies catch in hyacinth bowls.
PERCY BYSSHE SHELLEY (1792–1822)

Honeysuckle has been much loved through the centuries for its sweet scent which pervades the air in summer gardens, and in woods and hedgerows where it grows wild. Honeysuckle is one of the oldest English flower names, dating to at least the early 8th century, deriving from its honey-sweet fragrance, the inspiration of many poets and writers. Its old name woodbine describes its twining habit, scrambling through woods or garden arches with seemingly inexhaustible energy, for it blooms throughout the spring, summer and autumn. The Chinese believe that prolonged use of honeysuckle increases the lifespan. In other cultures it was known as the herb of immortality because it flourishes even when severely cut back.

Its clinging nature symbolizes, in the language of flowers, 'we are united in love', and bonds of devoted affection. Its sweet fragrance symbolizes a sweetness of disposition while the heady perfume of wild honeysuckle that might turn a maiden's head is a symbol of inconstancy of love. Many parents used to forbid their teenage daughters to bring honeysuckle into the house as it was said to evoke erotic dreams.

The name Lonicera honours Adam Lonicer, a German botanist of the 16th century. Goats (Latin: *capra*) are fond of honeysuckle, which itself climbs as nimbly as a goat, hence its name caprifolium. Periclymenum comes from Periclymenus, one of the Argonauts from the Greek myths who had the power of changing his shape at will. The honeysuckle flower changes shape and colour daily to attract butterflies and night-flying moths to assist in pollination.

Herbal remedy

Twelve species of honeysuckle, out of about a hundred, are used medicinally. The leaves and flower buds are rich in salicylic acid, meaning that they can be used for symptoms that may be relieved by aspirin, such as colds and flu, fevers, headaches, aches and pains, arthritis and rheumatism. The leaves have anti-inflammatory properties and contain antibiotic substances active against staphlococci and coli bacilli making honeysuckle a useful remedy for respiratory and gastro-intestinal infections. Honeysuckle's antispasmodic and expectorant effects can remedy spasm and phlegm in the respiratory system, as in asthma, croup, whooping cough and bronchitis.

When used for respiratory problems, honeysuckle is generally given as a syrup of the flowers, but a tea or tincture of the leaves can also be taken. The leaves and flowers have diuretic properties and relieve fluid retention, urinary stones and gout. The leaves have an affinity for the liver and spleen; they benefit the digestion and make a gentle laxative. (The berries are best avoided as they are purgative and cathartic and nauseatingly bitter.) The plant has a calming effect on the nervous system and is useful where anxiety or tension gives rise to symptoms such as asthma, headaches or stomach cramps. The Russians apparently prepare an oil from the wood which they use for tumours and chronic pain.

Homeopathic remedy: LONICERA

L. periclymenum (leaves) is used only for irritability, and violent outbursts of temper while L. xylosteum (berries) is used for profuse vomiting and diarrhoea, spasms and convulsions.

The flower essence

Honeysuckle is a Bach Flower Remedy particularly suited to those who live in the past and cling to pleasant memories of events gone by, unable to enter fully into the present. Honeysuckle people tend to glorify the past, only remembering the good things and wish that the good old days could return, or feel unhappy that they can not. They may find it very hard to get over the loss of a loved one, particularly if they are elderly, closing themselves to the possibility of new relationships; they may yearn for their old home after a move, or for younger days when they were happy and successful; honeysuckle children may suffer from homesickness. Honeysuckle people may also get stuck in regretful feelings about the past, about missed opportunities or unhappy occurrences or about growing old. Honeysuckle helps to bring such people into the present and help them to let go of the past, or bring it into perspective so that they can benefit from lessons learned from experience.

147

Tiger lily

The flower of resurrection

I like not lady's slippers
nor yet the sweet pea blossoms,
Nor yet the flaky roses,
Red or white as snow;
I like the chaliced lilies,
The heavy Eastern lilies
The gorgeous Tiger lilies,
That in our garden grow
  THOMAS BAILEY ALDRICH (1836–1907)

The lily is one of the oldest and most beautiful flowers in the world and has been the inspiration of poets and artists alike for thousands of years. Lilies have been found painted on the walls of Ancient Greek palaces where the white lily was the personal flower of Hera or Artemis, the moon goddess. According to Greek legends, two drops of milk fell from the lips of Hercules when he was feeding at the breast of Juno, his mother. One drop spread across the sky and became the milky way, and the other fell to the earth where it bloomed as the white madonna lily. To the ancients lilies were a symbol of fertility and also of purity and innocence. Their perfect form was a manifestation of the spirit of creation and satisfied our ancestors' innate longing for symmetry and harmony. Homer when describing the skin of Ajax said it was as delicate as the lily and in his hymn to Demeter he said the lily was 'a wonder to behold'.

With the coming of Christianity, the lily was used by artists as an emblem to depict the marvels of paradise. The white lily became known as the madonna lily because in Renaissance art the Archangel Gabriel holds a spray of lilies at the Annunciation to Mary, telling her she is to be the mother of Christ. It was dedicated to the Virgin Mary in honour of her purity. Lily was also a sign of the resurrection and so used in Church decorations at Easter. It was said that after Mary died, three days later her tomb was visited and found empty apart from lilies and roses.

In contrast to the pure white madonna lily are many brightly coloured varieties including the tiger lily, introduced by William Kerr, a plant collector, to Europe from Japan via China in 1804. It is native to China, Japan and Iran. Like other lilies its exotic flower releases a powerful and haunting scent, but its form is quite different. It was said in folklore that if you plant lilies in your garden, it will keep your house free of ghosts and other unwanted intruders. Also that if you accidentally tread on a lily your lover is being unfaithful. In the language of flowers, the tiger lily says, for once may pride befriend me.

Herbal remedy

Tiger lily bulb was once a popular remedy for problems affecting the female reproductive system, relating to its old associations with purity, virginity and fertility. It was recommended for nausea and vomiting of pregnancy and was used for pain and congestion in the pelvic organs, painful and heavy periods and uterine prolapse. It was also used for heart symptoms, including a rapid and irregular pulse, angina and palpitations, and for arthritis. The little bulbs that grow in the axils of the leaves were prescribed for intestinal problems such as wind and colic.

Homeopathic remedy: L. TIGRINUM

Lilium tigrinum has an affinity, like the herb, for the female reproductive system and the heart. It is prescribed for sharp pain in the ovaries, a bearing down sensation in the uterus, and burning pain in the abdomen. A Lilium woman may suffer from painful or absent periods, prolapse, vaginal discharge and experience increased sexual desire. There may be dull pain in the heart area, fluttering, a feeling as if the heart is squeezed in a vice, or violently throbbing. She may feel depressed, weepy, apprehensive, constantly in a hurry, inclined to swear, envious of others and unable to be alone. She may feel despairing or tormented about her salvation and while the emotional symptoms predominate the uterine symptoms are relieved.

The flower essence

Tiger lily is a feminine remedy, good for over-aggressive, rather tense women, who easily feel threatened by others or in competition with them. It helps to engender a sense of inner calm and security and to ease relationships with others, establishing harmony and co-operation, and an ability to work together for the common good.

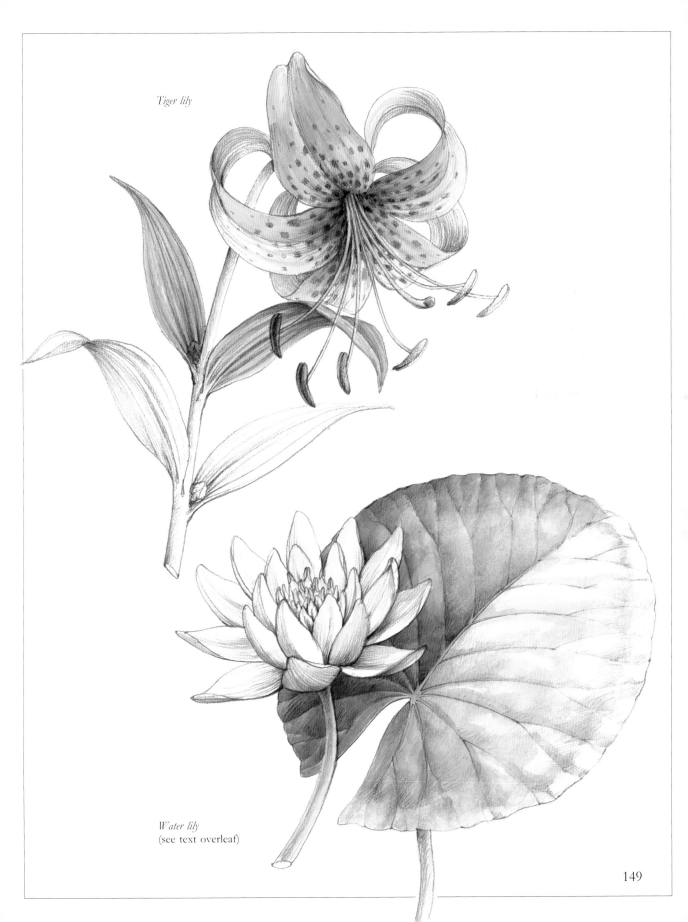

Tiger lily

Water lily
(see text overleaf)

149

Water lily

The flower of secrecy

Now folds the lily all her sweetness up
and slips into the bosom of the lake;
so fold thyself, my dearest, thou and slip
into my bosom, and be lost in me.
ALFRED, LORD TENNYSON (1809–92)

The Lady of the Lake is not in fact a lily, but is just
as exotic-looking as the most beautiful of lilies, with
its large flower like a crown on green leafy thrones
like velvet. It flourishes in slow rivers, ponds and
lakes and is native to America and England. Like the
lily, the water lily has inspired many an artist and
writer to capture its elegance and sense of quiet tran-
quility in paintings. The tales of Beatrix Potter would
be all the poorer without the lily pads to act as fish-
ing rafts for Jeremy Fisher the frog.

The water lily derives its botanical name
Nymphaea from Nymphe, the Greek water nymph
and goddess of springs, as water lilies were found
growing where the nymphs were said to play. Like
the white lotus flower, the water lily was held sacred
by the Ancient Egyptians as a symbol of purity. In
medieval Germany, where the water lily was a symbol
of female purity, country people believed that water
lilies were nymphs disguised as flowers to escape the
attention of over-amorous men. Apparently ladies
used to carry a water lily in their hands as an
antidote to the effect of love potions designed to
threaten their purity. It was called by some 'the one
sinless flower'. The flowers open as the sun rises and
gradually close after a few hours, being tightly closed
at midday and at night. This pattern was interpreted
as the flower's ability to keep hidden and intact her
innermost secrets, invulnerable to hopeful invaders.
In the language of flowers, the water lily means
purity of heart.

Herbal remedy

Culpeper said that the water lily was 'under the
dominion of the moon and therefore cools and
moistens like the former ... the leaves both inward
and outward are good for agues, the syrup of flowers

procures rest and settles the brain of frantic persons'.
The long association between water lilies, female
purity and the reproductive tract is illustrated by the
plant's use for a variety of gynaecological problems.
The native Americans used it for vaginal discharge,
uterine inflammation, and vaginal problems both
internally and locally. In Europe it was used for calming excessive sexual desire, and for relieving period
pain and heavy periods. It was a good remedy for
vaginal infections such as thrush and was used to
treat venereal infections such as gonorrhoea.

Water lily was popular in beauty preparations. The
fresh juice of the root was mixed with lemon juice
and dabbed on the skin to remove freckles and
blotches from the skin, and to soothe skin irritations
and sunburn and clear pimples and boils. It was only
used on unbroken skin. The juice was also rubbed
into the scalp in the hope of stimulating the skin and
circulation to it, to prevent falling of hair.

Homeopathic remedy: N. ODORATA

Nymphaea odorata is prepared from a tincture of the
root of the water lily. It is a lesser known remedy
used for back pain, weakness in the lumbar region,
urinary incontinence, or a feeling that urine was not
all passed. It is indicated by excessive sexual desire,
weak and aching lower limbs, erotic dreams, heavy-
headedness and a sore throat with a runny nose.

The flower essence

The water lily, with its shy and secretive nature, is a
remedy for people who are so intensely shy that
social interaction is almost painful. It is particularly
recommended for those who are shy about their bodies and their sexuality, and have psychological inhibitions preventing them from enjoying intimacy and
sex. Water lily is called the Kama Sutra among flower
essences. It not only helps one to feel more
confident with others, and to be more outgoing, but
it also helps to release fear around sexuality and
allows heightened sensuality making for greater enjoyment of intimacy and sex.

see drawing on previous page

Mahonia aquifolia

Oregon grape
The flower of acceptance

Oregon grape is an attractive ever-green shrub with fragrant flowers. The stoneless berries used to be made into jams, and were valued as a remedy for malaria and intermittent fevers. The plant was imported into England in 1823 for its ornamental value in winter gardens.

Oregon grape was used by indigenous mountain people of California as a treatment for chronic degenerative diseases, particularly cancer and arthritis. In the Spanish-American tradition it was known as *yerbe de la sangre*, herb of the blood, as it was a blood purifier, used as a diuretic and laxative, and for anaemia as it releases stored iron from the liver. It has been used as a cleansing remedy for many centuries; the Egyptians used the berries for pestilential fevers.

Herbal remedy Oregon grape root is an excellent remedy for the liver and gall-bladder. The bitters stimulate the flow of saliva and digestive enzymes, awakening the appetite, improving digestion and absorption, and activating a sluggish liver and gall-bladder. It remedies slow, painful digestion and constipation, removing stagnant food from the system and thus acting to detoxify the body. It thereby improves general health, increases strength and stamina and helps relieve fatigue and lethargy, particularly that associated with anaemia, poor absorption and during convalescence. Oregon grape treats conditions associated with a toxic system and sluggish liver function, including skin conditions, particularly dry scaly problems, gout and headaches, rheumatism and arthritis. Its diuretic properties aid cleansing by enhancing the elimination of toxins via the kidneys.

Oregon grape has a cooling and drying effect in the body, clearing

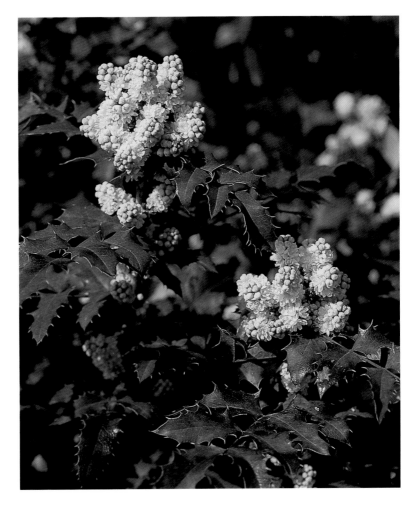

heat involved in inflammatory problems, and phlegm. Berberine in oregan grape is an immune enhancer, active against a wide range of microbes, and inhibiting tumour development. It is a helpful remedy when treating hepatitis and gall-stones. Oregon grape also acts to reduce congestion in the venous system and improves varicose veins and haemorrhoids, and heavy periods and period pain caused by uterine blood congestion.

Homeopathic remedy Berberis aquifolium is used to treat a range of symptoms associated with poor liver function, such as nausea, bilious headaches, lethargy, skin conditions, heat in the face, bitter taste in the mouth, ravenous hunger

even after eating, burning in the stomach and constipation. It will also help to relieve intermittent fevers and catarrhal conditions with greenish-yellow phlegm.

The flower essence Oregon grape is a cooling remedy for fiery people who are perfectionistic, critical, self-critical, dissatisfied and bitter. They feel their imperfections too strongly and fear being unloveable and unloved. They tend to see the world around them as hostile and may suffer from paranoia. Oregon grape helps to transform self-criticism into self-love and acceptance of who one really is. It reduces the tendency to be judgemental of oneself and others and helps to engender a feeling of trust and goodwill.

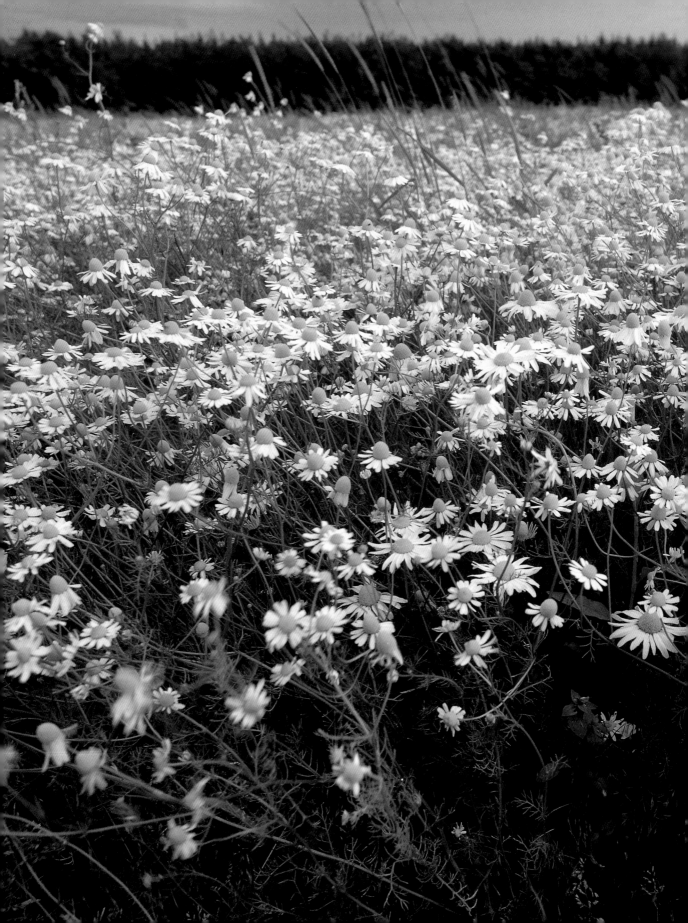

Chamomile

The flower of equilibrium

Whilst some still busied are in decking of the
bride, some others were again as seriously
employed
In strewing of those herbs at bridals used that
be, which everywhere they throw, with
bounteous hands and
The healthful balm and mint from their full laps
do fly free
The scentful chamomile, the verdrous costmary.
MICHAEL DRAYTON (1563–1631)

Chamomile is a favourite among garden herbs and
has been for over 2000 years. It was well known to
the Greeks who thought its scent resembled that of
fallen apples and so called it *khamaimelon* meaning
earth apple (from *kamas*: on the ground, and *melon*:
an apple). The famous physician Dioscorides recommended it as a medicine for fevers in 900BC. The
Spaniards must also have likened it to an apple for
they called it *manzanilla*, meaning little apple. The
Egyptians revered chamomile for its medicinal
virtues, particularly its power to cure 'ague' and dedicated it to the sun god Ra as it was considered an
effective remedy for fevers. It was one of the nine
sacred herbs of the Saxons who used it widely as a
sedative and calming medicine for the stomach. It
was highly valued as a remedy for hysteria, insomnia,
nightmares, convulsions, delirium, tremors of
alcoholics, melancholy and a whole range of other
nervous afflictions, especially of women.

In the language of flowers, chamomile is a symbol
of energy and patience in adversity, because of its
great ability to restore equilibrium and support the
nervous system. Not only does chamomile benefit
ailing people but it has also been used traditionally to
cure sick plants and was known as the plants' physician. Chamomile tea can be added to a vase of
drooping flowers to revive them and chamomile can
be planted in the garden to remedy ailing plants or
to prevent disease.

In the Middle Ages chamomile was highly valued
as a strewing herb and was also burned as incense to
keep foul smells and infection at bay. It was hung in
bunches over babies' cots to protect them and keep
them healthy. Chamomile was traditionally used in
love potions and at weddings, and to wash the face

and hair to attract the beloved. It was also respected
by our ancestors as a grave plant, to ease the passage
of the dead into the world to come.

Two kinds of chamomile are used medicinally:
German chamomile (*Matricaria chamomilla* or
Chamomilia recutita) and Roman chamomile (*Anthemis*
or *Chamaemelum nobilis*). Their properties are fairly
identical but German chamomile may be preferable
as it is less bitter. Roman chamomile was well known
for planting lawns, paths and arbours where it releases its pleasing fragrance when trodden on.
Shakespeare apparently grew it in his garden and Sir
Francis Drake is said to have played his famous
game of bowls on a chamomile lawn. There is a saying, 'like a chamomile lawn, the more it is trodden,
the more it will spread'. It has been called the herb
of humility because it grows best when walked on.

Chamomile prefers well-drained, either slightly
acid or alkaline soil, in a sunny position. Perennial
chamomile can be propagated from rooted offsets as
it has a creeping habit, while the annual German
chamomile is easily grown from seed in the spring.

Herbal remedy and Aromatherapy oil

The main constituent of chamomile is a beautiful
blue volatile oil containing azulenes which gives it
such a distinctive fragrance. It is a wonderful relaxant, particularly to the nervous system and the digestion and is a perfect remedy for babies and children.
It calms anxiety and nervousness and is excellent for
tense, stressed people who tend to be hyperactive
and highly sensitive, prone to digestive problems and
allergies. The tea makes an excellent addition to
baths for tired, fractious children, soothing irritability
or over-excitement and ensuring a restful sleep. It is
recommended for restless or hyperactive children and
can be given in a bottle or on a teaspoon to small
babies for teething, as it helps relieve pain.

Chamomile has the marvellous ability to relax
smooth muscle throughout the body. In the digestive
tract it relieves tension and spasm and is
recommended for colic (particularly in babies),
abdominal pain, wind and distension. By regulating
peristalsis it can treat both diarrhoea and constipation. Chamomile is a famous remedy for soothing
all kinds of digestive upsets, especially those related

to stress and tension such as nervous indigestion, heartburn and acidity. Chamazulene in the volatile oil is anti-inflammatory, helping to relieve gastritis and peptic ulcers, colitis and irritable bowel syndrome. The bitters in chamomile stimulate the flow of bile and the secretion of digestive juices, enhancing the appetite and improving a sluggish digestion. Bisabolol in the volatile oil has been shown to prevent and to speed up the healing of ulcers both internally and externally, making chamomile an excellent remedy for gastritis, peptic ulcers and varicose ulcers on the legs.

Chamomile is very useful in all fevers and infections. By inducing a restful sleep it encourages natural recovery, particularly in children for whom rest is probably the best medicine. Its volatile oil is a powerful antiseptic, active against bacteria, including staphylococcus aureus, and fungal infections, including thrush (*Candida albicans*). Hot chamomile tea will help bring down a fever and can be given for colds, flu, sore throats, coughs and digestive infections such as gastro-enteritis. Its antiseptic oils are excreted via the urinary system where it will soothe an inflamed bladder and relieve cystitis.

The Greeks and Romans considered chamomile one of the best remedies for menstrual disorders. The name matricaria comes from *matrix* meaning mother or womb, indicating its value as a remedy for women's ailments. It has been used for hundreds of years as a digestive remedy for nausea and sickness in pregnancy, to relax spasm and relieve painful periods, to reduce menopausal symptoms, relieve mastitis, premenstrual headaches and migraines, and absence of periods due to stress or psychological problems such as anorexia nervosa. Chamomile tea has been drunk throughout childbirth to relax tension and lessen the pain of contractions. Dilute chamomile oil can be used for massage and for inhalation and can be wonderfully effective when pain seems intolerable during childbirth.

As a general pain reliever, chamomile can be taken for headaches and migraine, neuralgia, toothache, earache, aches and pains during flu, cramps, rheumatic and gout pains. Its anti-inflammatory properties also help resolve inflammatory conditions such as gout and arthritis. Chamomile has long been used as a remedy for asthma and hay fever. Recent research suggests that chamomile is a natural antihistamine. It has an anti-allergic effect by reducing the body's response to allergens such as pollen and house dust in those who are sensitive to them, and by reducing the severe allergic reaction, anaphylactic shock. Its relaxant effect on the bronchial tubes helps to reduce broncho-constriction in asthma. Its profoundly relaxing and balancing effect helps to deal with emotional problems underlying such allergies.

Externally, chamomile is an excellent healer. The oils exert a soothing and anti-inflammatory effect on the skin, and stimulate tissue repair. These benefits in conjunction with its antiseptic properties explain its long tradition of use as a wound healer. Dilute oils, or compresses of chamomile tea, can be applied to ulcers, sores, burns and scalds.

Steam inhalations will help relieve asthma, hay fever, catarrh and sinusitis. Chamomile tea makes a good mouthwash for mouth ulcers and inflamed gums, and a gargle for sore throats. It can also be used for sore nipples and as a douche for vaginal infections including thrush. Sitting in a bowl of chamomile tea is wonderfully soothing for cystitis and haemorrhoids. It makes a good antiseptic eyebath for sore inflamed eyes as in conjuctivitis, and a lotion for inflammatory skin conditions.

Dilute oil of chamomile when massaged into painful, inflamed joints will bring relief as it will help to relieve pain such as trigeminal neuralgia or sciatica. It will also help repel and soothe the pain of bites and stings. A wash of chamomile tea used as a hair rinse after shampooing imparts golden highlights.

Homeopathic remedy: CHAMOMILLA

Chamomilla is particularly suitable to people with great sensitivity to pain, which is often bought on or aggravated by emotions such as anger and irritability, as well as by teething in babies and toddlers, and too much tea or coffee. Chamomilla is particularly recommended for a woman in labour when the pain feels unbearable.

The flower essence

As a remedy of the sun, chamomile helps to ease emotional problems and soothe anger and conflict to bring out a sunny disposition. It is best for those who are moody, changeable, easily upset, irritable, impatient and angry. It will soothe tension and anxiety, and stop it from accumulating through the day to cause restlessness, insomnia or nightmares. Inner tension and disharmony may also cause stomach problems in both children and adults, as well as depression, hyperactivity, poor concentration and learning problems. Chamomile will help one to stand back from the day-to-day things that irritate and annoy, and upset one's superficial equilibrium, and to find a place of calm and serenity where light, like the sun behind the clouds, is always shining.

Olive

The flower of peace

The olive is one of the oldest cultivated plants of the Mediterranean and is thought to have been grown at least 5000 years ago in Egypt and on Crete for its highly valuable oil. According to archeological finds, the olive played an important part in the culture of these early civilizations. In the Palace at Knossos in Crete the olive press room and the enormous oil jars dating from Minoan times can still be seen. The first pressing was used for eating, the second for making ointments and liniments and the third made a good oil for lamplighting.

The olive was mentioned frequently in Christian literature. 'And thou shalt command the children of Israel, that they bring thee pure oil olive beaten for the light, to cause the lamp to burn always' (Exodus 27: 20). Jesus spent his night in the Garden of Gethsemane, whose name means 'the garden with the olive press', in the vicinity of an olive tree.

Olive oil was considered in early times the purest of all vegetable oils and became a symbol of purity. The olive tree also represented peace and goodwill as well as life and hope. When the dove returned to Noah's Ark for the second time, it carried in its beak a fresh branch of olive so that Noah knew the flood waters had abated, and peace and quiet had returned to the earth.

As a symbol of peace an olive branch would be carried by those asking for a cessation of hostilities and it is still used for such purposes today: the olive branch features on the United Nations flag. Perhaps the reason why the olive is a worldwide symbol of peace is that in cultivation, decades passed between planting the seed and harvesting the fruit, so that unless a man was desirous of a long and peaceful life he would not plant an olive grove.

To the Greeks the olive is a symbol of wisdom. It is said that olives are the goddess Athena's gift to humankind. She won an island from Poseidon, the sea god, by presenting the inhabitants with the gift that would be of the greatest benefit to them – the olive tree. The olive is also an emblem of victory; an olive branch was used to crown winners of the Olympic Games. Athletes would rub olive oil into their skin from head to foot before a race or contest to keep their muscles and joints supple.

Herbal remedy

Olive oil has been used historically as folk remedy and employed extensively in pharmacy and in the preparation of liniments, ointments and plasters until the present day. The pale greenish-yellow oil is highly nutritious and was used to provide extra nourishment for babies by rubbing it into the skin. It also kept the skin smooth and free from irritation.

The sweet fruity-tasting oil is highly mucilaginous. Its demulcent (soothing) properties have been employed for treating a variety of digestive problems including wind, indigestion, heartburn, gastritis and peptic ulcers. It soothes irritated and inflamed conditions of the lining of the digestive tract such as colitis and has a slightly laxative effect. If poisoning by alkalis or corrosive substances occurred olive oil was given freely as gastric lavage to soothe the irritated mucous membranes and hasten the elimination of poison from the body. An enema of warm olive oil was a common remedy to relieve severe constipation, as it helps break up the faeces.

Olive oil has also been used to soothe irritated conditions of the respiratory system: harsh dry coughs, laryngitis and croup. It was also given to reduce catarrh. When rubbed over the whole body it is well known as a remedy for febrile eruptive diseases including scarlet fever and even the plague.

Traditionally olive oil has been taken internally as a remedy for the liver and gall-bladder for it stimulates the flow of bile into the intestines, and still today makes an excellent remedy when alternated with lemon juice to dissolve and encourage passing of gallstones. For a sluggish liver, gallstones and gall-bladder colic as well as bowel problems, 1 tablespoonful of cold-pressed olive oil can be taken first thing in the morning before eating. During attacks of either renal or gall-bladder colic, olive oil was once given a wineglass at a time, sipped slowly until the pains were gone.

Recent research into olives and olive leaves has suggested that those who consume most olive oil have a longer life expectancy. The leaves act as a vasodilator, relaxing blood vessels and lowering blood pressure. They have been recommended for high blood pressure, angina pectoris and a wide variety of circulatory problems. The leaves have also been shown to lower blood sugar levels and are helpful in management of diabetes. They can be taken as a tea, prepared by soaking 1 oz (25 g) of leaves in 1 pint (600ml) of cold water for 6–8 hours. Bring to the boil and then leave to infuse for half an hour. This should be drunk freely through the day. Taken hot this increases sweating and reduces fevers.

The cold pressed oil, high in oleic acid, also benefits the heart and circulation. Taken regularly it has been shown to reduce the harmful low density lipoprotein cholesterol and reduce the tendency to atherosclerosis, heart attacks and strokes. Olive oil also helps to reduce blood pressure and reduces the tendency for the blood to clot. Research suggests that olive oil may also reduce the development of cancer and retard the ageing process. The anti-oxidants it contains make cell walls more stable and less susceptible to destruction by free radicals.

Externally, the soothing effect of olive oil on the skin helps to protect it from irritation, to soothe sore and inflamed areas, and to make the skin more supple and flexible. It also has astringent properties and has often been used to treat minor cuts and abrasions, and as a wash to protect the skin from corrosives. It can be applied to boils and abscesses, eczema, cold sores, chapped skin, and is included in many beauty preparations for the skin. It will relieve the pain of burns and speed healing, particularly if mixed with an egg, and relieve insect bites and stings. The oil mixed with alcohol is a valuable hair tonic when massaged into the scalp; the oil is good for cradle cap on babies to soften the crusts. It can also be rubbed into the nails to make them less brittle.

Warm olive oil dropped into the ear will help soften an accumulation of wax and can be used as a vehicle for essential oils such as lavender to drop into the ear to relieve earache. It will also help retrieve an object accidentally inserted into the ear: fill the ear with oil and it should float out.

An infusion of the leaves can be used for cleansing cuts and wounds, as well as sores and ulcers, and promote healing. It is also used as a mouthwash for bleeding and infected gums.

Olive oil can also be used to soothe irritated conditions of the mouth and throat. It can be mixed with equal parts of myrrh tincture and used as a gargle for sore throats, a mouthwash for ulcers and inflamed gums. Mixed with grated garlic, olive oil makes an excellent liniment for joint pains, gout, neuralgia and sprains.

The flower essence

The symbol of peace and harmony, olive the Bach Flower Remedy has the power to restore peace to a distressed and tired mind, and give strength to an exhausted body. It is especially beneficial for people who have suffered from stress, trauma or illness for long periods of time; such people have often become very depleted and drained of the strength they need to carry on.

Equally well, olive can be used by those who have very full and busy lives and set aside little time for rest and relaxation. Gradually their energy goes, they begin to tire easily, and no longer enjoy their work and activities and lose interest in their lives where formerly they were happy and stimulated. The smallest job such as washing-up can seem an insurmountable obstacle to an olive person who has reached the end of their resources.

Olive helps to bring 'peace after the storm' and enables people to assess the cause of their utter exhaustion, often a case of using vital energies incorrectly. People may deplete themselves at the personality level where one's energy is limited, rather than drawing strength from higher sources. People in a positive olive state are able to rely on inner strength and guidance and cope with extreme demands with seemingly inexhaustible energy and joy.

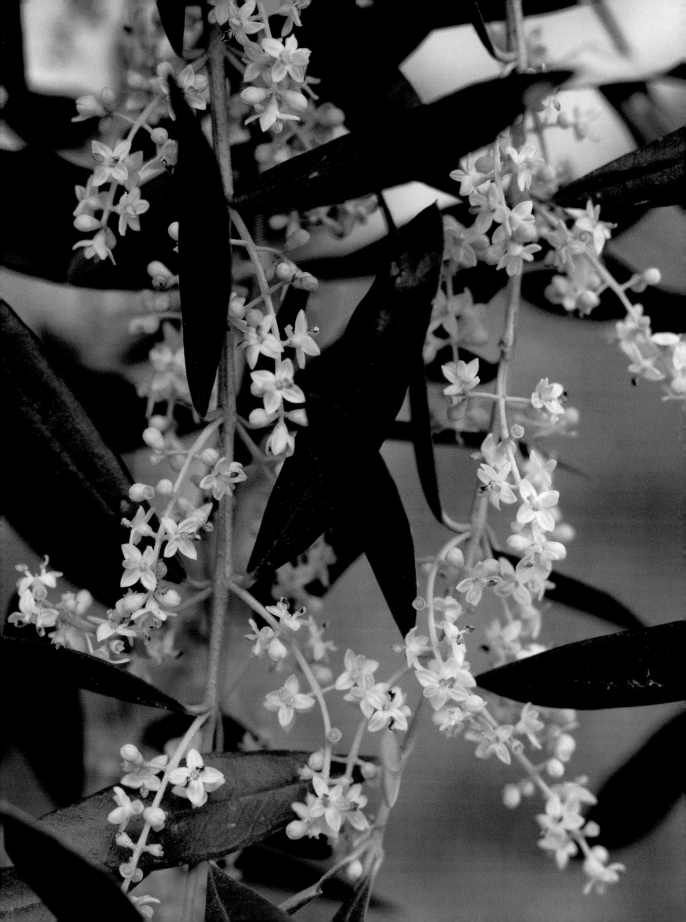

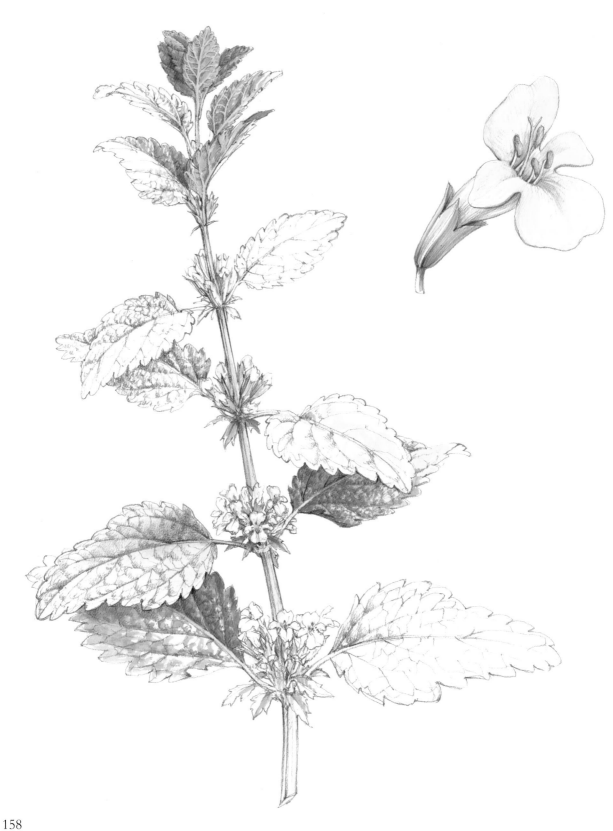

Lemon balm

The flower of bees

This delightful lemon-scented plant is a relative of mint and sage and a favourite in cottage gardens. Native to the eastern Mediterranean, the Arabs were among the first to extol its virtues. It featured in Middle Eastern remedies for epilepsy and mental illness, apoplexy, lethargy and melancholia. Paracelsus said that 'essence of balm given in Canary wine every morning will renew youth, strengthen the brain, relieve languishing nature and prevent baldness' while John Evelyn said, 'Balm is sovereign for the brain, strengthening memory and powerfully chasing away melancholy'. Lemon balm is an excellent plant for attracting bees into the garden. It was called Melissa by the Greeks, as the word means honey bee. Bee keepers still rub their hives with balm to attract bees.

Herbal remedy

Lemon balm influences the limbic system in the brain which is concerned with mood and temperament. While being sedative, enhancing relaxation and inducing natural sleep, calming tension and anxiety, and even mania and hysteria, lemon balm is also restoring. It lifts the spirits, improves memory and helps tired brains to concentrate. It can be taken as tea frequently through the day and also at night for insomnia. The dried leaves are a frequent component in sleep pillows. A strong infusion in a warm bath at night will help calm excitable children.

Lemon balm has particular affinity with the digestive system, calming and soothing stress-related problems. The bitters provide tonic support and gently stimulate the liver and gall-bladder. A mild infusion is excellent for children's nervous tummy upsets.

Lemon balm also influences the heart. Carmelite water, made from lemon balm with lemon peel, nutmeg and angelica root makes a useful remedy when nervousness, agitation or depression cause heart pains, palpitations or an irregular heartbeat.

In the reproductive system, lemon balm relaxes spasm causing menstrual pain and relieves irritability associated with premenstrual tension. It also helps to regulate periods. During the weeks prior to delivery it helps prepare for the birth, to ease and speed the process and reduce pain. Lemon balm can help relieve menopausal depression. It relaxes spasm in the kidneys and urinary system, and relieves headaches, migraine, vertigo and buzzing in the ears.

Lemon balm has a cooling and cleansing effect. In hot infusion it causes sweating, reducing fevers and making a good remedy for childhood infections, colds and flu, coughs and catarrh. Its relaxant and mucous-reducing properties are helpful during acute and chronic bronchitis, as well as harsh irritating coughs and asthma. Its antiviral action is effective against herpes simplex, mumps and other viruses. The oil is antibacterial and antihistamine, helpful for treating hay fever and allergic rhinitis. Its ability to destroy bacteria makes it useful for surgical dressings.

Aromatherapy oil

Melissa oil calms and slows the heart, relieving palpitations and reducing high blood pressure. While it has relaxant properties it also acts as a tonic and rejuvenator. It can be used to calm nervousness and anxiety, release tension and tension headaches, and relieve insomnia. It makes a good digestive particularly in stress-related problems such as colic and indigestion. Its antihistamine action is helpful for allergy sufferers and it can be used in creams for allergic skin conditions. As an antiviral remedy the dilute oil can be massaged into the skin in mumps and cold sores, and relieves wasp and bee stings. It is cooling for fevers and makes an antimicrobial inhalant for colds, catarrh, coughs and chest infections. Its antispasmodic action relieves harsh irritating coughs and asthma. Massaged into the lower abdomen it relieves period pains, and generally relaxes muscles and eases tension pain. It will help joint pain and neuralgia. The oil can be used in eardrops for infections and in mouthwashes for gum infections and toothache.

The flower essence

Just as Paracelsus recommended lemon balm to renew youth, strengthen the brain and relieve a languishing nature, so too the flower essence can help to renew health and vigour, lift the spirits and balance the emotions. It is excellent for those whose health and strength have been depleted by stress or overconcern for other people, restricting their lives and inhibiting their spiritual growth. Restoring and relaxing, it gives support during emotional difficulties and increases inner strength and courage.

Peppermint

The flower of refreshment

Then went I forthe on my right honde
Down by a little path I fonde
Of mintes full and fennel green.
GEOFFREY CHAUCER (1340–1400)

There is probably no other herb that can rival the popularity of mint. The Ancient Egyptians grew it for cooking, medicines and perfumes, and the Ancient Chinese and Japanese were equally fond of it. Mint was an essential ingredient in refreshing perfumes made in Ancient Greece, where athletes would massage the oil into their muscles before competitions. The Greeks and Romans scented their bathwater and their bodies with mint and used it as a restorative. They also wound it into crowns used in religious ceremonies, rather like the Jews who used it to strew the floors of synagogues. Garlands of mint were thought by the Romans and Greeks to stimulate clear thoughts, concentration and inspiration. The name mint comes from the Latin *mente*, meaning thought, in reference to the Romans' respect for mint as a brain tonic. In the language of flowers, mint represents eternal refreshment. Pliny said, 'the very smell of mint restores and revives the spirit just as its taste excites the appetite'. The Arabs have for centuries drunk mint tea to stimulate their virility and to them it was a symbol of friendship and love.

Spearmint, horsemint, garden mint and pennyroyal all have similar virtues but are milder than peppermint in taste, smell and medicinal action.

Herbal remedy and Aromatherapy oil
Peppermint is both cooling and warming, depending on how and where it is used. Internally it induces heat and improves the circulation. As a heart tonic it relieves palpitation, stimulating the action of the heart, and dispersing blood to the surface of the body, causing sweating. Hot peppermint tea makes an excellent warming remedy to ward off and relieve winter ailments, and it checks mucus production. Peppermint oil is a good inhalant for colds, catarrh and sinusitis. Its stimulant action makes a good general tonic to recharge vital energy and dispel lethargy, useful during chronic illness and convalescence.

The refreshing taste of mint is followed by a cooling and numbing effect in the respiratory tract and can be felt on the skin. Peppermint oil added to massage oils cools hot, aching muscles, and swollen feet. It is a powerful analgesic, and when the fresh bruised leaf is applied or the oil added to lotions it relieves general aches and pains. When taken internally peppermint has a relaxing effect, calming anxiety and tension, relieving pain including menstrual pain and spasm as in the bronchial tubes in asthma, and helping insomnia. In the digestive tract mint relaxes smooth muscle and relieves conditions associated with pain and spasm: stomach aches, colic, flatulence, heartburn and indigestion, hiccoughs, nausea, vomiting and travel sickness. The tannins help protect the gut lining from irritation and infection, and relieve griping during diarrhoea, spastic constipation, Crohn's disease and ulcerative colitis. The bitters account for its use in liver cleansing and gallstones.

The volatile oils are antiseptic, antiviral, and antifungal, can neutralize the TB bacillus, treat herpes simplex, and ringworm. It makes a useful gargle for sore throats and a mouthwash for gum troubles and mouth ulcers. It relieves toothache and earache, and is used extensively as an antiseptic and flavouring in toothpastes, cough and cold preparations, chewing gum, throat lozenges and indigestion remedies.

Homeopathic remedy: M. PIPERITA
Mentha piperita like the herbal remedy and aromatherapy oil is refreshing and revitalizing, good for mental dullness in the morning. It has an affinity for the respiratory tract, relieving dry, painful coughs aggravated by cold and smoke, flu, dry and painful throats and earache. It also helps digestive problems, notably colic and wind. It relieves pain in the neck, in shingles, toothache, earache and headache.

The flower essence
Peppermint helps those who feel sluggish, lethargic and mentally cloudy or apathetic, often with digestive or metabolic imbalances. Such people may crave food which then makes them feel sluggish or sleepy. Peppermint improves digestion and absorption and frees energy, helping to keep the mind alert and clear for higher purposes. It helps to dispel mental laziness and poor concentration, and awakens the mind. It is an excellent remedy for students.

NB Peppermint oil should always be used diluted and should be avoided in pregnancy. Do not use on babies or small children

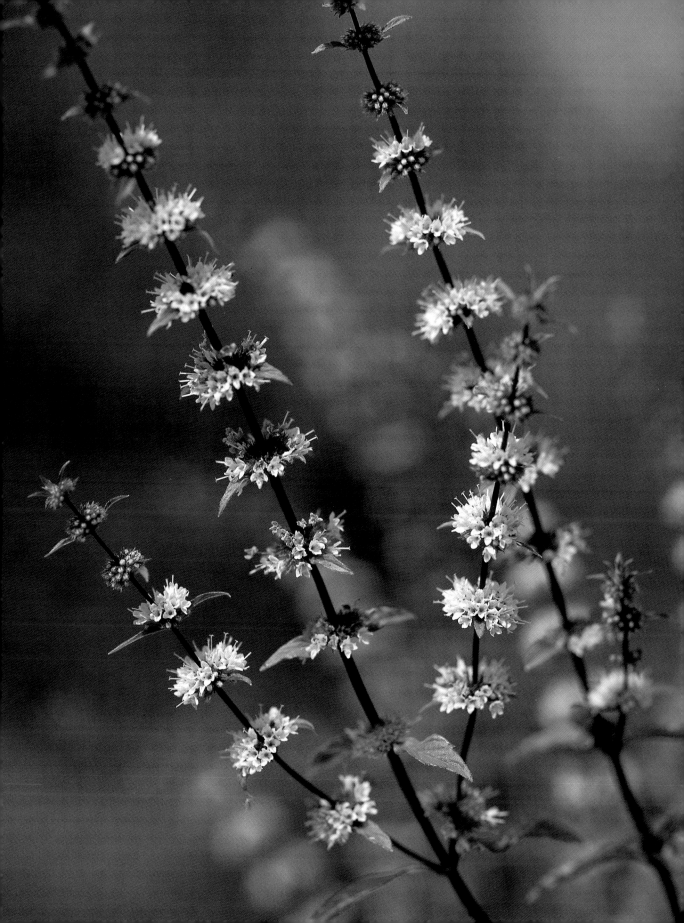

Catnip, Catmint
The flower of cats

Catnip or catmint derives its name from the well-known fact that cats love its scent. They rub themselves on the plant and eat it, reputedly in recognition of its medicinal virtues. It is hard to grow in a garden where cats roam as it will be eaten to the ground unless well protected, but apparently only if it is transplanted into the garden as a plant. If grown from seed cats are said to leave it alone.

The cultivated variety of this attractive Labiatae, which is cousin to mint and pennyroyal, is familiar to all gardeners, as a lovely herbaceous edging plant which blooms in early summer. The wildflower is found in fields and hedgerows, particularly on chalk or gravel soil in Europe, North Africa, North America and temperate Asia. It can be grown from seed very easily in most soils, or propagated by root division in the spring.

Catnip tea has a refreshing taste and was enjoyed by country people long before China and Indian tea were imported. In France it has been grown among kitchen herbs for seasoning. It was also planted around houses to keep out rats, for they hate it.

There is an old belief that if the root is chewed, it will turn the mildest nature fierce and quarrelsome; perhaps this refers to the stimulating and tonic properties of the plant. Culpeper said that catnip was a herb ruled by Venus, perhaps because in healing catnip has an affinity for women.

'Tis hot and dry. 'Tis chiefly used for obstruction of the Womb, for Barrenness, and to hasten Delivery and to help Expectoration', said John Pechy in *The Compleat Herbal* of 1694. 'Nep is much used of women, either in baths or drinkes to procure their feminine courses', according to John Parkinson's 1629 *Paradisus*. Parkinson also said that it was used 'to help those that are bruised by some fall or other accident', while Pliny said, 'Nep also is powerful against Serpents, for the smoke and the perfume of this herb they cannot abide, but will flie from it: which is the cause that such as bee afraid of Serpents strew Nep under them in the place where they mean to repose and sleepe'.

Herbal remedy

Catnip is an invaluable remedy for respiratory infections; taken as a hot tea it stimulates the circulation, increases perspiration and effectively brings down fevers. It acts as a decongestant for catarrh and should be taken frequently at the first signs of colds and flu. Catnip is also helpful in bronchitis, asthma, and eruptive infections such as chickenpox and measles. A wonderful remedy for babies and children, it is calming and relaxing and will induce healing sleep, and is used to stop their nightmares.

The relaxant effect of catnip is also felt in the digestive tract where it relieves tension and colic, wind and pain: an excellent remedy for babies who have wind or colic or trouble sleeping. A strong infusion will relax headaches related to tension, and soothe pain.

Catnip's relaxant effects are also felt in the uterus. It can be used to relieve period pains as well as tension or stress prior to a period. It can also be taken for irregular, delayed or suppressed periods.

Externally, a hot infusion makes a good antiseptic inhalant for sore throats, colds, flu and coughs, a decongestant for catarrh and sinusitis, and a relaxant for asthma and croup. The tannins speed tissue repair and staunch bleeding of abrasions and cuts, they aid healing of burns and scalds, piles and insect bites, as well as inflammatory skin problems.

Homeopathic remedy: CATARIA

Cataria is mainly used as a remedy for babies or children for colic and abdominal pain. The baby or child may be seen to draw their legs up or twist their body around in pain. It is also recommended for nervous headaches, anxiety, crying, even hysteria. It is similar in action to Chamomilla.

The flower essence

Catnip is a mint and belongs to the Labiatae family, the same family as peppermint. Its flower essence has parallel actions to peppermint and these are described on page 160.

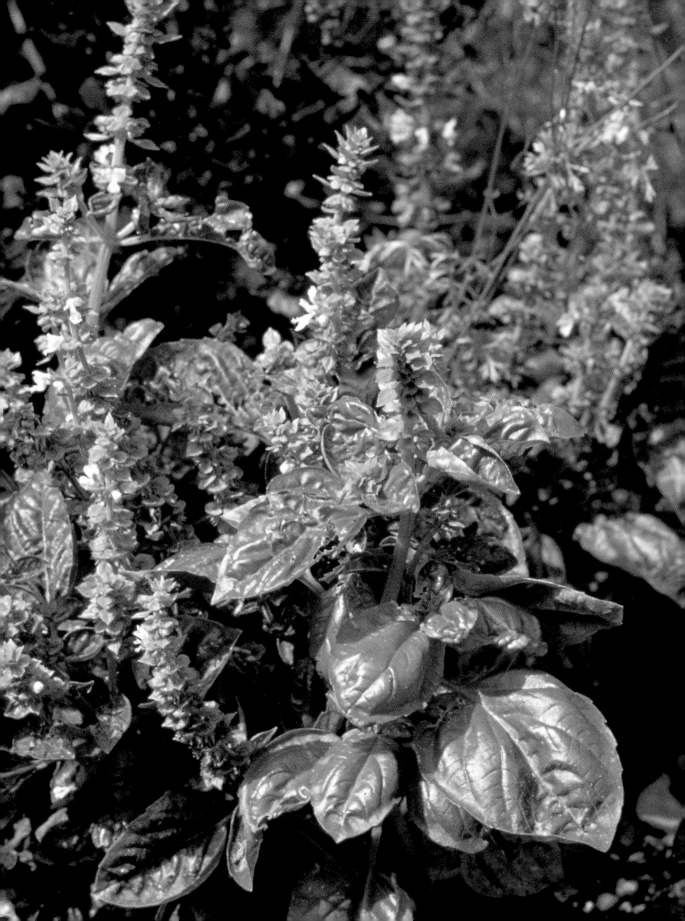

Basil

The flower of Vishnu

This beautiful plant with its wonderful sweet and pungent aroma is a native of India and has been grown throughout the Mediterranean for thousands of years. It was only introduced into western Europe in the 16th century, reaching England in 1573. The name basil, or basilicum, comes from the Latin *basilisca* or from the Greek *basilikon*, both meaning royal, either because it was considered king of herbs or because in India it was held sacred to one of the gods of the Hindu trinity, Vishnu the preserver. A leaf is traditionally laid on the chest of the dead to open the gates of heaven for them. In Egypt basil is scattered over graves and was an embalming herb for mummies. In Greece it is a symbol of mourning, and was believed to antidote the venom of the basilisk, a fabulous reptile whose breath or glance was fatal.

Basil has also been associated with the need for courage in times of great difficulty. The Greeks carry it on journeys for safety and it was thought to aid the journey of the soul after death. In Tudor England it was customary to present departing guests with a pot of miniature basil to help their journey.

Basil is revered for its ability to open the heart and the mind, to engender love and devotion, and to strengthen faith, compassion and clarity. In India basil is grown in domestic courtyards for three months and then worshipped with offerings of rice, flowers and lighted lamps. In Crete bush basil is a symbol of 'love washed with tears'. In Italy it was worn by courting peasants in remote areas as an emblem of love and fidelity. Basil is often planted on window ledges to purify the air. In India wherever it is planted is a place of peace, piety and virtue.

Herbal remedy

Basil makes a good cleansing remedy for treating infections and to clear phlegm from the nose and chest. Use it in hot infusions for colds, fevers, flu, catarrh, sinusitis and as an expectorant for coughs. The volatile oils have an antispasmodic effect, particularly in the digestive system, making it a good remedy for stomach cramps, wind, nausea, diarrhoea and vomiting and constipation related to tension. It also relieves travel sickness. It relaxes spasm in the bronchi and is used for whooping cough and asthma.

Basil has an affinity for the nervous system and helps to strengthen the nerves, release tension and lift the spirits. It imparts clarity of mind, improves concentration and sharpens the memory. It can be used to relieve headaches, neuralgia and rheumatism and for stress-related problems such as indigestion, back pain and migraine. It has been used since ancient times as a tranquilizer and aid to digestion.

Aromatherapy oil

Sweet basil's wonderfully penetrating sweet, almost pungent aroma helps to calm and strengthen the nerves, clear and stimulate the mind and lift the spirits. It is refreshing and reviving when feeling tired and yet calming when feeling tense or anxious. It is particularly helpful for those studying for exams as it relieves intellectual fatigue and exam nerves. It can be used for many stress-related problems, such as headaches, migraine, exhaustion, indigestion, nausea and muscle pain. When feeling tired, weak and vulnerable, basil is strengthening and revitalizing and when vulnerable to infection, its antiseptic properties can help protect against illness.

Basil can also be used to reduce fevers and treat infections such as colds, coughs and flu. It aids digestion and relieves indigestion, nausea, colic and flatulence. Externally the oil can be rubbed in massage oils into tired, aching muscles and painful joints and it makes a good insect repellent.

Homeopathic remedy: OCIMUM CANUM

Ocimum canum is prepared from the leaves of Indian basil and is used predominantly for urinary problems. It treats prolapse, engorged breasts, pain on breast-feeding and vulval irritation as well as for fevers and arthritis, vomiting and diarrhoea.

The flower essence

Basil helps those who cannot reconcile their physical sexuality with their ideas of spiritual purity, seeing them as opposing forces. They are fearful of their sexuality, or disgusted by it and want to hide it but are often drawn to illicit or illegal sexual activities. Basil helps to bring a greater understanding of our nature and to harmonize our emotional, sexual and spiritual lives so that we can perceive both sexuality and spirituality as part of a sacred whole.

Evening primrose
The flower of silent love

The glimmering cups of waking evening
primrose
Filled the dusk now that the scent of the rose
was done.
   JOHN SQUIRE (1884–1958)

Evening primrose is a tall elegant plant with large
fragrant cup-shaped yellow flowers that generally
open at dusk (or on very cloudy days), attracting the
night-flying moths and insects which pollinate them.
Evening primrose flourishes throughout Europe, and
both North and South America. It grows wild on
disturbed ground, and makes a colourful plant for
the back of garden border.

Evening primrose was known to the Ancient
Greeks, and Theophrastus (350BC) gave the flower
its generic name which is derived from *oinos* meaning
wine and *thera* meaning hunt, in reference to the
plant's power to stimulate a desire for wine, or its
power to dispel the effects of over-indulgence. Pliny
said, 'it is an herbe good as wine to make the heart
merrie. ... Of such virtue is this herbe that if it be
given to drink to the wildest beast that is, it will
tame the same and make it gentle.' In the language
of flowers evening primrose symbolized both inconstancy and silent love, perhaps because of the opening and closing of its flowers.

Traditionally evening primrose was valued as an
edible wild plant. The seeds were used as food by
native Americans in Utah and Nevada and the young
leaves have been enjoyed in salads. Evening primrose
is a biennial, and in the first year it grows a fleshy
root which was boiled as a nutty-tasting vegetable.

Herbal remedy
The outer flower stems and leaves are highly
mucilaginous and make a lotion to soothe skin eruptions, and internally soothe an irritated digestive tract
and treat diarrhoea. A mild sedative, it relieves nervous indigestion and colic. Its antispasmodic effects
help with asthma and whooping cough.

Until recently the leaves and outer stem were the
only parts used medicinally, apart from the root that
was eaten. Since then a vast amount of research has
been done on the medicinal effect of the oil extracted from the seeds which has made evening primrose

one of the most valuable remedies from nature. The
oil is a good source of Omega 6 fatty acids, vital for
healthy functioning of the immune, nervous and hormonal systems. It is one of the few oils that contain
gamma linoleic acid (GLA), a fatty acid that is normally produced in the body as an intermediate step
during the metabolism of linoleic acid, a fatty acid
from other sources such as sunflower seeds. A
breakdown in the production of GLA from linoleic
acid is related to problems such as eczema and PMS,
and thus evening primrose oil provides an excellent
way to remedy such metabolic errors. Evening primrose oil has been found to be extremely valuable in
the treatment of PMS, breast and menopausal problems, hyperactivity in children, eczema, acne, asthma,
migraine, metabolic disorders, arthritis and a whole
range of allergies. It counteracts the effect of
alcoholic poisoning and encourages regeneration of a
damaged liver. It can help with withdrawal from
alcohol and alcoholic depression. Further studies
indicate a role in treating multiple sclerosis, high
blood pressure and to help prevent high cholesterol,
clotting of the blood and coronary artery disease.

Homeopathic remedy: OENOTHERA BIENNIS
The fresh flowers, leaves and stems of Oenothera
biennis are used in homeopathic preparations and
treat watery diarrhoea that passes without effort and
is accompanied by exhaustion. There may be abdominal and other cramps. The symptoms also indicating
oenothera include dizziness, light-headedness, great
weakness, numbness and pricking of the skin, fluttering in the heart, and fever with rigors.

The flower essence
The flower remedy *O. hookeri* is recommended for
people who suffer from feeling rejected or unwanted,
often due to childhood problems; perhaps they
lacked proper emotional support or love or did not
bond closely with their mother during infancy.

Such people tend to avoid close emotional
contact, intimacy and committed relationships, due to
fear of rejection. Evening primrose helps to heal feelings of rejection and feeling unlovable and enables
one to be more open emotionally and to form
deeper relationships.

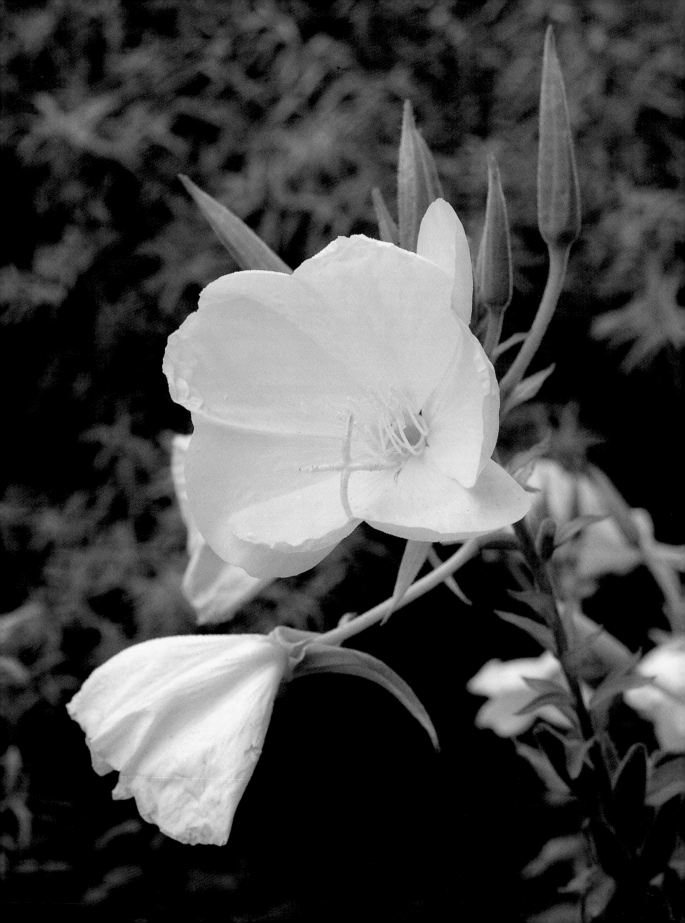

Sweet marjoram

The flower of honour

Marjoram is one of the most ancient and versatile healing flowers. The botanical name Origanum comes from the Greek words *oros* for mountain and *ganos* for joy, making 'joy of the mountain' which conjures up a lovely picture of wild marjoram carpeting a mountainside and scenting the warm air. In Greek mythology marjoram is the creation of Aphrodite while in Roman myths it was a flower of Venus, and sacred to her. A symbol of honour, love and fertility, marjoram was woven into wreaths for crowns to bestow good fortune and long life on newlyweds in both the Greek and Roman traditions. There are several different marjoram plants, all highly aromatic and a delight to cooks, particularly the Greeks and the Italians. *O. marjorana* or sweet marjoram is half-hardy, and the most sweetly scented. It will grow in most sunny places in well-drained soil. Wild marjoram (*O. vulgare*), like pot marjoram (*O. onites*), has a sharp, warm flavour. All marjorams have similar healing properties, although the more sun the plant has the greater the concentration of essential oils, and so the more aromatic and powerful it is.

For the Ancient Greeks marjoram comforted the bereaved and was planted on graves to help the dead sleep in peace. If found growing wild on a grave it augured well for the happiness of the departed in the next world. Marjoram was also associated with Thor and Jupiter, and it was said to invoke their protection against thunder and lightning. English dairymaids would hang it in the dairy or near pails of new milk, to stop it from curdling in thundery weather.

The Greeks also used marjoram extensively in medicine, notably to nourish the brain and the digestive organs, for narcotic poisoning, convulsions and dropsy. In Tudor and Stuart times marjoram was valued as a strewing herb for its pungent aroma and for its ability to protect against disease and infestation. The spicy juice made a furniture polish, the oil a hair tonic and the dried leaves snuff and tobacco as well as a stuffing for sleep pillows and sweet-bags.

In the language of flowers, marjoram symbolized consolation.

Herbal remedy and Aromatherapy oil

The essential oil in sweet marjoram, rich in camphor, borneol, terpinene and sabinene, is an excellent antimicrobial, effective against bacteria and viruses. It will help to protect against infection in the winter, and will also clear phlegm, soothe coughs and relieve sinusitis and fevers.

The warming, relaxing properties of marjoram oil can be felt when massaged into stiff, painful joints, aching and tense muscles, sprains and strains. By stimulating the circulation and clearing toxins, it relieves poor circulation, chilblains, arthritis and gout. It aids elimination of wastes via the urinary system.

In the digestive tract marjoram's antispasmodic and warming properties will relieve indigestion, improve appetite, calm wind and colic, reduce nausea, diarrhoea and constipation.

Marjoram's wonderfully relaxing effect will help to relieve both mental and physical tension. It has been used traditionally to calm unwanted sexual desire and to treat problems of the reproductive tract. In aromatherapy it is used particularly for its emotionally warming and calming properties for lonely people, and those who live alone. It is comforting to those who have recently lost someone they love, and has a long history of use to comfort the heart. In medieval monasteries, monks grew marjoram in their herbariums for use as an anaphrodisiac and to benefit 'nervous problems', and Gerard recommended it 'for those who are given to over-much sighing'. The presence of antioxidant in marjoram helps to minimize damage from free radicals and to protect the body from the impact of the ageing process.

Homeopathic remedy: *O. MARJORANA*

O. marjorana has an affinity for the reproductive system, and can be used to remedy sexual over-excitement, inappropriate sexual desires, or both. Like the herbal remedy and aromatherapy oil, the homeopathic remedy also helps people who are alone, not involved in a close relationship and thus feel unable to express themselves as they would want to sexually.

The flower essence

Marjoram is comforting, calming, soothing and greatly supportive in times of grief, sorrow, and vulnerability. It helps one let go of fear of being vulnerable, of being alone, and helps one to be more self-reliant and find inner strength.

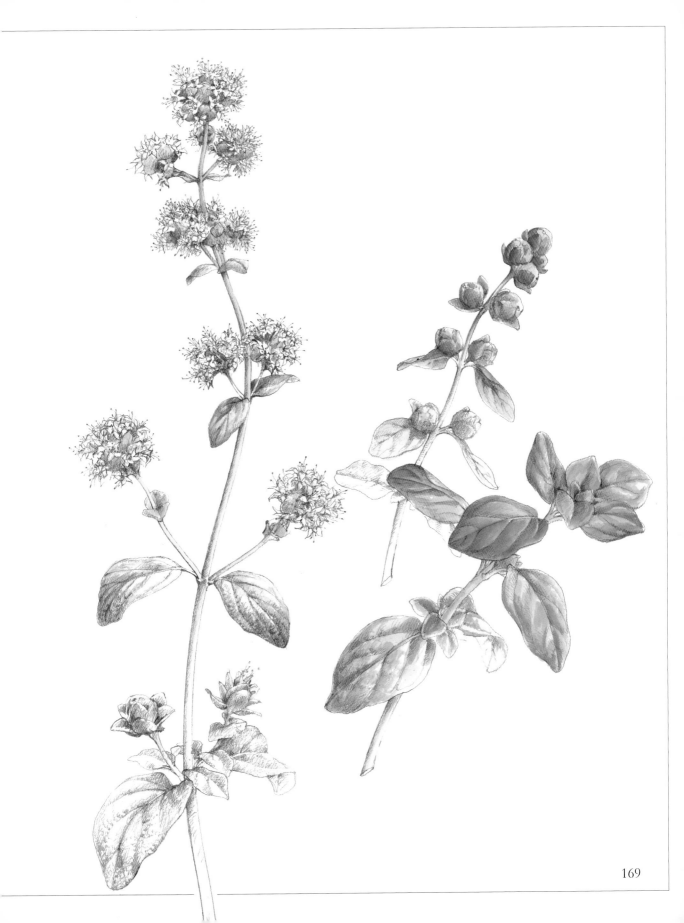

169

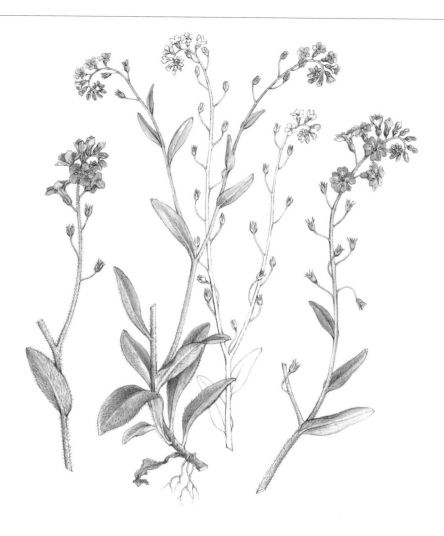

Myosotis symphytifolia

Forget-me-not

The flower of remembrance

This pretty little blue flower has long been a symbol of love and remembrance. It was traditionally given to a loved one so that the giver be remembered. Forget-me-nots were planted on graves of departed loved ones, and exchanged by friends on leap year day, 29 February.

A story tells how Adam named all the flowers in the Garden of Eden, but one flower forgot the name it had been given, and Adam renamed the flower forget-me-not. The name Myosotis comes from the Greek *mus* (mouse) and *otos* (ear) in reference to the leaves.

Herbal remedy The leaves and flowers of forget-me-not have soothing demulcent properties which can be put to good use in the respiratory system for harsh, irritating coughs. The expectorant and astringent properties reduce and expel chest phlegm. It is an old remedy for chronic bronchitis and TB.

Homeopathic remedy: Myosotis is given for chronic and obstinate coughs, for coughs with profuse purulent phlegm, for gagging and vomiting with a cough as in whooping cough, and for chronic bronchitis and TB.

The flower essence Forget-me-not is used for enhancing relationships not only with others living on earth with us, but also with those in other dimensions who have left their physical bodies, and with whom we have a strong connection. This may be important for people in the early stages of grief after a bereavement, enabling them to maintain their connection and continue the loving relationship which began on earth. Forget-me-not may also help those unable to resolve the grief or loneliness of a childhood bereavement. It may enable a deeper understanding of current relationships with children, friends or family.

170

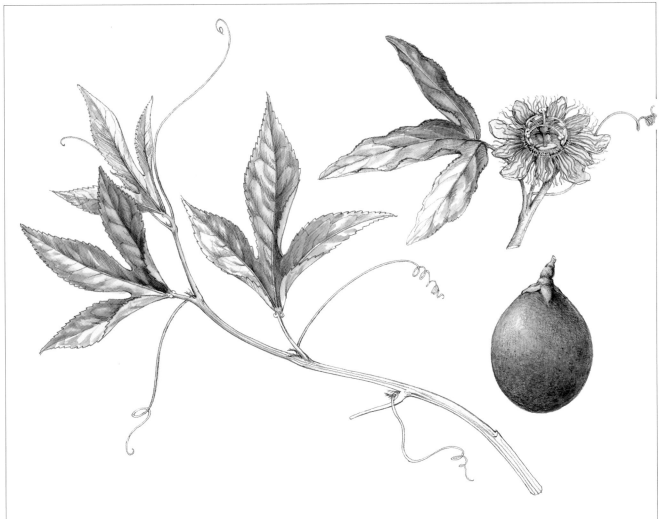

Passiflora incarnata

Passionflower

The flower to pacify the spirit

Passionflower is a fast-growing climbing vine with one of the most striking and remarkable flowers in the plant kingdom. It was sent to Pope Paul V in 1605 from a mission in Peru, with the suggestion that the beautiful corona and petals resembled and therefore represented the crown of thorns, and the Passion of Christ.

Herbal remedy The flower and the vine of passionflower make a wonderfully relaxing remedy. It is one of the best tranquilizing herbs for chronic insomnia, whether from overwork or exhaustion, and relieves many stress-related symptoms. It is non-addictive and allows you to wake refreshed and alert in the morning. Being both sedative

and antispasmodic, it relaxes spasm and tension in the muscles, calming the nerves and lessening pain as in neuralgia, shingles and Parkinson's disease. It pacifies the spirit.

Passionflower exerts its beneficial effects on the nervous system by improving circulation and nutrition to the nerves. Its cooling properties help relieve symptoms related to excess heat in the system. Its relaxing effects in the chest soothe irritating and nervous

coughs, and relieve spasm. It also relieves painful spasm in the gut.

Homeopathic remedy Passiflora is for symptoms characterized by restlessness, agitation, over-excitement, pain and spasms.

The flower essence Passionflower helps us get in touch with our inner selves, also called our 'Christ consciousness'. It eases tensions within and calms the spirit, and is said to open the throat and heart chakras. The throat chakra is associated with taking responsibility for one's personal needs and for nourishing one's inner self. The heart chakra is the centre through which we love. The more open it becomes the greater our capacity to love an ever-widening circle of life.

171

Peony

The flower of radiance

As quickly as white milk with rennet thickens, likewise the blood in the wounds of Ares became, Because of Paeon's herbs.

HOMER

This beautiful and exotic-looking flower comes from a family of 33 different species, native to Europe, China and North America. The peony is one of the most popular garden flowers – *P. lactiflora*, with its red, white or pink scented flowers was cultivated in China as long ago as 900BC. The peony is frequently depicted in Chinese art, often with peacocks and lions, decorating temple and palace walls as a motif.

The name peony derives from the mythical Paeon, physician to the Greek gods, and the god of healing. Leto, Apollo's mother, gave him the peony on Mount Olympus where he used it to heal the wounds of Pluto, god of the underworld, and Ares, god of war, as recorded above in Homer's *Iliad*.

The Greeks certainly regarded the peony as a sacred flower, with the power to keep evil spirits at bay. In other parts of Europe seeds were collected and threaded together on to white thread to wear around the neck to ward off evil. The roots were dried and carved into amulets in pagan times, and into beads for rosaries when Christianity arrived.

Although Culpeper said the peony is ruled by the sun, it was earlier thought to have been created by the moon goddess and to reflect her light through the night. It was said to ward off any unpleasant associations with darkness and was used for nightmares and melancholy dreams. In the Middle Ages many nervous diseases were considered manifestations of lunacy, and peony, as an emanation of the moon, was the sovereign remedy. The lunatic was often covered with peony plants as he lay down and arose with his senses fully restored. Both Dioscorides and Pliny mention the use of peony for nightmares and hysteria. In the language of flowers, peony was also a symbol of shyness or bashfulness.

Herbal remedy

Since the days of Dioscorides and Theophrastus, peony has been used for nightmares, hysteria, and pains of the womb. The dried root was given to women after childbirth to help expel the placenta and aid recovery. Culpeper recommended the fresh root for falling sickness (epilepsy) and the root or seeds for cleansing the womb after childbirth. He said the black seeds taken morning and evening would cure nightmares and melancholy dreams.

Peony acts to stimulate the uterine muscles and will aid contractions in childbirth and expulsion of the placenta. Through the centuries peony has been used for kidney stones, and a liver and gall-bladder remedy for gallstones. By relieving stasis of blood it can be used for varicose veins and haemorrhoids. As a tonic to the nervous system, it was used for spasm, epilepsy, nervous twitches and St Vitus's dance.

In China peony root has been used as a medicine for thousands of years. *Bai-shao* (cultivated root) is used for wounds, hypertensive headaches and poor circulation. It is helpful for diarrhoea, period pain, fevers and night sweats, and gastric ulcers. It has antibacterial, antiviral and anticonvulsive properties. It is calming and anti-inflammatory. *Chi-shao* (wild harvested root) is prescribed for pains in the chest, heat in the blood, absent or painful periods, dysentery and boils.

Homeopathic remedy: PAEONIA

Paeonia is prepared from fresh peony root and used for symptoms of congestion of the blood. It is prescribed for ulcers, haemorrhoids, headaches, varicose veins, and griping pains in the abdomen associated with trembling and anxiety. Paeonia people are prone to nightmares and nervous oversensitivity, are easily frightened, depressed and excited.

The flower essence

Peony is now available as a flower essence and looks promising as a remedy for tense, fearful people who have nightmares and are easily affected by negative influences. It has an affinity for the moon, 'lunacy' and dispelling the forces of darkness, so appears an ideal remedy for emotional problems related to women's monthly cycles such as PMS or menopausal depression. As a great healer, as the flower that healed Pluto the god of the underworld, peony is a good strengthener for unconscious fears, our 'underworld' that gives rise to disturbing dreams or apparently irrational fears. Peony is a remedy of light.

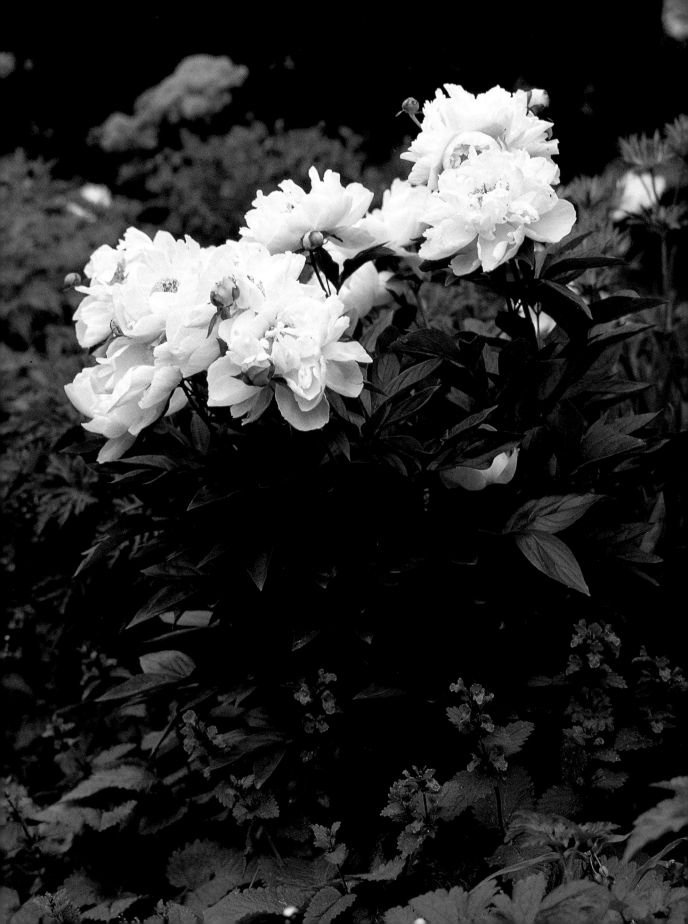

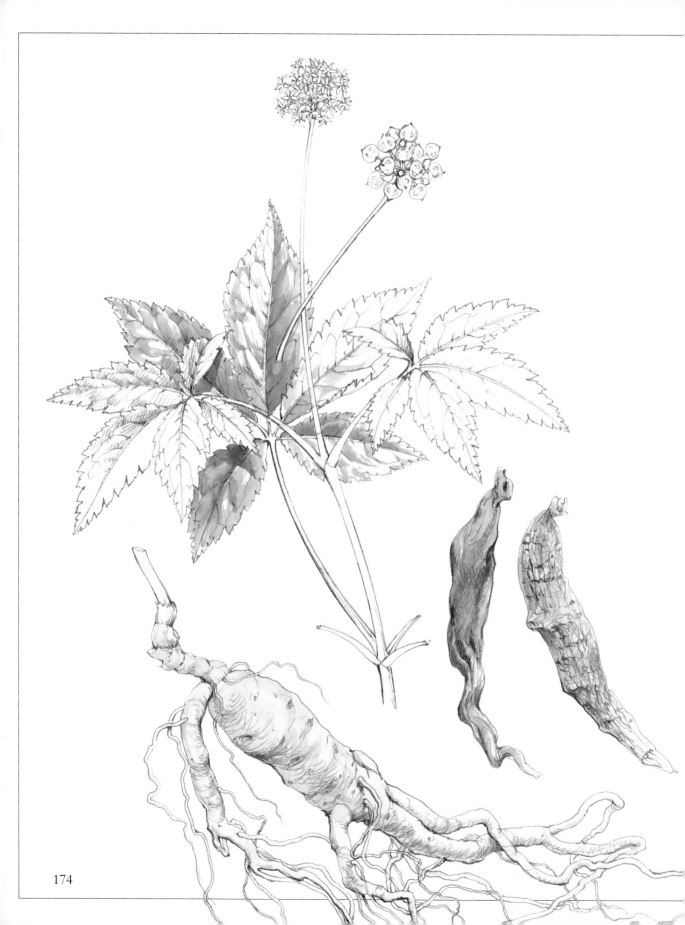

Ginseng

The flower of unity

Ginseng is familiar to many as a wonderful tonic to increase energy and vitality, improve mental and physical performance and protect against the effects of stress. The name ginseng is used for a number of different plants including *Panax ginseng*: Chinese or Korean ginseng, *Eleuthrococcus senticosus*: Siberian ginseng, and *Panax quinquefolium*: American ginseng.

Ginseng and its other Chinese names are all different transliterations of the same Chinese ideogram, meaning 'essence of the earth in the form of a man', or 'man-root', so-called because the root of ginseng resembles that of the mandrake and has a human form. To the Chinese, *Panax ginseng* is the king of tonics. For centuries in the East top grade roots have been valued more highly than gold.

In Northern China *Panax ginseng* grows in the mountainous forests, allegedly only where lightning has struck a clear stream. It was noted in 1709 by Father Petrus Jartoux, a Jesuit missionary in North China. He said that if this wonder plant were to be found anywhere else in the world it would be in Canada where the forests and mountains resemble those of North China. Another missionary, Père Joseph Francois Lafitau, discovered *Panax quinquefolium* growing outside his Montreal cabin in 1716. Very soon American ginseng was being shipped from Canada to China. The practice continues to this day.

Herbal remedy

The word Panax comes from the Greek *pan* meaning all, and *akos* meaning cure, referring to ginseng's traditional use as a cure-all or panacea. In China this famous tonic has been used for Qi deficiency associated with debility, insomnia, weakness and breathlessness, which may be caused by stress, illness, or ageing. Over the past 50 years nearly 3000 scientific studies have demonstrated ginseng's amazing ability to increase resistance to mental and physical stress in many different forms. It has been described as an adaptogen, having a normalizing action in the body, which may for example be relaxing in a person feeling tense and anxious, and stimulating in someone feeling tired and lethargic. Ginseng acts on the pituitary gland and stimulates the adrenal glands, normalizing their function during the challenges of stress. By increasing the efficiency of nerve impulses,

ginseng increases mental performance, sharpens memory and diminishes fatigue. It improves physical performance, increasing stamina locally in the muscles. It reduces wheezing and shortness of breath.

By increasing white blood cell action ginseng acts as an immune enhancer. It reduces blood sugar, which is useful for diabetics, improves the appetite and digestion, lowers harmful cholesterol and decreases allergic responses. The saponins stimulate sexual function in both men and women, and increase sperm production in men. Ginseng also helps the liver resist hepatotoxins and radiation and reduces the depression of the bone marrow in those on anti-cancer treatment. Ginseng thus raises resistance to stress, increasing the threshold over which stress is challenging and becomes damaging. It can be taken on a short-term basis for 3–4 months during a particularly stressful period. It can also be taken by the elderly as a rejuvenating tonic – the presence of antioxidants in ginseng will support this action.

American ginseng is more tranquilizing and cooling than *Panax ginseng*. It has been used in America for treating TB and more generally it can be used to strengthen one in the aftermath of a high fever when feeling weak, thirsty and debilitated or when suffering from after-pains after childbirth.

Homeopathic remedy: PANAX

Ginseng gives a sense of joy, vigour and elasticity of the limbs and clearness of mind in cases of physical and mental fatigue. It has an affinity for the lower part of the body and is specific for lumbago, sciatica, chronic rheumatism and sexual over-excitement.

The flower essence

The root of American ginseng has a human shape, and the flower essence imparts a strong awareness of what it means to be a human being. It engenders a blending of both male and female energies, creating a unity within. It is in every way a strengthener – mentally, emotionally and physically. It protects against the effects of stress and has a beneficial influence on the endocrine system. When used in massage oils ginseng increases physical stamina, and helps to connect the spiritual side of oneself to the physical. It is a great tonic.

NB Avoid in acute inflammatory conditions and bronchitis as it may aggravate the symptoms

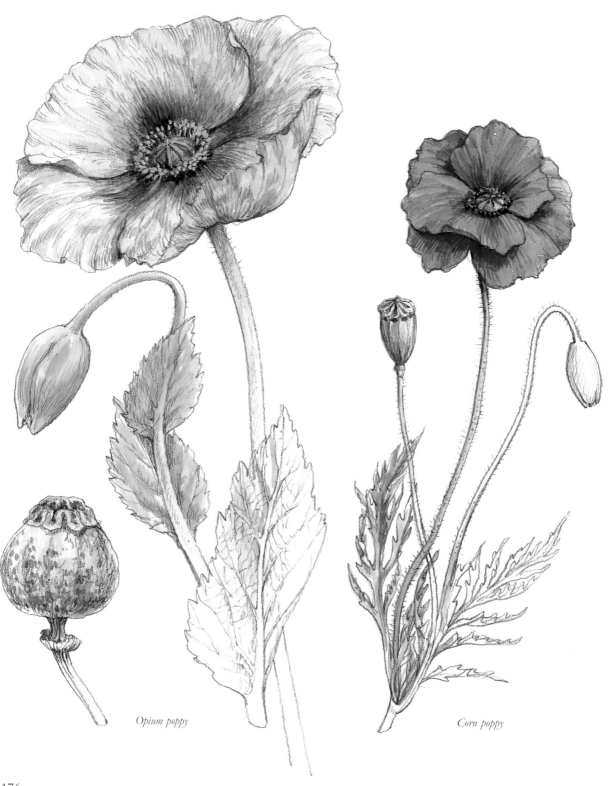

Opium poppy

Corn poppy

Opium poppy
The flower of the underworld

The bright red corn poppy is a familiar sight in un-sprayed wheatfields and likes to grow on disturbed land, such as ploughed or battle ground. From European battles of the 17th century until the First World War, the appearance of poppies on the battle-field has given rise to the idea that they spring from the blood of the fallen.

In Greek mythology, the opium poppy was an attribute of the goddess Demeter, who was called Ceres the corn goddess by the Romans. Demeter was so grief-stricken when Hades took her daughter Persephone away to the underworld that she turned to the soporific effects of the opium poppy (whose Greek name *nepenthes* means 'that potent destroyer of grief') to ease her pain and soothe her to sleep. Zeus persuaded Hades to let Persephone return from the underworld after each winter for two-thirds of the year, when the seeds were sprouting and the flowers were coming out, to live with Demeter, the earth goddess who bestowed fertility on fields. Thus the poppy came to represent the renewal of life, regener-ation, and activity after sleep. The fact that the poppy seed head contains an enormous number of seeds was another reason for its reputation for giving life and its association with fertility and Demeter. Because of its association with sleep and the under-world, the Greeks also consecrated the poppy to Nyx, goddess of night and Morpheus, god of dreams. In the language of flowers the red poppy means extravagance and consolation; the opium poppy means sleep.

The twin themes of sleep, and of blood and circu-lation, run through the use of the poppy in healing. Opium extracted from the seed capsule latex contains the powerful alkaloid morphine. No other plant drug has played such a role in world events, underlying wars and world-wide organized crime. Morphine is still used for pain relief, particularly post-operatively and in cancer. It acts on the circula-tion by engorging the blood vessels of the brain. In small amounts this has a transitory exhilarating effect as the mind floats free and the imagination has full play. With repeated or larger doses, it produces sleepiness and eventually stupor. Thus it takes away the awareness of pain. It also affects the muscles of the body, in small doses causing relaxation while in larger quantities causing paralysis, so that for example it can relieve griping and diarrhoea, but can lead to bowel inertia.

Herbal remedy
The opium poppy is unsafe for internal use because of its highly addictive nature. The red corn poppy also has soporific qualities, but its main ingredient rheadine, while soothing and sedative, is not addic-tive. Cooks use the seeds for seasoning bread; the red petals and seeds can be used to aid relaxation, calm excitement and induce sleep. They make a good gargle for sore throats and tonsillitis, and an expecto-rant for chest complaints. The leaves soothe and relax spasm in the chest, act to sedate the cough reflex and are helpful in irritating coughs, croup and whooping cough, bronchitis and pleurisy. They soothe and relax spasm in the stomach and intestines, and relieve pain of nervous origin such as headaches, shingles and neuralgia. Their astringent properties are useful when treating diarrhoea.

Homeopathic remedy: OPIUM
Opium is used for insensitivity of the nervous system, painless symptoms, sleepiness, lethargy, lack of vital reaction, even stupor. It has also been used for cases of typhoid, cholera infantum and stroke.

The flower essence
Opium poppy can be used to help find a balance in daily life between activity and rest, the spiritual and the physical, evolution and being.

The oriental poppy is used for escapists who find it hard to face up to the realities of life and tend to live in the world of the imagination and dreams. It helps you find strength to live in the present. The field poppy is for those who are fearful of expressing strong emotions such as anger. It lends courage to assert yourself, to express your feelings in all their colours, and to shine like the bright red poppy.

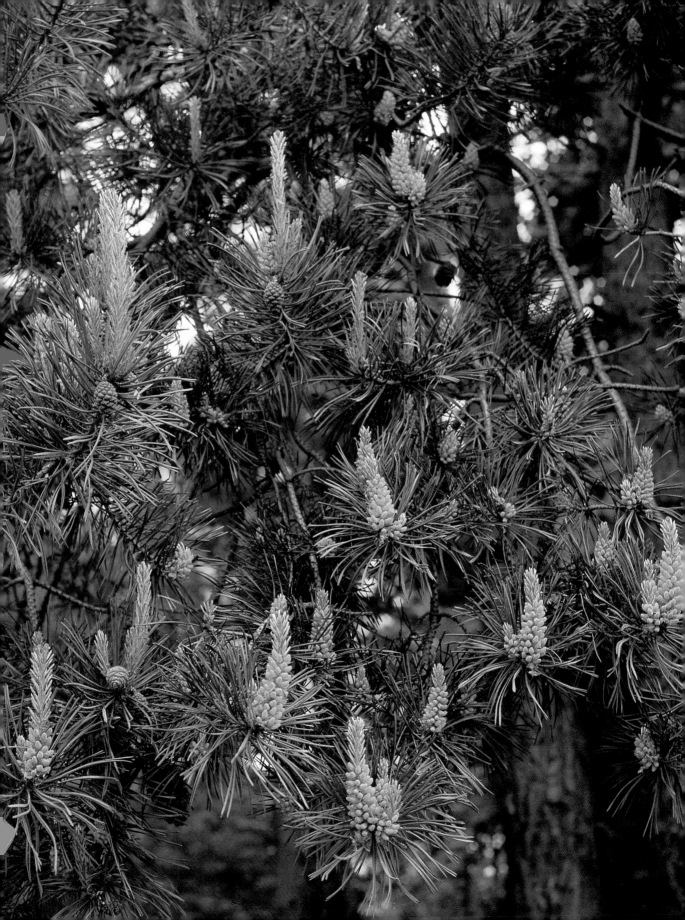

Pine

The flower of pity

But of all the Pines, Mount Ida bears the best
By Cybele prefer'd above the rest.
This plant a lovely boy was heretofore,
Belov'd by Cybele, upon whose score
He sacrific'd to chastity, but now
His fruit delaying Venus now excites,
His wood affords the torch which Hymen
lights.
   ABRAHAM COWLEY (1618–67)

The majestic evergreen scotch pine has been revered
for centuries in many parts of the world for its symbolic significance and medicinal value. It also has
great economic value as the straight long trunks
make excellent timber, its resin and turpentine oil are
good solvents and are used in paints and varnishes.

In Greek mythology the pine tree belongs to the
goddess Cybele, mother of the gods. Her consort
was a shepherd named Atys, the guardian of her
temple from whom she obtained a vow of celibacy.
However, Atys fell in love with another, named
Sangaris. Cybele turned him into a pine tree to prevent him from killing himself and afterwards sadly
mourned the loss of her unfaithful lover under the
branches of the tree, until Zeus promised her that
the pine would remain forever green.

As an evergreen tree the pine symbolizes immortality and the undying spirit and was often used in
funerary and mourning rites. In China pine trees are
planted on graves to strengthen the soul of the
deceased and save their body from corruption.

The Greeks also dedicated the pine tree to others
of their gods, to Zeus and Artemis, Jupiter and
Venus, to Neptune because the first boats were made
of pine, to Bacchus as pine cones were put into vats
to flavour Greek wine, and to Pan. Pan seduced one
of his nymphs, Pitys, who preferred him to Boreas,
god of the North wind. Boreas in a jealous fury
flung her about, crushing her limbs, and so Gaia
transformed her into a pine tree to escape his wrath.
Since then pine has been a symbol of pity.

The pine also symbolizes uprightness, straightness,
vitality, strength of character, and because it grows
so high, the connection between earth and heaven. It
is an emblem of Confucius to the Chinese and represents longevity, courage, faithfulness and constancy

in adversity. With the plum and the bamboo it is one
of the three friends of winter in Japan, used in New
Year celebrations:

Hear the Pine: may your prosperity be as constant as the greenness of my mantle, and may
your friends stand as I do, steadfast against the
adverse winds of the world.
Hear the Bamboo: may your lifetime be as long
as mine and may you know the joy of living
abundantly.
Hear the Plum: may your hopes rise fresh and
strong like the young shoots that spring from
my rugged trunk and may your life flower with
loveliness.

In cold winter months, particularly, the pine is a
favourite subject of Japanese artists in association
often with the crane and the tortoise. In flower decorations the thick gnarled branches are used to represent a strong and happy old age. In Indo-European
symbolism, the pine cone represents good fortune
and fire, the masculine creative force and fecundity,
and the cones were carried to increase fertility and to
bring a vigorous old age.

Herbal remedy

Pine is an excellent remedy for the lungs. It liquifies
and helps to expel bronchial phlegm and clears the
head of congestion. Its antiseptic and anti-inflammatory action is recommended for treatment of respiratory infections, colds, coughs, flu, sore throats, bronchitis and pneumonia. It has also been used for
tuberculosis. Its antispasmodic action in the chest
will help relieve asthma and a harsh, tight cough.
Pine also strengthens the digestion, and has a tonic
revitalising effect generally. It can be given to those
suffering from mental, physical or sexual depletion
and from adrenal insufficiency as it has a stimulating
effect on the adrenal medulla and cortex.

Pine is also a good remedy for the urinary system;
it helps to remedy infections and the discomfort that
accompanies cystitis. By aiding the elimination of
toxins via the kidneys it will help in arthritis and
gout, and due to its anodyne properties it may help
to relieve headaches and toothache.

179

Externally, the resin and oil have been used in liniments to rub into painful joints and aching muscles and to increase the circulation. The tar is used in lotions for skin problems, such as ringworm.

Aromatherapy oil

Pine oil, obtained from steam distillation of the needles, is used much like the herbal remedy. It can be added to massage oils and rubbed into arthritic joints and will help to detoxify the body through its diuretic effect. It makes an excellent inhalant for respiratory infections, coughs, colds, catarrh and sinusitis. It can be used preventatively to keep infections at bay. Its antiseptic action extends to the urinary system where it can be used for urinary infections – pyelitis, cystitis and prostatitis.

When used in the morning, pine's tonic and invigorating properties will help wake you up, enliven the mind and alert the senses. At the same time pine is calming and refreshing and can be used for exhaustion, debility, anxiety and stress-related problems. It is warming and strengthening, particularly in winter as it stimulates the circulation. Rubbed into the skin, pine will act as a good insect repellent and deodorant. It has a particular application to excessive perspiration. It can also be rubbed into the hair to clear headlice, and into the skin to repel fleas and scabies, but only when diluted in a base oil as it can sometimes cause irritation if used neat.

Homeopathic remedy: PINUS

Pinus works particularly on the bronchial and urinary systems and the joints. It is prescribed for feelings of oppression in the chest and a sensation that the chest wall is thin and could easily give way. There is burning in the sides of the chest. There may be swollen glands and fever with chilliness and a pale face, alternating with heat and flushing. There may be burning on urination and difficulty passing water. Pinus is also indicated by rheumatic, gouty or paralytic pains in the limbs, bones and joints, with stiffness. There may be emaciation in the lower limbs, and weak ankles in children who tend to be late walking. A Pinus person may feel anxious or despondent, the mind feels dull and they are unable to think clearly. They may undertake many things which they don't finish. They tend to feel worse on exertion, from touch, in the morning and in the evening.

The flower essence

Pine is the Bach Flower Remedy for guilt and for those who feel guilty either about recent events or for just being alive. Such people cling to their guilty feelings which can affect their whole outlook on life, taking away their *joie de vivre*, and their energy. They tend to set high standards for themselves and feel dissatisfied when they cannot live up to them perfectly. They blame themselves for not doing better; they can even blame themselves for the mistakes of others. The pine child will be the scapegoat in the class who uncomplainingly accepts punishments for the misdemeanours of others. Unable to forgive themselves, pine people unconsciously put themselves in situations designed to punish them, such as unrewarding relationships with inconsiderate partners or friends.

The flower remedy helps people to accept their faults and not cling to them. It enables a greater understanding of human nature which is not perfect and allows light back into the lives of people who can learn to forgive themselves.

Cowslip

The flower of keys

Whilst from off the water fleet,
Thus I set my printless feet,
O'er the cowslip's velvet head,
That bends not as I tread.

JOHN MILTON (1608–74)

This pretty cousin of the primrose grows on chalk and limestone grassland and downs throughout Europe and Britain. While it was once a common feature of the countryside in spring, the cowslip has become more rare because of overpicking and the use of herbicides – it is now a protected plant. The flowers have certainly been picked in enormous quantities in the past, as the many recipes from the 17th to 19th centuries show. Cowslip flowers were used in making wine, mead and cordials, syrup and vinegar, pickles and conserves, cheese, cakes, tarts, creams and puddings.

Cowslip flowers threaded on a string and bunched tightly into a ball made a 'totsie', which was tossed to and fro in a game. Girls used these balls as a love oracle, throwing them from one to another saying: 'Titsy, totsy, tell me true, who shall I be married to?' Cowslip flowers were a valued ingredient of love potions used by Saxon women. The petals were collected in the morning before the dew had dried on them and placed in a pot with fresh rainwater and left all day in the sunlight. The flower essence was then sprinkled on the pillow of their sweetheart whose heart was expected to melt within the following month. The plant was exchanged by courting couples and the flowers sold on the streets of London for good luck.

In Norse mythology the cowslip was dedicated to the goddess Freya, the key virgin. The flowers were believed to open the lock to her treasure palace, hence the old name keyflower. Freya was the ruler of fate, the stars and the heavens, and she was a symbol of sexual love (her other name, Frigg, descended into slang). The god Odin is said to have learned all his magic and divine powers from the goddess Freya.

With the coming of Christianity, cowslips were dedicated to the Virgin Mary, and called Our Lady's keys. Their appearance was said to resemble a bunch of keys which would open the gates of heaven, so they were also named Peterkeys, Peterwort and Peterkin, as well as keys of heaven, and dedicated to St Peter, to whom Jesus had promised the keys to the gates of heaven.

The name cowslip derives from the belief that they grew up wherever a cow left a cowpat, and so they were called *cuslyppe* or *cuslop*, the old English word for cowdung. It then became cowslop, and a little later cowslip. A garland of the flowers was hung around the necks of cattle to increase milk production. In Russia its name *Pervo-Tzuet* means first flower of spring, and cowslips are indeed one of nature's signs of renewed life unfolding, to reveal treasures as yet unknown. In some traditions girls would exchange posies of cowslips in May as a symbol of trust and friendship.

Another name for cowslip is fairycup, as fairies are supposed to like nestling in the drooping bell of cowslip flowers.

Herbal remedy

Both the root and flowers have been used for centuries for the nervous system. They are relaxing and sedative and can be taken for anxiety, tension, insomnia, stress headaches, and as a general tonic to the nervous system. They have a reputation for lifting the spirits and so are recommended for negativity and depression. They are cooling and decongestant, and have been used traditionally for nervous problems associated with excess heat and congestion, such as irritability and hysteria, inflammatory and painful nervous conditions such as neuralgia and neuritis, as well as vertigo. Cowslip syrup was an old country remedy for palsy (paralysis), hence another of its names, palsywort. The Greeks called cowslips *paralysio*. Culpeper said the flowers could be used successfully to relieve 'all infirmities of the head coming from heat and wind as vertigo, false apparitions, phresnies, falling sickness, palsies, convulsions, cramps, pains in nerves'. Cowslips were also used to improve the memory and strengthen the brain.

An infusion of the flowers makes a good detoxifying remedy, and has a diaphoretic effect, bringing down fevers, and an expectorant action. It makes a good remedy for babies, children and the elderly for fevers, colds, flu, sore throats and coughs. Its combined sedative action will soothe dry, irritating coughs and induce restful sleep, very useful when hacking coughs can disturb a good night's sleep. By bringing blood to the surface of the body cowslips relieve heat and also bring out eruptions, explaining why cowslips were an old country remedy for children's measles.

The root is particularly high in saponins which account for the plant's expectorant action, and can be used for chest infections, bronchitis and whooping cough. The salicylates also in the root have an anti-inflammatory action – particularly useful for swollen joints in arthritis and gout. In old herbals cowslip is known as *Radix arthritica*.

Externally, cowslip flowers can be used in lotions and ointment for skin problems such as eczema and acne, and to soothe sunburn. In the past they were also used as a beauty aid. Culpeper said they 'taketh away spots and wrinkles of the skin, sun burnings and freckles' and add 'beauty exceedingly'. According to the doctrine of signatures, the freckles on the petals denoted the flower's value for removing blemishes and freckles on the skin. Certainly Shakespeare thought so:

In their gold coats spots you see,
These be rubies: Fairy favours,
In those freckles lie their savours.

Perhaps this is why for some the cowslip flower is a symbol of grace and beauty. Certainly the beautiful cowslip has been the inspiration for many a poet.

Homeopathic remedy: PRIMULA VERIS

The same themes run through the homeopathic use of cowslips. They are prescribed wherever there is heat and for symptoms characterized by burning. They have an affinity for the nervous system, useful in headaches, migraine, vertigo, tinnitus, anxiety and febrile excitement. They are specific for 'threatened apoplexy (stroke) arising from psychic depression' (Clarke) and cerebral congestion associated with neuralgia, and headaches which are associated with heat in the face and are better from pressure. They also help to relieve hot burning skin conditions, such as eczema, itching scalps, burning pains in the throat and chest, palpitations, cystitis (where the urine smells of violets), burning in the stomach with a tendency to vomiting and diarrhoea, and burning in the joints, particularly the right shoulder joint, and stiff neck and back. The symptoms tend to diminish in the open air, but are worse from stooping, movement and being indoors in stuffy rooms.

The flower essence

A relative of the cowslip, the oxslip (*Primula elatior*), which is very similar in appearance, was well known to the Ancient Greeks. It was called *dodekatheon*, meaning plant of the twelve gods, and was used as a panacea, as a remedy with twelve constituents. The flowers were gathered by the dryads at new moon and administered particularly for melancholy. Cowslip flowers were traditionally woven into funeral wreaths and put on graves, and were worn pinned to clothes as a sign of bereavement. They have been used to ease the grief of separation or the breakdown of a relationship, leading to negativity, depression, grief, loneliness and feelings of abandonment.

Another relative of cowslip, the primrose (*Primula vulgaris*) is the remedy for both unexpressed and unresolved emotions. It is helpful for seasonal affective disorder (SAD) and also for those who have an unrealistic view of love and relationships. This view can inhibit the development of more grounded, intimate relationships.

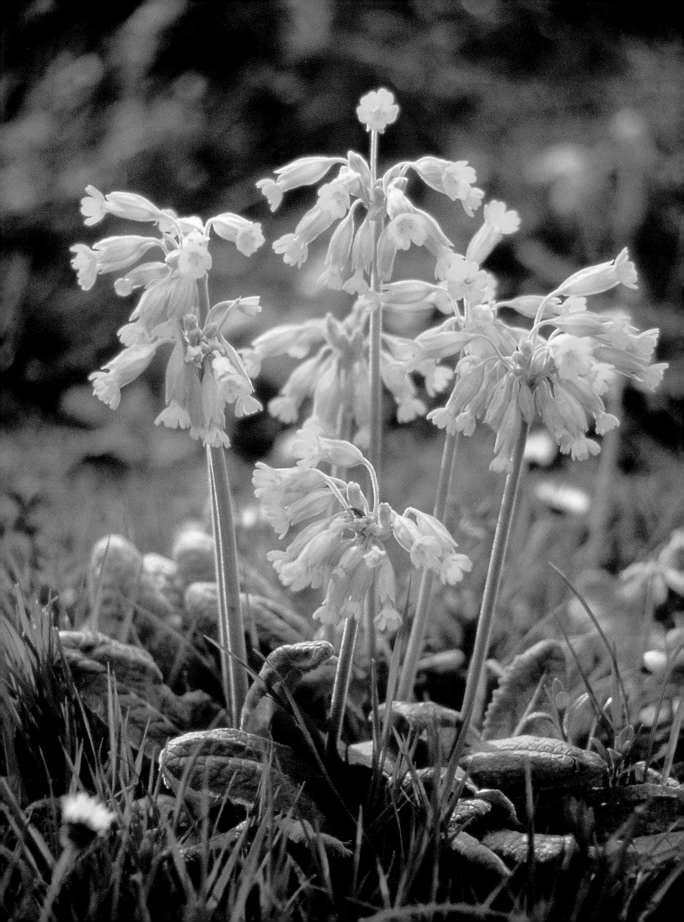

Aspen

The flower of sensitivity

Aspen or white poplar is an attractive tree with catkins in the spring followed by silver-lined leaves that rustle and quake even when the air seems still. Its continuously trembling leaves also explain the Latin name for the American poplar, *P. tremuloides*. The leaves of the white poplar tree are dark on one side and light on the other and so the tree has come to symbolize night and day, and the passing of time. To the Chinese poplar leaves represent yin and yang, moon and sun, and life in all its duality.

In Greek mythology the aspen was dedicated to Hercules who wore a crown of poplar on his descent into Hades. Groves of white poplar trees were planted in his honour and represented the Elysian fields while the black poplar denoted Hades. Aspen was associated with funerals. It was said that Jesus' cross was made of poplar and the trembling of the leaves is linked to the shivering of the tree whose wood was cursed by his death.

Twigs and branches of aspen were used in the past for making arrows and hence had divinatory virtues. The buds and leaves were carried to attract money and apparently used by wizards in flying ointments. According to Pliny the aspen turns its leaves towards the opposite side of the sky immediately after the summer solstice, and when the leaves showed their undersides it heralded wet weather.

Herbal remedy

The flower buds, leaves and bark have been used as a bitter tonic, to stimulate the appetite and enhance digestion and absorption. They can be taken for digestive problems including flatulence, acidity, colic and diarrhoea, as well as liver disturbances. They make a good remedy for conditions associated with poor digestion or a weak liver, such as headaches, irritability, lethargy and debility. Aspen is good as a tonic after illness or when feeling weak and tired from stress or overwork, or from chronic diarrhoea.

Aspen contains salicylic acid and so has an action similar to aspirin. It can be taken for headaches, nerve pain and fevers and was used in the past as an alternative to Peruvian bark for intermittent fevers or malaria. It will help to relieve urinary problems such as cystitis and irritable bladder and acts as a diuretic. It is a good remedy for painful, inflamed joints and due to the presence of astringent tannins, it can be used for weakness of the vaginal and uterine muscles, predisposing to prolapse.

Externally, aspen tones the skin and makes a good anti-inflammatory for cuts and grazes, eczema and ulcers and an astringent for excessive perspiration.

Homeopathic remedy: POPULUS TREMULOIDES

Populus tremuloides can taken for digestive problems such as acidity, nausea, vomiting, heartburn, indigestion and flatulence. It has a particular affinity for the bladder, relieving cystitis with tenesmus of the bladder and urine containing mucus and pus. It is a good remedy also for prostate problems and for night sweats and intermittent fevers.

The flower essence

Aspen is the remedy for those who suffer vague or acute fears for no apparent reason. Such people are more sensitive than most – they rustle even in the slightest breeze like the leaves of the tree. They are easily affected by the collective unconscious and the realm of archetypes, by superstition, myth and legend, and by concepts of life and death and religion.

Anxiety and apprehension can creep up on aspen people both during the night and day. They may awake in the night in terror, and may dread going to sleep again. Their fears are often connected to thoughts of death or religion or a sense of disaster impending. The fear can be so intense as to become terrifying and cause trembling, sweating and butterflies in the stomach.

The flower remedy increases inner strength and confidence, and helps to still fears and anxieties. It enhances the awareness of a higher power behind and above all existence, and the ability to trust more in the divine power of love, encouraging one into a wider range of experiences and adventures without fear holding one back.

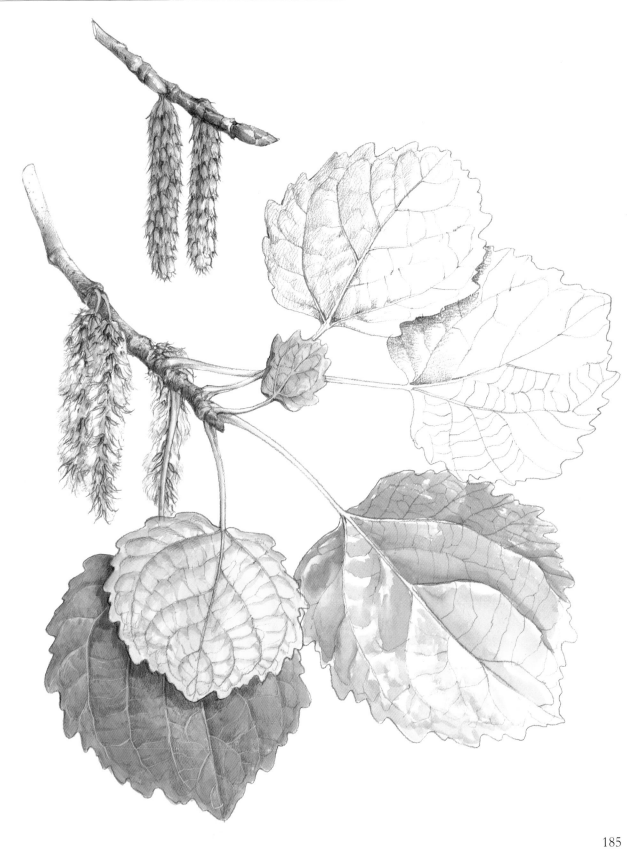

Self-heal

The flower of confidence

Self-heal is a pretty member of the mint family, much loved by bees, and which grows all over Europe in pastures, woods and clearings. It has found its way to North America where it is called heart of the earth and blue curls. The name Prunella was originally *Brunella* or *Brunellen*, a name given to it by the Germans as it was used to treat *die Breuen*, an inflammatory mouth and throat problem, common to soldiers in garrisons. Self-heal was commonly used for throat complaints according to the doctrine of signatures, for its corolla was seen to resemble a throat with swollen glands.

Self-heal has also been called carpenter's herb and hook heal because the corolla, when seen in profile, is shaped like a bill hook. Thus, according to the doctrine of signatures, self-heal was used to heal wounds inflicted by sharp-edged tools. Gerard said, 'the decoction of Prunell made with wine and water, doth join together and make whole and sound all wounds, both inward and outward, even as Bugle doth'. It was commonly used by country people and labourers for cuts and wounds, and a saying went 'no one wants a surgeon who keeps self-heal'. It was seen as one of the best herbs to grow for home use.

Herbal remedy

Self-heal can be used as an astringent gargle for sore throats and a mouthwash for mouth ulcers and bleeding gums. The tea can be used, or the fresh plant rubbed on to the skin to stop bleeding from cuts and reduce swelling from bites and stings. Self-heal can also relieve inflammatory skin problems, piles, varicose veins and ulcers, as well as inflammation of the eyes that include conjunctivitis, blepharitis and styes.

Culpeper said that self-heal was under the dominion of Venus, and explained the name: 'self-heal whereby when you are hurt, you may heal yourself'. He also said 'the juice used with oil of roses to anoint the temples and forehead is very effectual to remove the headache, and the same mixed with honey of roses cleaneth and healeth ulcers in the mouth and throat'.

Taken internally self-heal can be used for headaches, particularly where they are related to tension, vertigo, over-sensitivity to light and high blood pressure. It has an affinity for the lymphatic system and can be taken for swollen glands, mumps, glandular fever and mastitis. An astringent, it can be taken for diarrhoea and colitis.

Self-heal, although largely neglected by western herbalists, is an important herb in Chinese medicine. The bitters have a stimulating action on the liver and gall-bladder, and self-heal is prescribed for symptoms of jaundice and liver problems. It is also recommended for gout.

Homeopathic remedy: PRUNELLA

Prunella is sometimes prescribed for colitis and similar bowel problems.

The flower essence

Self-heal, as the name suggests, is used to enhance our own healing powers. The body possesses an inherent healing ability, which enables a cut to heal, inflammation to resolve and infection to subside. We are also able to heal ourselves emotionally and we can be healed spiritually.

Self-heal increases confidence in our ability to heal ourselves. It is particularly recommended for those who doubt their innate recuperative powers, or who cannot face the responsibility of looking after themselves and hand over the responsibility of their physical health or emotional, mental or spiritual welfare to healers, counsellors and gurus.

It may be needed by those who are unwell or unhappy, who have lost belief in their own capacity to be well, for addicts dependent on external factors for their feeling of wellbeing, and for those facing crises in their lives. Self-heal helps to reduce dependence on others, and to inspire motivation and a belief in your own inherent healing powers.

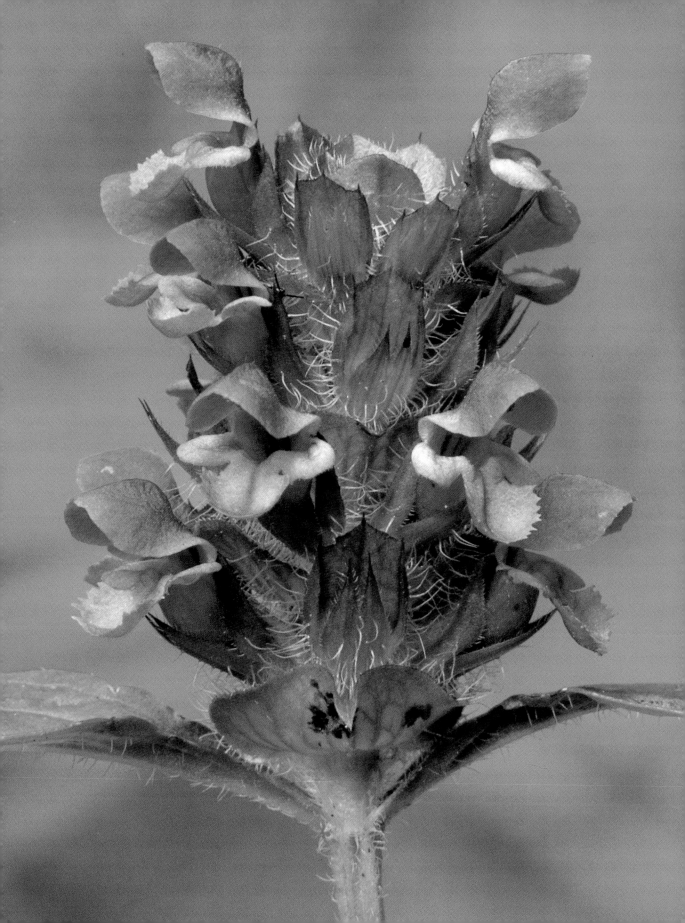

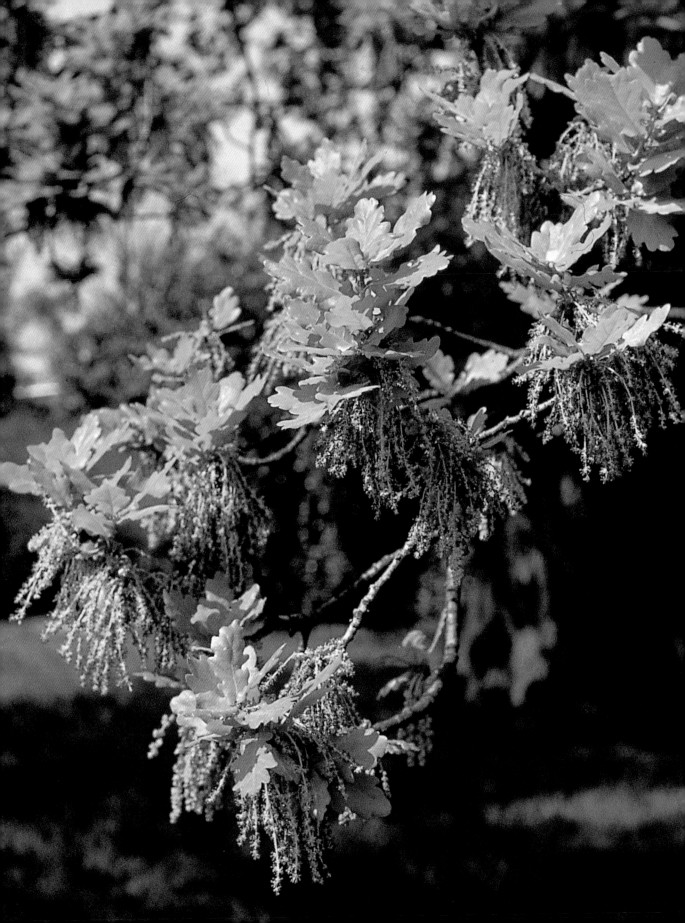

Oak

The flower of the Druids

The oak is the most majestic of trees, and although it grows all over Europe it is regarded as being peculiarly English. The Common or British oak is intricately linked to British history since the time of the Druids. An oak twig featured on British coins until replaced by the British lion. The oak is well-known both for growing slowly, and for growing to a huge size. It may take 500 years in growing, 500 years in maturity and 500 years declining. As a result the oak is symbolic of how the British liked to see themselves: strong, proud and steadfast. The acorn is a symbol of effort and great achievement; we say 'great oaks from little acorns grow' and sing proudly of being like 'heart of oak'.

Oak timber, renowned for its toughness and durability, is also strong and elastic, making it excellent for building houses and ships. So the oak also symbolizes durability, courage, protection and truth. To the Chinese and the Druids it symbolizes masculine strength. In Christianity it denotes Christ as strength in adversity, steadfastness in faith and virtue. The oak was often called the Gospel oak, as psalms and gospel truths were uttered in its shade.

The Druids planted sacred groves of oak, and it was believed to ward off lightning – another reason for using the timber in building, especially if the tree it came from had already been struck, as lightning was said never to strike the same place twice. Acorns were carved on bannisters to deter lightning, and carried to ward off illness and ensure potency and long life. The acorn symbolizes the cosmic egg, whence all life springs, and of immortality. To the indigenous people of California, the oak was the world tree or cosmic axis, sacred to the earth mother.

Herbal remedy

The astringent properties of oak bark, provided by the tannins, have been well known since the time of Hippocrates. A decoction of acorns and oak bark was added to milk and taken to resist the effect of poisons and infections in the digestive tract, and to heal infection and inflammation in the bladder.

The tannins have a toning effect on the mucous membranes throughout the body and protect them from irritation, inflammation and infection. Thus oak bark makes a good remedy for catarrh, sinus congestion and post-nasal drip. It reduces excessive menstrual bleeding and tones pelvic and abdominal muscles, very useful for prolapse. In the digestive tract it aids digestion and absorption, and also makes an excellent remedy for diarrhoea and dysentery. By toning muscles throughout the circulatory system it is useful for varicose veins and haemorrhoids.

Oak has been valued as an antidote to the effects of alcohol, and to control alchol craving. It was taken daily in small doses for withdrawal symptoms.

Externally, it makes a gargle for tonsillitis, pharyngitis and laryngitis. As a mouthwash it is good for bleeding gums and mouth ulcers. As a lotion it relieves chilblains, varicose veins, ulcers, haemorrhoids, burns and cuts, and as a douche or lotion treats vaginal discharges and infections.

Homeopathic remedy: QUERCUS

Quercus is a predominant remedy for the effects of alcoholism, and excess alcohol consumption, such as liver problems, ascites, gout, enlarged spleen, skin flushing, diarrhoea, irregular heartbeat, trembling hands, tottering gait, nervousness, depression and craving for alcohol.

The flower essence

An oak person has great strength and powers of endurance, tremendous willpower and courage, devotion to duty and high ideals. However, they can become rigid in their approach to life, stuck in high achievement stress. They are hard-working, reliable, often plodding, but do not allow time to relax, have fun or allow creative interludes. Their inner life may become impoverished while the oak person keeps working, gradually becoming increasingly tired, even to the point of exhaustion. In illness or exhaustion, an oak person struggles bravely on, never complaining or showing others how they feel, as they do not like to appear weak, or unable to support others. The Bach Flower Remedy oak helps to reduce the inner pressure to achieve and keep going. The pleasure in life returns – you feel more able to relax and let go, as well as fulfilling your commitments in life. Oak allows the vital energies to flow naturally through the body, as the rigid fighting spirit begins to let go, and makes it possible to be as strong as an oak tree.

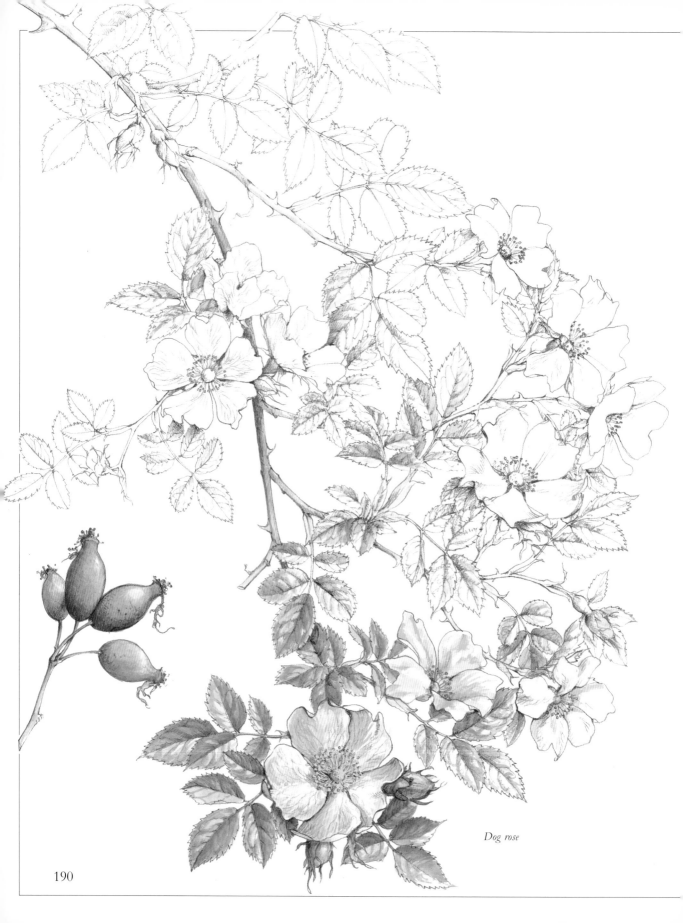

Dog rose

Rose

The flower of love

This beautiful, most sensuous and romantic of flowers has inspired poets and artists for centuries as the symbol of love and beauty. Its praises have been sung and its beauty depicted in art since the days of the early Greeks; a rose in a Minoan fresco dated 1500–1600BC is probably the gallica rose, often called the damask rose and the one most often used in apothecary.

The rose, of all flowers, is probably the one most steeped in legend and symbolism. According to Greek myth, the goddess of flowers, Chloris, one day found the body of a beautiful nymph and asked the help of the Three Graces to create a very special flower out of the lifeless body of the nymph. The Graces gave the flower joy, brightness and charm. Then she asked Aphrodite the goddess of love to give the flower beauty, Dionysus the god of wine to add a special nectar to create a beautiful perfume, and Zephyr the wind god to blow away the clouds so that the precious flower could open her petals to the sun. Thus the rose was born and was crowned the Queen of Flowers, the emblem of Venus, and the symbol of love.

According to Eastern traditions the original rose was stirred into life by the first rays of the rising sun in the Great Garden of Persia, and since then its seeds have been carried over and spread to all lands. When a soul knocked at the door of the next world and all material things had to be left behind only the red rose was allowed to accompany that soul over the threshold.

There are other legends telling how the red rose obtained its colour. The Romans said that Venus blushed when Jupiter caught her bathing and the white rose turned red in her reflection. The Greeks tell how Aphrodite and Persephone were both lovers of Adonis, and when Aphrodite wanted to prevent Adonis from returning to her rival Persephone, she asked Ares, God of war, to help; so Adonis was attacked by a wild boar while out hunting, and flying to his aid Aphrodite scratched herself on a white rose. Red roses sprung up where Adonis and Aphrodite's blood had spilled, and the white roses turned red in sympathy.

According to the Persians, a nightingale began to sing when roses first bloomed, and overcome by their heady perfume it dropped to the earth. Its spilled blood stained the petals, turning them from white to red.

In early Christianity the red rose became the symbol of martyrs' blood, and life after death, and the white rose the symbol of innocence and purity, spirituality and virginity, dedicated to the Virgin Mary. At first the rose was unacceptable to the Christians because of its association with Venus, the goddess of carnal love, but gradually it was taken on as the emblem of divine love and heavenly joy. The rose was depicted in Christian paintings of the garden of heaven, along with the lily and the pink.

The perfection of the rose symbolized all that was ideal and from paradise. It was also emblematic of the heart or mystic centre of being. The philosophers and alchemists who founded the secret society the Rosicrucians, in the 15th century, had a rose mounted on a cross as their symbol.

The birthplace of the cultivated rose was probably Northern Persia, now Iran, from where it was taken to Turkey, Greece, Italy and the rest of Europe. Roman emperors would fill their swimming baths and fountains with rose-scented water.

The Romans decorated their banqueting halls with roses, and strewed the floors with them to fill the place with their enchanting scent. Brides and bridegrooms were crowned with roses; they were scattered on the marriage bed, and worn as garlands at feasts, apparently to prevent drunkeness. They were associated with joy, merriment and wine, but they were also scattered on graves of the dead at funerals, and white and red roses were planted on lovers' tombs, perhaps to compare the short span of human life to the quick-fading life of the rose.

Since those early days the rose has been extolled not only for its beauty and perfume but also for its medicinal virtues. Greek doctors used the champagne rose as a tonic. Pliny listed 32 medicines prepared from roses.

Avicenna in the 10th century praised the rose and was the first to make rose water. He used rose jelly to cure spitting of blood. Around the turn of the 16th century otto or attar of roses was discovered in Persia, now a major ingredient in perfumes and soaps, and widely used in aromatherapy.

NB Rose can stimulate the uterus so the herb and oil should be avoided in pregnancy

Herbal remedy and Aromatherapy oil

Both the leaves and petals of roses have a cooling effect and have been used in tea to bring down fevers and to clear toxins and heat from the body which produces rashes and inflammatory problems. They also enhance immunity, helping to restrain the development of infections by clearing heat and toxins from the system. An infusion of rose petals can relieve cold and flu symptoms, sore throat, runny nose, as well as blocked bronchial tubes. An infusion or syrup of the petals or hips strengthens the lungs in their fight against infection. Roses help fight infection in the digestive tract and help re-establish the normal bacterial population of the intestine when it has been disrupted by antibiotics or faulty diet.

Rose hips, rose petals and rose oil have an uplifting and wonderfully restoring effect on the nervous system. They calm the nerves, relieve insomnia, lift depression, dispel mental and physical fatigue and soothe irritability, grief and anger. Their calming effect on the heart eases palpitations. Oil of roses is used in aromatherapy for depression and anxiety, for all problems of the heart and for those who lack love in their lives.

Rose petals have a decongestant action in the female reproductive system. They have been used to relieve uterine congestion causing pain and heavy periods, as well as for irregular periods, infertility and to enhance sexual desire – perhaps this is why roses have always been associated with love. In men they have been used to treat impotence. In aromatherapy oil of rose is used to treat a wide variety of reproductive ailments, as well as emotional stresses which are related to sexuality causing, for example, frigidity or impotence. Rose makes a good remedy for premenstrual syndrome and for emotional difficulties around the menopause. It makes an excellent remedy for women who feel insecure about their sexuality, and lacking in confidence in loving, intimate relationships.

Like the seeds, rose petals have a diuretic effect, relieving fluid retention and hastening elimination of wastes through the urinary system. They have been used for stones and gravel in the kidneys and bladder. They contain tannins which have an astringent effect throughout the body, staunching bleeding, drying phlegm and arresting discharges. In the digestive system this helps reduce hyperacidity and overactivity bringing excessive hunger and thirst and often mouth ulcers. An infusion makes a useful remedy for diarrhoea, enteritis and dysentery.

The hips of the wild rose, *R. canina*, were found just before the Second World War to contain one of the most abundant sources of vitamin C in the plant kingdom. They are also rich in vitamins A, B and K. They were made into rose hip syrup which was then rationed in Britain in wartime to ensure children's resistance to infection. This syrup or a decoction made from the empty seed cases makes a remedy for diarrhoea, stomach and menstrual cramps, nausea and indigestion. They are used as a laxative, for kidney problems and as a detoxifying agent.

Externally, rose water has been used to cleanse and tone the skin, to prevent and smooth out wrinkles, to clear skin blemishes and inflammation such as acne and spots, boils and abscesses. It can be used to bathe sore, tired or inflamed eyes, and to promote tissue repair. It helps to prevent infection of minor cuts and wounds, and to reduce the swelling of bruises and sprains. An infusion of rose petals can be used as a mouthwash for mouth ulcers or inflamed, bleeding gums, a gargle for sore throats and a douche for vaginal discharge.

Rose oil or ointment makes a good lipsalve and an infusion of rose petals in wine or vinegar added to the bath relieves arthritis and rheumatism.

The flower essence

The rose is the symbol of love. The red rose increases confidence in those feeling insecure about their sexuality and who suffer from feelings of shame or timidity about their bodies. It helps you to open up to love and bring your desires into action.

The white rose is quietly inspiring and strengthening, renewing energy and joy in your life. The white rosebud can be given to infants and children to help them grow up, keeping a sense of heaven on earth.

The wild rose is the remedy of independence. It is traditionally said to mean 'pleasure and pain' as it brings pleasure to the eyes and heart when found blooming in the wild, but pain from its sharp prickles if you try to pluck it. Wild rose warms the heart and softens the emotions, engendering an easy-going feeling to enhance sensuality.

Rosemary

The flower of loyalty

Even to smell the scent of the leaves
keep one youngly.
    BANKES

Rosemary is an aromatic perennial, native to the Mediterranean and many parts of Europe, especially coastal areas; it derives its name from the sea – Rosmarinus means dew of the sea. Rosemary is traditionally the herb of friendship and remembrance, and has played an important part in ceremonies associated with marriage, love and death through the ages. It was believed to bring luck and joy, so artisans wove it into royal crowns for kings and emperors, and into posies and veils for brides. It was also a symbol of love and loyalty, sacred to Venus or Aphrodite, the goddess of love who rose from the sea.

Anne of Cleves, fourth bride of Henry VIII of England, is said to have worn a circlet of gold and precious stones intertwined with sprigs of rosemary, though it did not bring her much luck. It was traditionally known to strengthen the memory, perhaps explaining its use as a symbol of fidelity, particularly in Italy and in Portugal where rosemary was placed in the slippers of the bride and groom so that they would remain loyal to each other. Shakespeare refers to rosemary's association with memory, for Hamlet tells Ophelia, 'Here's rosemary for remembrance .... I pray you love remember'. A sprig of rosemary was given to mourners at funerals, as a symbol of immortality, fidelity and fertility in the next life, to place in the coffin before it was lowered into the ground. The pharaohs of Ancient Egypt put rosemary in their tombs, a custom the Welsh continue today. Some say that rosemary was used to protect a man's soul throughout eternity from evil, and so it was placed in the hands of the departed as they lay in their coffin.

Herbal remedy

Like other aromatic herbs, rosemary contains volatile oils which are antiseptic with antibacterial and antifungal properties, and which enhance the function of the immune system. Because of this, rosemary was believed to protect from pestilence and disease, as well as from evil and witchcraft. Nurses brewed rosemary tea as an antiseptic wash in delivery rooms to protect mother and baby from infection and to sterilize the instruments. Tubfuls of dried rosemary leaves mixed with juniper berries were burnt to fumigate hospitals and dispel the foul air of disease and death there and in the homes of the sick. In the streets ladies of delicate health carried fresh rosemary to disguise bad odours and protect against disease.

Gerard advised a garland of rosemary to be worn around the neck to relieve 'stuffing of the head and a cold brain'. A hot tea can be taken for chasing away colds, sore throats, flu, coughs and chest infections. By causing sweating, and increasing circulation to the skin, it will bring down fevers. It used to be the remedy for tuberculosis, and smoked for coughs and flu or *la grippe*. Culpeper advised 'leaves shred small and taken in a pipe, as tobacco is taken, helpeth those that have any cough, phthisick or consumption'. The warming and stimulating effects of rosemary help clear phlegm from the head and chest, indicating its old use as a remedy for catarrh, coughs, wheezing, bronchitis and whooping cough. Its relaxant effects help relieve spasm in the bronchial tubes in asthma.

Rosemary has long been considered a wonderful tonic particularly to the heart, brain and nervous system. The Renaissance herbalist of Strasbourg, Wilhelm Ryff, said of rosemary: 'The spirits of the Heart and entire body feel joy from this drink which dispels all despondency and worry'. By increasing the flow of blood to the brain, it stimulates the brain and heightens concentration and may account for the belief that rosemary improved the memory. It has been used as a folk remedy for fainting, nervousness, anxiety, exhaustion, lethargy, depression, insomnia, during convalescence and for the elderly. It has been said to cure apoplexy, dim sight, dizziness, drowsiness, drooping spirits, feebleness, palsy, convulsions, and even insanity. It was worn in a linen cloth tied around the right arm to make the wearer 'light and merrie'. It was also reputed to have aphrodisiac powers. John Evelyn found that rubbing his closed eyelids with rosemary in wine strengthened his sight as well as the rest of his senses.

By stimulating blood flow to the head, and relaxing tense muscles, rosemary when taken frequently makes an excellent remedy for preventing migraines and headaches. It has a warming effect throughout the body as it also stimulates the heart and general circulation. It dispels cold and the winter blues, and the lethargy and weakness associated with it, warms cold hands and feet and prevents chilblains. It has been used for varicose veins, tendency to bruising, and arteriosclerosis.

Rosemary's warming and invigorating qualities improve vitality, and have a stimulating effect on the digestion, relieving flatulence and distension, enhancing the appetite and increasing the flow of digestive juices. It helps move food and wastes efficiently through the system, removes stagnant food, improves sluggish digestion and helps the absorption of nutrients so that maximum benefit is derived from the diet – so it is not just taste that makes rosemary such a wonderful aid to cooking. The bitters in rosemary stimulate the action of the liver and gall-bladder, increasing the flow of bile and aiding digestion of fats. By enhancing liver function rosemary will help to clear toxins from the system that may account for headaches, lethargy, irritability and general malaise. It used to be sold in apothecaries as a cure for hangovers, and was considered excellent for jaundice, gallstones, 'liverishness', and, by cleansing the system of impurities and wastes, for gout, arthritis and as a remedy to clear the skin.

Rosemary also helps the elimination of wastes through the urinary system as it works as a diuretic, increasing the flow of urine. Rosemary was the main ingredient of Hungary water, an old recipe apparently given in the 14th century to Izabella, Queen of Hungary by a hermit, whom she later believed to be an angel. She was aged 72, 'infirm of limb and afflicted with gout' and after one year of using the preparation she recovered her health, strength and beauty to the extent that the King of Poland wanted to marry her. She had prepared the Hungary water from alcohol and rosemary flowers and taken 1 dram once a week, and washed her face with it each morning and rubbed it on her limbs. From this story and many before it, rosemary has gained the reputation of slowing the ageing process, when taken regularly. Recent research has shown that it is a powerful antioxidant and may therefore do just that.

The tannins in rosemary leaves have an astringent effect, checking bleeding and reducing excessive menstruation. Its relaxant effect in the uterus relieves period pains and helps to regulate periods.

Externally, a bath with a few drops of rosemary oil makes an excellent pick-me-up when aching or feeling tired at the end of the day. It is stimulating and relaxing at the same time, so it makes a good

early morning bath too. A dilute oil rubbed onto the skin is warming and invigorating, and by bringing blood to the skin speeds healing and helps resolve inflammation. It can be used for cuts, wounds, sores, chilblains, scalds and burns, and as a general tonic to the skin. As a beauty aid a rosemary lotion can be used to reduce wrinkles and puffiness under the eyes. The oil massaged into painful swollen joints will bring relief; rubbed into the scalp it will check hair fall and condition the hair. It is frequently made into shampoos and hair conditioners for this reason. It has been used to treat scabies and lice.

Rosemary tea can be used as a douche for vaginal infections and discharge and used as a mouthwash for bleeding gums and loose teeth.

The fresh leaves can be chewed to sweeten the breath and to combat infection of the teeth and gums. The oil rubbed into the temples relieves tension and headaches and can be inhaled to dispel drowsiness and increase concentration. A wreath of rosemary was often worn round the heads of students to enhance memory and concentration.

Aromatherapy oil

The essential oil of rosemary reflects the use of the herbal remedy. It is a wonderful tonic to the nerves, the heart, circulation and digestion. Its refreshing and invigorating aroma is stimulating, awakening and strengthening, good for tiredness, lethargy, nervous debility, weak memory and poor concentration. It wakens the senses and clarifies the mind, and has an uplifting effect emotionally, helping to dispel low spirits and depression. It can be used to rekindle energy at the end of a long day, to enhance concentration during mental work, and to help clarify the mind during meditation. It has also been used where there is diminishing of the senses, such as loss of smell or dimness of sight. It also has analgesic properties and helps to dull pain, as in arthritis, rheumatism and neuralgia. It is a rejuvenative oil.

The flower essence

The colour blue represents heaven and eternity, wisdom and truth and blue or purple is associated with the crown chakra, related to inner peace and ecstasy. The blue-purple flowers of rosemary bring clarity of mind, and peace and balance to the emotions, enabling a meditative state. The remedy increases sensitivity both physically and emotionally, and enhances creativity. It symbolizes the blooming of higher thought forms in the midst of activity.

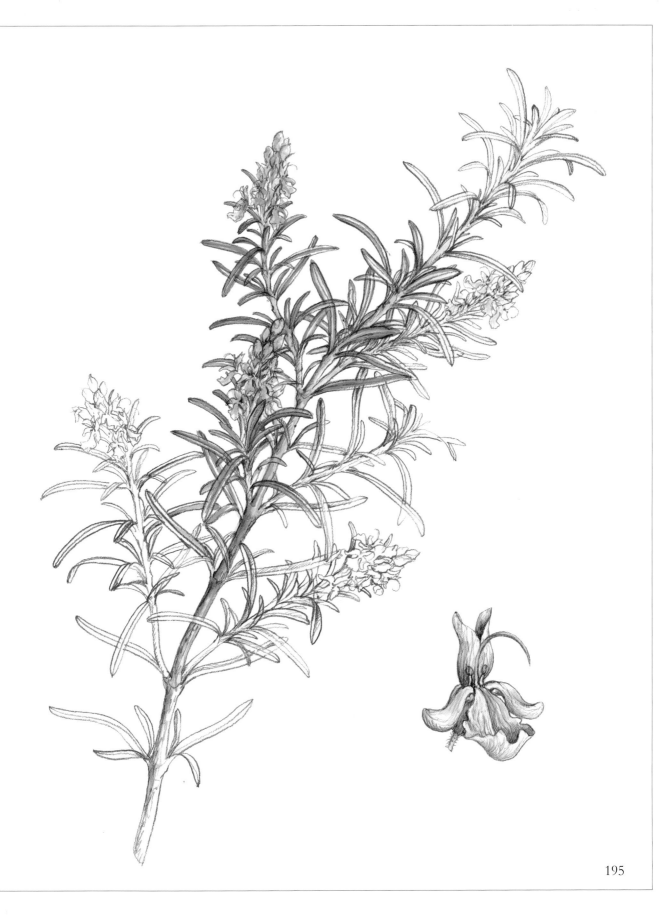

195

Castor oil plant

The flower of vitality

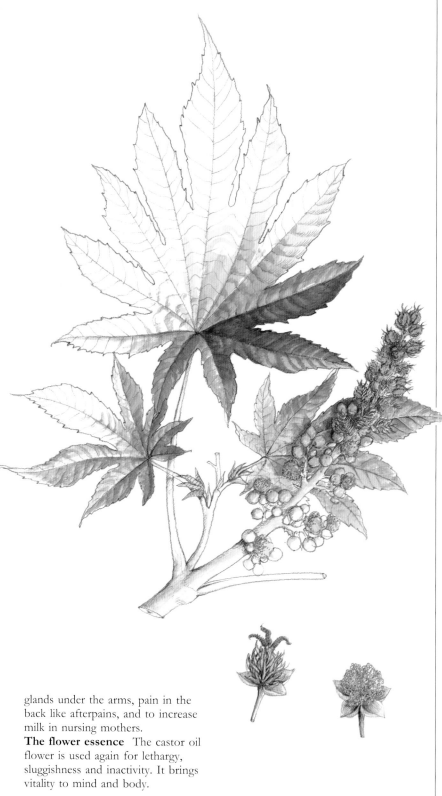

This handsome perennial has seeds containing a pale yellow almost colourless oil, which has been used as medicine for thousands of years. Seeds have been found in Egyptian tombs dating back 4000 years. It was used as a purgative by the Ancient Egyptians; the Greeks used it similarly and externally for sores and abscesses. Turner and Gerard used it externally in skin diseases, to relieve irritation and itching of the skin as in ringworm, and even recommended it for leprosy.

Herbal remedy Castor oil was considered one of the most useful and indispensable medicines for clearing the bowels, for acute constipation, and to remove irritant toxins from the bowel. It relieves colic and diarrhoea caused by indigestible food, or from infection, as well as in the early stages of dysentery. The leaves are used in India to stimulate breastmilk, when applied to the breasts or taken internally.

Castor oil clears the bowel thoroughly with one dose, and produces a semi-soft stool within 2–8 hours. When it reaches the intestine it releases irritant acid which stimulates the whole of the intestines, producing its aperient action. The lubricating oil produces an effortless bowel movement without any griping. It should only be used for acute problems and never over a long period, for its initial purgative action is followed by a binding one causing constipation. Nor should it be taken after treatment for worms.

Externally, castor oil can be applied to sore, dry, cracked skin or lips and sore nipples. It relieves itching of haemorrhoids.

Homeopathic remedy Ricinus is used specifically for the symptoms that indicate cholera or other severe bowel disorders. It is also given for swollen and painful breasts, swollen glands under the arms, pain in the back like afterpains, and to increase milk in nursing mothers.

The flower essence The castor oil flower is used again for lethargy, sluggishness and inactivity. It brings vitality to mind and body.

Clary sage
The flower of elation

Clary sage is a large, aromatic plant with velvety leaves, native to Syria, Italy, southern France and Switzerland. It has been used for its medicinal virtues since the time of the Ancient Greeks. Its name Clary comes from the Latin *sclarea*, derived from *clarus* meaning clear. One of its popular names is clear eye because the highly mucilaginous seeds in decoction will soothe eye irritation caused by foreign bodies. It is associated with the ability to see, in the widest sense. It can inhance inner perception, helpful in meditation.

Herbal remedy Clary sage is a relaxing tonic to the nervous system, and excellent for many stress-related problems. These include asthma, headaches, migraine, insomnia and indigestion. Its antispasmodic action can relieve muscle tension, abdominal pain and constipation, reduce period pains and ease childbirth. At the same time clary sage is strengthening, valuable for convalescents and mental and physical exhaustion. It can help lift the spirits in depression, including postnatal depression. It also relieves excessive perspiration.

Externally, clary sage has been applied to the skin to draw out boils, inflammation and infection.

Aromatherapy oil Clary sage oil can produce a heightened state of elation or euphoria in some, and in others can be deeply relaxing and sleep-inducing. It is highly recommended for relieving muscle tension, anxiety and stress-related problems. It can be used to relieve pain, such as headaches, gripping abdominal pain and pain during childbirth. The oil is particularly suitable for women's problems. It has an oestrogenic effect and will help to balance the emotions during the menopause. It is also a good remedy for PMS and period pain. It acts as an emmenagogue, bringing on suppressed peri-

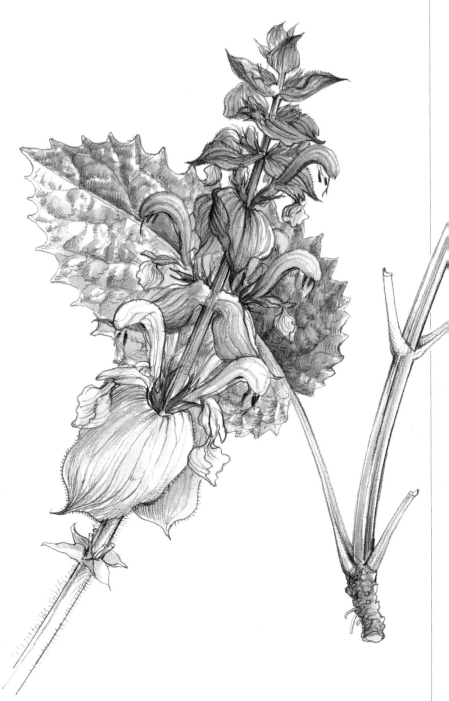

ods and stimulating the uterus, which is helpful in childbirth. Its relaxant effects help treat postnatal depression, and emotional and sexual problems, particularly when related to femininity and lack of

self-confidence. It encourages vivid dreams and can enhance creative work and imaginative ideas.

The flower essence The flower essence of sage, a close relative, is described on page 202.

Willow

The flower of strength in weakness

Thou are to all lost love the best
The only true plant found
Where with young men and maids distrest
And left of love are crowned.
  ROBERT HERRICK (1591-1674)

Of the 250 species of willow, the white willow and the black willow are most commonly used in healing. The white willow is a large elegant tree that grows by riverbanks and in damp places and can reach a height of 80 feet (24 metres). It can be found throughout Europe, North Africa and central Asia. The black or pussy willow is smaller, growing to around 20 feet (7 metres), also in damp areas, and is native to North America. It has a dark, rough bark. The name Salix comes from the Latin *saline* meaning to leap, for willows are very fast-growing. Small willow cuttings easily take root. For this reason, the white willow has come to represent purification and rebirth, and is an emblem of fertility. Branches from the tree were used in 'beating the bounds', an annual walk around parish boundaries, a springtime ritual of purification. In Ancient Greece, the willow was the emblem of Artemis, the moon goddess who governed fertility, pregnancy and childbirth, agriculture, rivers and streams. Culpeper described the white willow as being ruled by the moon, and in pagan traditions, wood cut from the willow was used to make wands for lunar magic. The white willow is also depicted in poetry and art as a symbol of peace, patience and perseverance. To the Taoists, willow represents strength in weakness. In Japanese legend, the spine of the first human was made from willow.

The black willow has been associated with sadness and grief. Being under the dominion of the fickle moon, the willow represents forsaken love, the symbol of the rejected lover in the language of flowers.

Herbal remedy

According to the doctrine of signatures, willow grew in damp, rheumy places so was used to treat rheumatic stiffness, as well as the aching in the muscles that accompanies flu and other infections. It was also used for its ability to bring down fevers, even in malaria. In 1763 the Reverend Edward Stone gave decoctions of the bark to rheumatism sufferers. He later isolated the active component salicin from the willow, from which is produced salicylic acid, the basis of aspirin. Willow bark is an excellent remedy for all the symptoms which are relieved by aspirin. Its astringent properties help to curb diarrhoea and dysentery, and to stem bleeding. It can be used for heavy periods, and externally to treat cuts and wounds. Willow can be made into gargles for sore throats, and mouthwashes for mouth ulcers and bleeding gums. As a diuretic willow reduces fluid retention and helps eliminate toxins from the body via the urinary system. Willow can be used for head colds, flu, fevers, and as a tonic to restore strength after illness. The willow is likely to be a good remedy for circulatory problems, because, like aspirin, it helps prevent rapid blood clotting. The black willow has very similar properties to the white willow, and acts as a sexual sedative. It helps to clear congestion and pain in the ovarian and uterine area, and helps take away or lessen sexual desire.

Homeopathic remedy: SALIX NIGRA

Salix nigra is said to moderate sexual passion and is prescribed for irritability of the genitals, pain in the testes and ovaries, painful periods, ovarian congestion and heavy periods, which are often related to fibroids. Salix is a good remedy, like the herb, for diarrhoea, sore gums, weakness after illness and aching muscles accompanying a fever.

The flower essence

Salix vitellina is used as a Bach Flower Remedy for people who tend to be bitter and resentful. Willow people tend to blame others for their perceived misfortune, and begrudge others their better fortune. Such people are unable to see that their negative and destructive attitudes have much to do with their disappointment. Willow people are quietly resentful and tend to sulk, spreading their negativity to others, and are not cheered by attempts to help them or lift their spirits, accepting them as their right. They take little interest in others' lives and can become increasingly isolated. Willow helps people to recognize their negativity and accept responsibility for it, so they can change their outlook on life, and shape their own destiny, rather than being a victim of it.

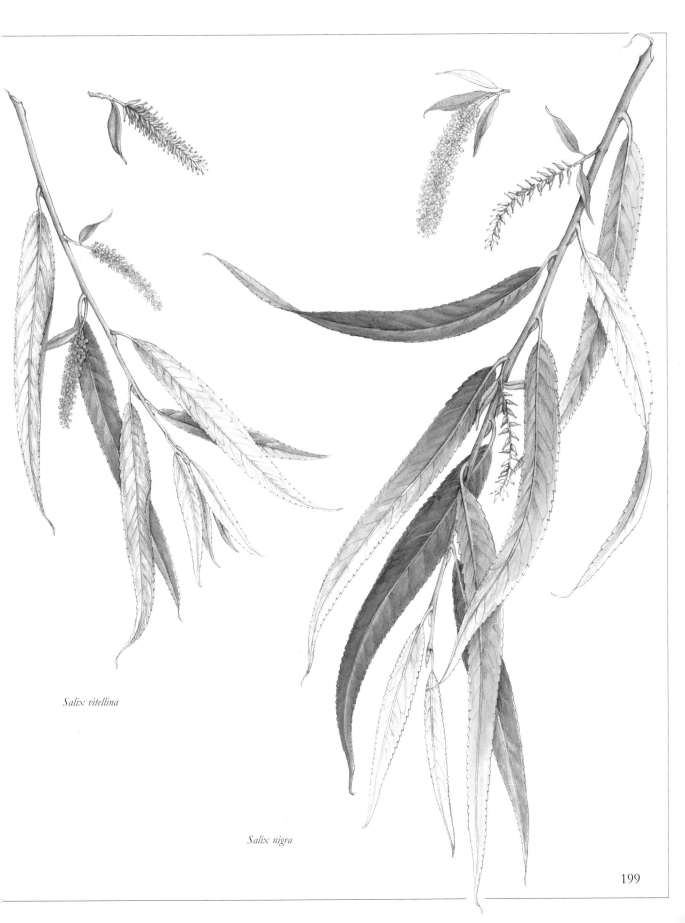

Salix vitellina

Salix nigra

Sage

The flower of immortality

He that would live for aye
Should eat sage in May.
OLD ENGLISH SAYING

Sage – the very word suggests wisdom and old age and it is these themes that permeate the use of this wonderful plant in its healing history. The Ancient Greeks considered sage could render man immortal and it became known as the immortality herb perhaps because it was seen to cure so many ills but also because it had the power to enhance inner wisdom which goes beyond the realm of our physical form. Theophrastus (c. 372–287BC) said it 'drove away the evils of illness and old age' and the Ancient Egyptians revered it as a giver and saver of life and used it for treating the plague. The Romans considered it sacred and prized it so highly that harvesting the leaves was an important ceremony, rather than an ordinary gardening activity. They gathered the aromatic leaves not with iron but with bronze and silver tools and harvesters were required to be barefoot, clean, and dressed in white tunics. Before it was harvested sacrifices of food and wine were offered to the gods. Like the Egyptians, they believed sage helped to give as well as protect life, and gave the herb as a fertility remedy to women wanting to conceive. In the Middle Ages sage had a wide reputation as a rejuvenating tonic. It was a major ingredient in prescriptions for longevity and elixirs of life. It was considered a brain and nerve tonic to strengthen the mind and the memory, enliven the senses, lift dull spirits, banish lethargy and restore failing virility. It was prescribed for depression, anxiety, nervousness, migraine, insomnia and nervous exhaustion. Sage was given during convalescence and to the elderly to reduce the signs and symptoms of ageing.

The botanic name Salvia comes from the Latin word *salvare* meaning to save or cure. In English sage means wise.

Sage can be propagated by seeds, cuttings, layering or root division. It will grow in most soil but likes good drainage, sufficient nitrogen and full sun.

Herbal remedy

Sage is highly antiseptic with antibacterial and antifungal properties. In the past it would have helped with intestinal and chest infections which could often have been fatal. Sage tea is an excellent remedy for colds, fevers and sore throats and can be taken at the first symptoms of any respiratory infection. It can be used for tonsillitis, bronchitis, asthma, catarrh and sinusitis. It is an old remedy for TB and other infections accompanied by night sweats. It can be used to enhance the immune system and prevent infection as well as for auto-immune disease. It has cleansing properties and acts as a diuretic making it useful in toxic conditions and for arthritis and gout.

Sage makes a good digestive remedy as it relaxes spasm and relieves colic and griping. It stimulates the appetite and improves digestion and has a beneficial action on the liver. It has been traditionally used in cooking with rich and heavy foods to aid their digestion. It can be given for anorexia, indigestion, wind, nausea, bad breath, excessive salivation, diarrhoea, colitis, liver and gall-bladder problems and worms.

Sage has a tonic effect on the female reproductive tract and can be used for scanty menstruation, irregular or absent periods, menstrual cramps and heavy bleeding. Its oestrogenic properties make sage excellent for menopausal problems, particularly as it has the added bonus of reducing sweating, and relieving hot flushes and night sweats. Its stimulating effect on the uterus can be put to good effect during childbirth and to expel the placenta. For this reason sage should not be taken during pregnancy. Neither is it recommended while breastfeeding as it stops the flow of milk, though making it useful when weaning.

Sage has a beneficial action on the central nervous system. In Ayurvedic medicine it is used to clear emotional obstructions from the mind and for promoting calmness and clarity. It curbs excessive desire and passions and calms the heart. Recent research has shown that sage has strong antioxidant properties, helping to delay the ageing process and reduce the harmful effect of free radicals.

Externally, sage is a first rate antiseptic and astringent for cuts and wounds, burns, sores, sunburn and ulcers. It makes a lotion for inflammatory skin conditions, and a liniment for painful joints. It is used as a gargle for sore throats and a mouthwash for mouth ulcers, inflamed gums and excessive salivation, and a douche to relieve vaginal infections such as thrush.

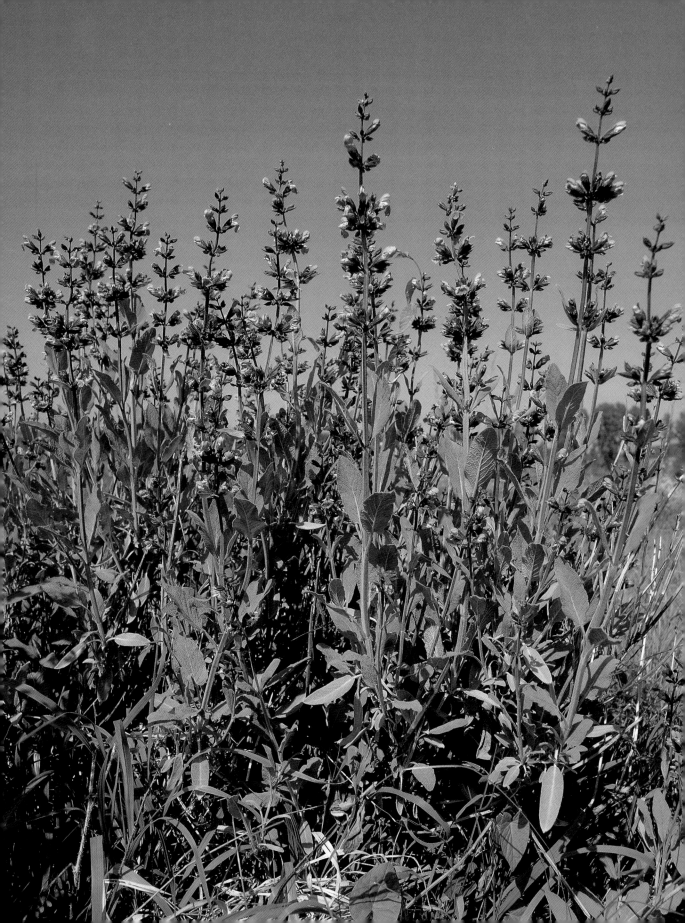

Homeopathic remedy: SALVIA OFFICINALIS

Sage is used for night sweats, particularly those in TB sufferers when associated with a tickly cough.

Aromatherapy oil

The essential oil of sage is used but only with great caution. The high proportion of thujone in the oil could, if used in large amounts, cause epileptic fits, convulsions or even paralysis. It is interesting that when used as a herbal remedy sage acts as a tonic to the nervous system and was a medieval cure for palsy, since the thujone is far less concentrated in the whole plant than in the extracted oil. In the uterus the use of the oil can stimulate contraction of uterine muscles, which can be useful during childbirth, but should be avoided during pregnancy because of the risk of miscarriage. It can also induce heavy menstrual bleeding. Sage's relative, clary sage, contains a much lower concentration of thujone and shares many of its properties; its use is preferred when treating women as it is a much gentler remedy.

Sage oil can be used in gargles and mouthwashes when diluted with water and alcohol to a low concentration (1 drop per 10 ml of liquid) or a few drops in a bowl of hot water can be used as an inhalation for coughs, colds and catarrh. It can also be used in massage oils for men – it is warming and penetrating to the muscles, particularly useful for men with muscles developed from taking part in sports or weight training.

The flower essence

Sage enhances the capacity for drawing wisdom from experience and is particularly recommended for people who find it hard to find purpose and meaning in life. They may feel resentful about events in their lives, seeing them as ill-fated or undeserved.

Sage is a remedy especially suitable for our later years, for helping to accept what life throws up for us in a calm and detached way. It helps to enhance the wisdom that comes naturally from years of experience. Such wisdom is natural to that end of life, enabling us to be in touch with our spiritual selves, to perceive a higher purpose in life and to experience inner peace. It is a remedy to use during changes and transitions, as it enhances the sage in all of us.

Elder

The flower of fairyland

The whole of the beautiful elder tree has been valued for its practical and medicinal uses for thousands of years. Elder has been considered sacred and magical in folklore and mythology, and has always been treated with great respect. The dryad that was said to live in the tree was consulted before any part of it was used. A Danish legend holds that if you stand under an elder tree on Midsummer's Eve you will see the King of Fairyland ride by attended by all his retinue.

Elder trees are found throughout the countryside along hedgerows, woods and in gardens in central and southern Europe, the British Isles, and North Africa. It was always grown near English cottages to grant protection against witches and evil influences. In some traditions, elder is regarded as holy wood and therefore is never struck by lightning; witches fear it for the same reason. Gypsies maintain that the whole plant is beneficial to man, so they never burn it. Perhaps this is why there are so many superstitions about bringing elder into the house, which is said to be unlucky. However, the Serbs used to take a stick of elder to wedding ceremonies to bring good luck, and in Poland it is customary to bury sins under an elder tree, where the tree's power will absorb them. In Russia it is thought that elder prolongs life; in other traditions elderberries are placed under the pillow to bestow peaceful sleep and a twig is carried to prevent the temptation to commit adultery. Pregnant women have been known to kiss the tree for good fortune for the baby.

The name elder derives from *ellar* or *kindlar*, because its hollow branches were used as blow tubes to kindle a fire. The botanical name Sambucus derives from the Greek musical instrument made of its wood, the sambuke, a kind of pan-pipe; nigra refers to the colour of the berries. When the masses of creamy-white fragrant flowers blossom in the countryside it is a signal that summer has arrived, and when the branches droop with purple-black berries, summer has gone the autumn has come.

Herbal remedy

Medicinally the elder tree has been called 'the medicine chest of the country people' and John Evelyn writing in 1664 said, 'If the medicinal properties of its leaves, bark and berries were fully known, I cannot tell what our countrymen would ail for which he might not fetch a remedy from every hedge, either for sickness or wounds'.

The flowers are principally used therapeutically and when taken in hot infusion they make a wonderful remedy for the onset of upper respiratory infections – colds, tonsillitis, laryngitis and flu – so characteristic of cold, damp climates. With the first signs of malaise – aching, sore throat, chills, restlessness and fever – elderflowers will stimulate the circulation and cause sweating, cleansing the system by elimination of toxins through the pores of the skin and thereby resolving the fever and infection. They are also recommended at the onset of eruptive diseases such as measles and chickenpox to bring out the rash and speed recovery. They also have a decongestant action, reducing and moving phlegm, and should be taken in hot infusion (often combined with yarrow and peppermint) for colds, catarrh, sinusitis, hay fever as well as bronchial congestion in chest infections and asthma. The relaxant effect of elderflowers is a bonus in respect of the latter, relieving bronchospasm and catarrh at the same time in the asthma sufferer.

Elderflowers enhance the action of the kidneys and so act further as a decongestant, relieving fluid retention in the body, eliminating toxins and clearing heat from the system via the urinary system. They have been used to reduce inflammation in rheumatism, gout and arthritis, especially that which is aggravated by cold, damp conditions. An elder twig used to be carried about in the pocket by country people to protect against rheumatism.

Elderflowers also have a long history of use as a relaxant, soothing nerves, allaying anxiety and lifting depression. A hot infusion at night-time will induce a restful sleep and is particularly useful for restless or irritable children at the onset of infections, to encourage healing rest, allowing the body to carry out its recuperative work.

Externally, elderflowers have traditionally been used to soothe inflammation and to heal ulcers, burns, cuts and wounds, either using the infusion as a lotion or when incorporated into an ointment. An infusion can be used as a gargle for sore throats, a mouthwash for mouth ulcers and inflamed gums, and an eyewash for conjunctivitis and sore, tired eyes. It also makes a good lotion for chilblains, skin eruptions, sunburn, any irritable skin condition and itching piles. Distilled elder water makes an excellent toning and cleansing lotion for the face.

Elderflowers can be made into deliciously refreshing summer drinks such as champagne and cordial. They also make an excellent addition to pancakes and fritters, jams, sorbets and cheesecakes. The delicious juicy berries make a tasty combination with stewed blackberries and apple, and can be eaten for their laxative effect. They are rich in vitamins A and C and used to be made into syrups and wines for preventing and treating coughs and colds and to bring down fevers, and into conserves for sore throats. They were also used to relieve neuralgia and sciatica. Until the end of the 19th century hot elderberry wine was sold on London streets on cold winter days and nights to cheer travellers and workers. Cinnamon was often added to elderberry syrups and drinks to enhance their warming effect. The Romans used the berries for dyeing their hair.

The leaves have a variety of uses in folklore when applied externally. When picked fresh and warmed, they can be laid on the temples to relieve nervous headaches. Bruised leaves used to be worn in a hat or rubbed on to the face to prevent flies and insects from settling or biting (sometimes the leaves can cause a reaction on sensitive skins). An infusion can be used as a lotion to keep away midges and mosquitoes, and as an astringent remedy for wounds, bruises, burns, sprains, swollen joints and haemorrhoids.

The root and bark of elder are both strongly aperient and laxative and should not be taken unless under medical advice. They are emetic in large doses, diuretic, useful in arthritis and gout, and help to regulate irregular periods. Externally, they make a useful ointment for eczema and psoriasis and a decoction can be used as a mouthwash or gargle for infection and inflammation of the mouth and throat.

Homeopathic remedy: *SAMBUCUS*

Sambucus acts particularly on the respiratory organs and suits people who are easily frightened or fretful. Such people are prone to anxiety, trembling and restlessness, and their physical symptoms tend to be characterized by spasms. Fright may give rise to suffocative attacks of coughing when the face turns blue, as in asthma, croup or whooping cough. A child may wake suddenly in the night around midnight, crying and unable to breathe.

Like the herbal remedy, Sambucus is used for catarrh, colds and blocked noses, particularly in babies and children, and also for hoarseness with tenacious phlegm in the throat, and for phlegm in the chest. Profuse sweating in the daytime tends to accompany such symptoms. Sambucus will also help relieve fluid retention which causes oedema that may contribute to this excess of catarrh in the system. Other urinary symptoms such as cystitis and nephritis may also call for Sambucus. Fevers, with the skin becoming dry and burning at night, but breaking out in a sweat in the daytime, fevers without thirst, preceded by a dry cough and accompanied by dread of being uncovered also indicate Sambucus.

The flower essence

The folklore of the elder is echoed in its application as a flower essence. It is recommended for its ability to impart inner strength and to increase self-esteem, making it ideal for times of challenge and change in life, and when in need of courage and fortitude. It helps to calm fears and anxieties and engenders a sense of being nurtured and supported by a strong and stable inner energy.

Elder is an excellent remedy for children as well as adults. As a protective remedy, it is given to people feeling invaded or over-dominated by others, or overcrowded by fears and anxieties. Elder stimulates energy, vigour, resilience and joy, and our innate powers of recovery and renewal of energy.

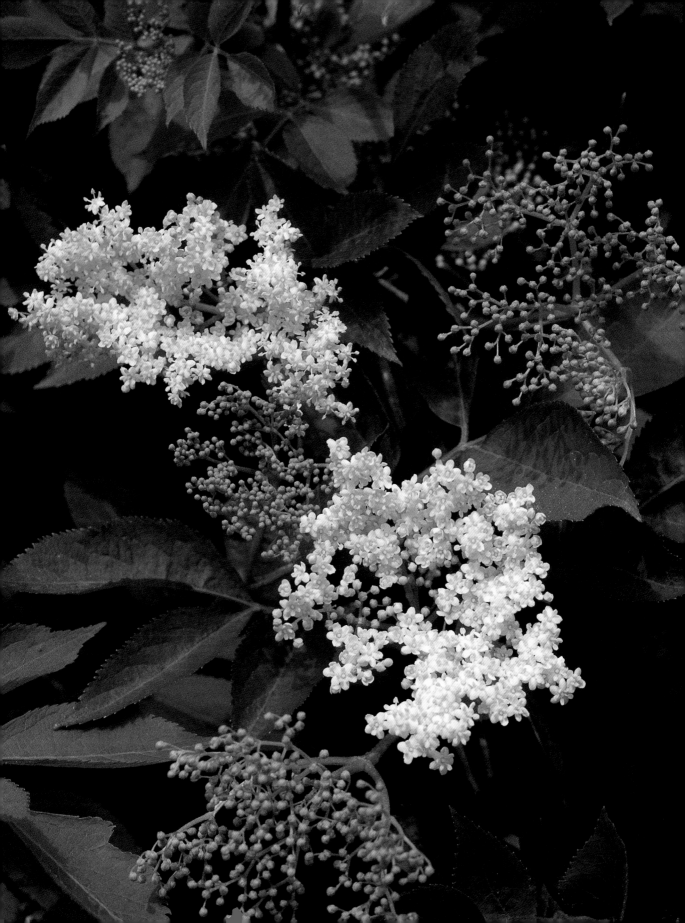

Skullcap

The flower of relaxation

Virginian skullcap, *Scutellaria laterifolia*, is indigenous to North America and grows in profusion in damp places, meadows and ditches, and by the sides of rivers and ponds. The name comes from the Latin *scutella* meaning a little cap which the calyx resembles, hence its common names hoodwort and helmet flower. Common skullcap (*Scutellaria galericulata*) and lesser skullcap (*Scutellaria minor*) are found in similar places in Britain. In America, Virginian skullcap is also known as mad-dog skullcap, or madweed, as it was said to cure rabies or hydrophobia, as well as every kind of nervous complaint in humans, even insanity. Traditionally, both the British and the American skullcaps have been highly valued for treating excitability, insomnia, epilepsy, convulsions, St Vitus's dance, hysteria, palsy, bites of poisonous insects and snakes and a whole range of other nervous symptoms. While they were held to cure infertility they were also recommended for people troubled by undue sexual desires.

Herbal remedy

Skullcap is one of the best nourishing tonics for the nervous system. The herbal remedy is made from the aerial parts of the plant. It is rich in minerals necessary for a healthy nervous system, and is greatly strengthening and supportive during stressful times. It is a wonderful remedy for all states of nervous tension, for headaches, agitation, anxiety, insomnia, hysteria, neurasthenia, exhaustion and depression. Its antispasmodic action is useful for twitching or jerking muscles, trembling, epilepsy (both petit and grand mal) cramps, menstrual pain and nervous heart palpitations. It is well worth using to aid withdrawal from orthodox tranquilizers and antidepressants, and is excellent when combined with hormone balancing herbs such as vitex or false unicorn root for PMS, and with sage, motherwort or both during

menopausal problems. Skullcap is an anti-inflammatory herb, and can be used for arthritis, particularly when aggravated by stress. The bitters help reduce fevers, enhance the digestion and stimulate the liver.

Homeopathic remedy: SCUTELLARIA

Scutellaria is a similarly wonderful medicine for a wide range of nervous problems. These include restlessness, excitability, being so tense one is unable to sleep or think, for hysteria, night terrors, heart irregularities and great agitation. It is prescribed for nervous debility after long illness, over-exertion, too much studying, overwork and for symptoms of a nervous breakdown. It is likewise used for epilepsy, convulsions, chorea, delirium tremens, nervousness or spasm in teething babies, and for a range of other stress-related problems including poor appetite, nausea, colic, hiccoughs, globus hystericus, muscle twitching, vertigo, cramps, nervous diarrhoea, frequent and scanty urination and severe headache, mostly at the back of the head.

The flower essence

Skullcap is used to benefit the nervous system and helps to alleviate the damage caused to the nerves by overuse of caffeine and drugs such as morphine and heroin. It can be used to help withdrawal symptoms from such drugs, and to remedy emotions often linked to drug addiction such as anxiety, low self-esteem, and a feeling of inability to cope with life. It is said to act on the pineal gland, enhancing the secretion of endorphins (natural opiate-like substances) and engendering a sense of physical and emotional wellbeing. Used in massage oils it helps to relax nerves and muscles, and a dab of the flower essence over the medulla oblongata is said to increase psychic healing ability, and to attune one to accepting healing more fully from others.

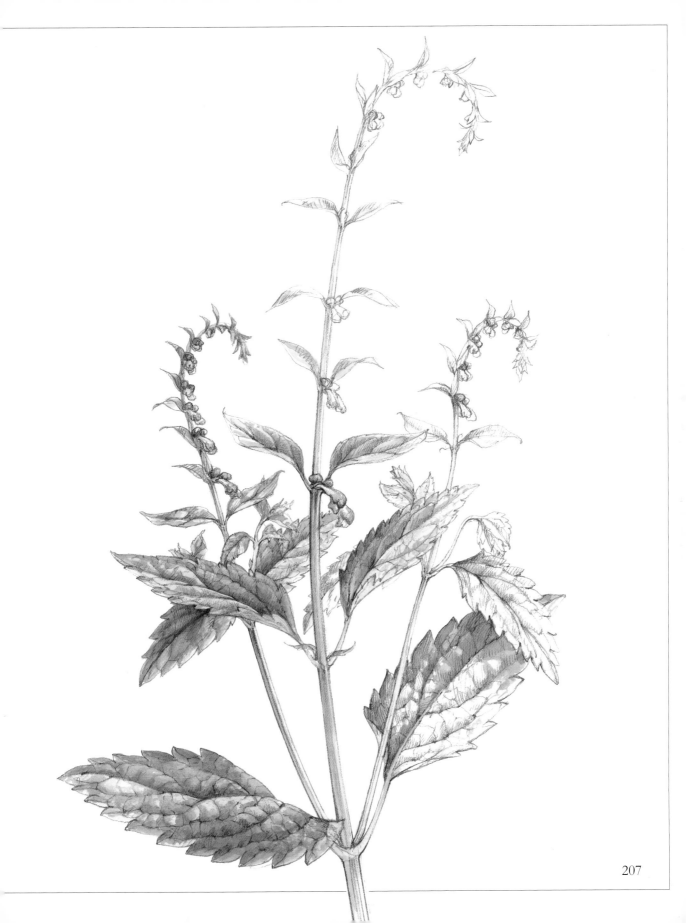

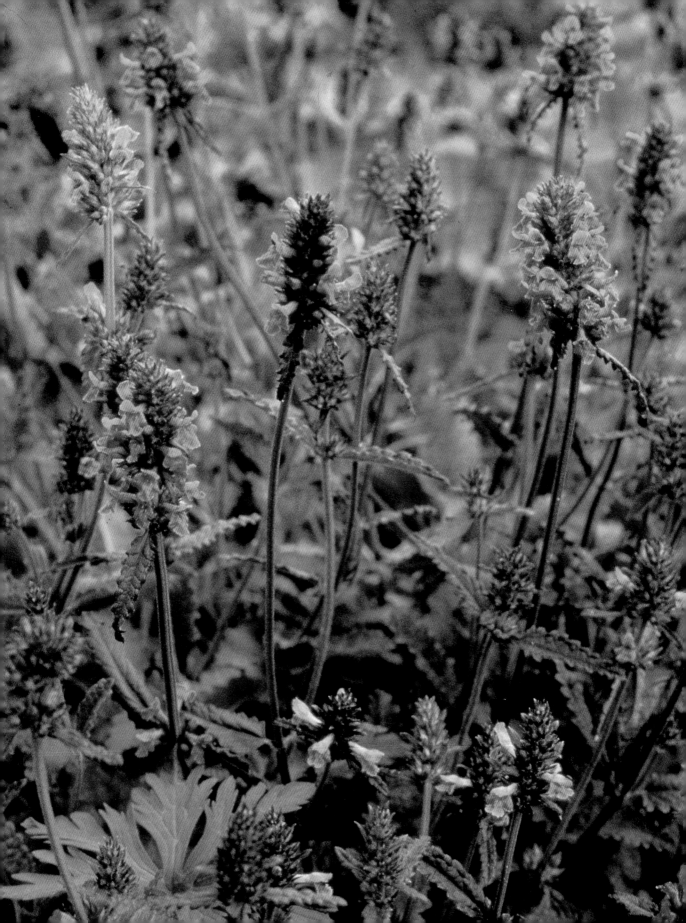

Wood betony

The flower of detachment

Wood betony grows in woods and copses, but can be found flourishing on heaths and moors, in meadows and country lanes. In the Middle Ages it was cultivated in the physic gardens of apothecaries and in monastery gardens as it was considered a panacea for all ills. It can still be found growing around the sites of ancient monasteries, as well as in churchyards, where it was planted for protection against evil. Wood betony was also worn around the neck as an amulet. Erasmus said it sanctified those who carried it about them and it was 'good against fearful visions', while the Ancient Greeks held, 'it is good whether for the man's soul or for his body; it shields him against visions and dreams, and the wort is very wholesome'. It was a religious herb of the Celts.

Few herbs have been more highly praised for their healing properties than wood betony. A whole treatise was written on its virtues by Antonius Musa, chief physician to the Emperor Augustus, showing it as a cure for no fewer than 47 diseases. Two old European proverbs illustrate the high regard in which wood betony was held. The Italians said, 'sell your coat and buy betony', while the Spaniards said of a good man, 'he has as many virtues as betony'.

Herbal remedy

The name betonica comes from the Celtic *ben* meaning head, and *tonic* meaning good – referring to its use for conditions associated with the head. The remedy, made from the aerial parts, has been used for inveterate headaches. It relieves those related to poor circulation to the head by improving the circulation; it helps those related to a sluggish liver by enhancing the liver's action, and those related to tension as it is a relaxant. It was taken internally, smoked and powdered as snuff for headaches, and when mixed with powdered eyebright, used to clear congestion in the head from colds and catarrh.

Wood betony acts as a tonic to the nervous system, relieving tension and anxiety, lifting depression and soothing pain, particularly nerve pain as in sciatica. It has also been used for arthritis, gout and rheumatism. It has a beneficial effect on the digestive tract and liver, useful for nervous indigestion, liver and gall-bladder problems.

Its astringent effect is also useful when treating diarrhoea, colds and catarrh. When taken as a hot tea, wood betony stimulates the circulation and helps to throw off colds and other infections – particularly those affecting the head. It contains trigonelline which lowers blood sugar, making wood betony useful to those suffering from diabetes.

Externally, the tannins make wood betony a useful astringent to stem bleeding, speed repair and repel infection of cuts and wounds, sores, ulcers, varicose veins and haemorrhoids. It can also be used for bruises, sprains and strains and was made into a lotion to beautify the skin.

Homeopathic remedy: STACHYS BETONICA

Stachys betonica is similarly used for problems affecting the head, and for colds and catarrh. It is prescribed for a feeling of fullness in the head and eyes, a heavy sleepy feeling, pain in the eyes and dizziness. These symptoms are relieved in the open air and aggravated by closing the eyes, moving or bending the head, looking at light, reading or thinking.

The flower essence

Wood betony relates to the head, and is said to enhance the function of the pineal gland, which secretes endorphins, natural opiates which engender a sense of physical and emotional wellbeing. It helps to bring inner calm and detachment, strengthening the desire for higher principles and goals, and has been used to help resolve conflicts between sexual desires and desires for greater enlightenment. A person using tantric practices in which sexual energies are potentially transformed into higher spiritual energies may gain help from wood betony, and the inner calm it brings should support a resolve of celibacy if that is the chosen path. It has been used for people of over-high sexual energy, and for those who are celibate through no choice of their own.

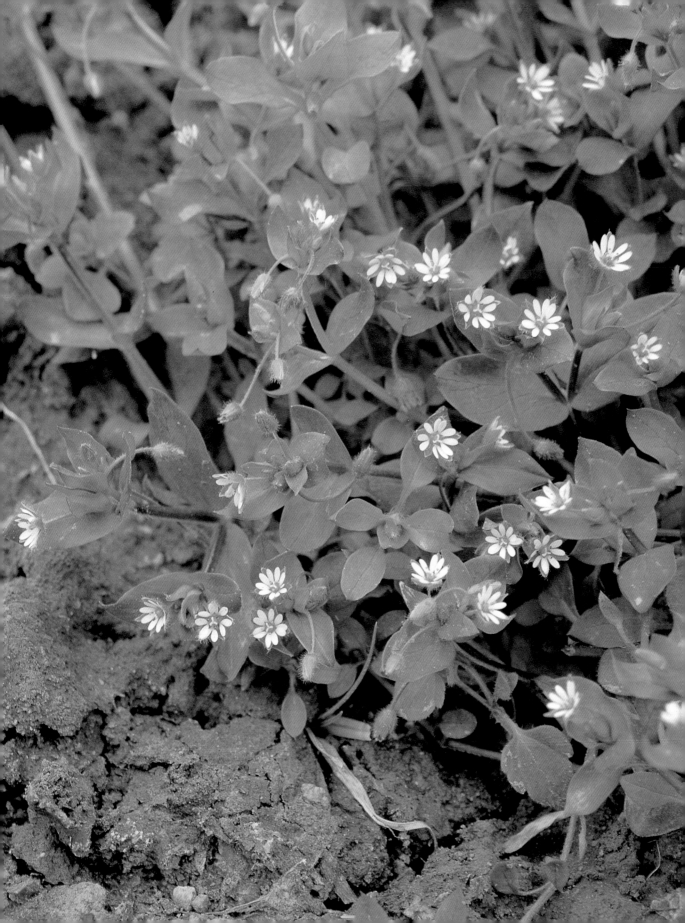

Chickweed

The flower of prediction

The small white star-like flowers of chickweed open regularly at nine o'clock in the morning on fine days, and are said to close at nine in the evening. The plant has been used to predict the weather in this way: if it opens fully into flower there will be no rain for four hours, but if the flowers remain shut you will need a raincoat. Chickweed grows wild in temperate regions, following the paths of settlers .

Birds and chickens are very fond of the plant and the seed used to be fed to caged birds, so it was also called bird-seed. The whole plant is highly nutritious, a good source of vitamins A and C, and minerals including iron and copper. It has been regarded traditionally as a delicacy in Europe and eaten in salads or cooked like spinach. It is said to be more tender than any other wild green. It was given as a blood tonic in the spring and during convalescence. The Swiss used to eat it to strengthen the heart. It was also said to improve eyesight – probably because of its vitamin A content – and was given to consumptives and undernourished children to build them up.

The name Stellaria derives from *stellar* meaning star-like, referring to the flowers. It was called winterweed because chickweed grows early in the spring, even when there is still frost on the ground.

Herbal remedy

The remedy is made from the aerial parts of the plant. Chickweed is an excellent cooling remedy for hot inflammatory skin conditions such as eczema, heat rashes, urticaria, sunburn, boils and spots.
It can be used as a lotion or made into ointment and cream, and also applied fresh to burns and scalds, ulcers, piles and abscesses. It has drawing properties and helps to bring poisons and pus to the surface. It makes a good remedy locally for hot, inflamed joints.

Culpeper referred to chickweed as a 'fine soft pleasing herb under the dominion of the moon'. He said, 'the juice or distilled water is of much good use for all heats and redness of the eyes, to drop some thereof into them'.

Internally, chickweed's cooling and soothing properties can be put to good use in hot inflammatory problems such as gastritis, colitis, acid indigestion, irritable bowel syndrome and excess heat in the liver and gall-bladder. It has an affinity for the respiratory system and can be given for sore throats, laryngitis, bronchitis, asthma, harsh dry coughs and pleurisy.

As a diuretic, chickweed can be taken to relieve fluid retention and to help elimination of toxins from the body via the kidneys. For this reason it can be taken for skin diseases, and for rheumatism and arthritis. Chickweed water was an old wives' remedy for obesity and can be given to cool the body and bring down fevers.

Homeopathic remedy: STELLARIA

Heat and burning characterize many of the symptoms calling for the cooling and moistening qualities of stellaria. There are burning pains in the liver area, hot inflammatory eye symptoms, flushes of heat in the face, burning on the lower lip with neuralgic pain and heat and dryness in the mouth. There may also be respiratory symptoms: short, dry, irritating cough, hawking of thick mucus, and a feeling of constriction in the chest.

Stellaria is also used for inflammatory problems, particularly of the joints and the liver. It is indicated by sharp rheumatic or arthritic pains which dart about all over the body.

A Stellaria person may be irritable and lethargic, with little energy to motivate themselves to work. They sleep well but wake unrefreshed and are generally worse in the mornings, from warmth, and better in the evenings and in cold air.

The flower essence

Chickweed is taken for unresolved emotional issues from the past that create tension or insecurity and stop one from entering joyfully into the present. Carrying around such unresolved feelings may affect one's health and energy, and may cause problems such as overweight, as the body adds protective layers to compensate for feeling vulnerable.

Chickweed helps one to let go of the past and relax into the present moment, able to respond freely to whatever arises, without feeling threatened or needing to be in control.

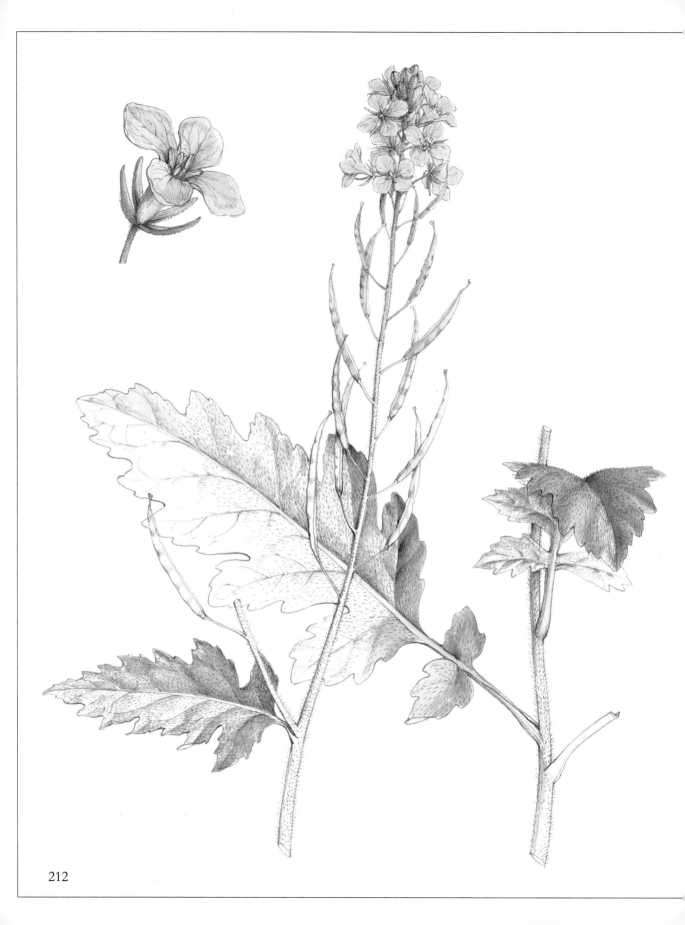

Mustard

The flower of fire

White and black mustard seeds have been used as medicines since earliest times. Pythagoras said mustard was excellent for curing scorpion bites when applied to the skin. Hippocrates advised the use of white mustard internally for digestive disorders and externally, when mixed with vinegar, as a counter-irritant to draw out inflammation. Pliny the Elder writing in Rome in the 1st century AD said that eating mustard made ideal housewives of lazy women. In the Middle Ages it was eaten as a vegetable and young seedlings are still grown today for salads. John Evelyn writing in 1699 said, 'mustard, especially in young seedling plants, is of incomparable effect to quicken and revive the spirits, strengthening the memory, expelling heaviness'.

In Denmark mustard seeds used to be strewn in the house to keep away evil spirits and the forces of darkness, and when mixed with ginger and peppermint increased sexual energy in women. In India black mustard is a symbol of fertility.

Herbal remedy

Mustard has been used as a condiment probably since Saxon times when the Romans took it to England to bring out the flavour of meat. An excellent digestive tonic, it also aids the digestion of meat.

White mustard seeds contain mucilage and were once fashionable as a laxative especially for old people with chronic constipation, and when infused in hot water they were used as a cure for hiccoughs. Black mustard seeds are more pungent than white, and both have an irritant and emetic effect, explaining their use as a folk remedy for poisoning.

The stimulating properties, particularly of black mustard, will ward off the effects of cold, such as poor circulation, chilblains, lethargy, colds and flu, and the winter blues. Many are familiar with mustard footbaths, the well-known folk remedy for sore and aching feet and for dispelling chills and colds.

An infusion of ground mustard seeds can also be used for chest infections, colds and flu, as well as rheumatism and arthritis. The volatile oils have been found to have strong antimicrobial properties, active against bacteria and fungi. An infusion can also be used as a gargle for sore throats and tonsillitis. Ground mustard used to be taken like snuff for

clearing the head, while the seeds were chewed for their painkilling properties to relieve toothache.

Mustard contains volatile oils which have a rubefacient or counter-irritant effect bringing blood to the areas of the body in contact with it. A hot footbath draws blood to the feet and relieves congestion in the head or lungs – this can be useful to relieve headaches, catarrh and sinus problems, and was an old remedy for bronchitis and pneumonia and other respiratory infections. In Russia the folk remedy for warding off colds was simply to dust woollen socks inside with dry mustard each day and wear them. The Latin name for mustard, Sinapis, refers to the *sinapisms* or hot mustard poultices that were applied externally near the seat of internal inflammation. They relieved congestion of the underlying organs and tissues by drawing blood to the surface. Such poultices were used for rheumatism, arthritis, lumbago, gout, sciatica, neuralgia, pain and spasm. Plasters were made with 1 part mustard to 4 parts wholewheat flour, mixed with water into a paste. An egg added to the mixture stopped any blistering of the skin caused by mustard's powerful irritant action.

It is best to use only mustard seeds or powder.

The flower essence

Mustard is the remedy for intense, black depression that descends like a dark cloud for no apparent reason, and lifts again as inexplicably as it came. It is for a hopeless, despairing feeling, shutting out all the joy and pleasure of life and causing a feeling of exclusion from the rest of the world. Daily life offers no interest, all thoughts are negative and turned in on oneself. This kind of depression can be particularly distressing because the sufferer has no control over its coming and going and tends to feel completely at its mercy.

However, the depression relieved by mustard often occurs before decisive steps are taken in life. Often one needs to experience darkness and pain to go through a period of accelerated learning, and come out the other side stronger and wiser. Mustard the flower remedy helps to transform darkness into light and helps to counter fluctuating cycles of depression by enhancing inner stability, joy and peace that is hard to shake or destroy.

NB Eat mustard in moderation as too much can irritate the stomach lining in those prone to an acid stomach or ulcers
Caution Mustard oil is toxic and should never be used undiluted. It is best avoided for domestic use 213

Thyme

The flower of bravery

Beneath your feet
Thyme that for all your bruising
smells more sweet.
　N HOPPER

Since ancient times thyme has been praised for its myriad virtues. According to legend, thyme grew where Helen of Troy's tears fell to the ground. The name thyme comes from the Greek *thumos* meaning to smoke or fumigate, as the Greeks burned it on their altars when making sacrifices to the gods, and it was made into an incense to drive away insects and infection. This name is also said to derive from the Greek *thumus* meaning courage, because of the plant's strengthening and energizing properties.

The Greeks used it as an emblem of bravery and action, and ladies in chivalrous days embroidered on scarves a bee hovering around a sprig of thyme to present to their knights when they left for battle, to imbue them with courage. The Romans slept on thyme, inhaling its sweet aroma to cure melancholy, while in other traditions thyme has been used to quell fears, nightmares, as well as convulsions, vertigo, ringing in the ears and migraine. John Gerard said it was 'profitable for such as are ferfull, melancholicke and troubled in mind'. Made into a soup it was said to cure shyness. Thyme's aroma was inhaled to strengthen the brain and increase longevity.

Wild thyme, called *serpyllum* because of its creeping habit, is also called mother of thyme, in allusion to its therapeutic effect on the womb which used to be referred to as the mother. Thyme has an affinity for the reproductive organs and because of its reputation for increasing strength and energy, it was naturally used as an aphrodisiac, a love herb. It was said to encourage wild times and was a beneficial medicine for those who had had too much of a wild time!

Culpeper said that thyme was ruled by Venus. It is as a bee plant that wild thyme is most well-known, however, as bees love it. Greek thyme honey is prized all over the world for its wonderful flavour. In this connection wild thyme came to symbolize sweetness. The sweetness of its perfume appealed so much to Bacon and the Elizabethans that it was grown where, being trodden underfoot, its scent would bring constant pleasure in the garden.

Herbal remedy

Thyme is most famous as a powerful antiseptic for both internal and external use. It enhances the immune system's fight against bacterial, viral and fungal infections. The main component of its volatile oil, thymol, has long been used in antiseptic cream, lotion, mouthwash and toothpaste. Thyme tea or tincture remedies infections of the respiratory, digestive and genito-urinary system – such as colds, coughs, flu, gastro-enteritis, candida, cystitis and salpingitis (infection of the fallopian tubes).

Thyme makes an excellent remedy, especially for children, for coughs whether they are caused by nerves and anxiety or an infection such as bronchitis, pneumonia or pleurisy. Its relaxant effect on the bronchial tubes relieves asthma and whooping cough, while its expectorant action increases the production of fluid mucus and helps shift phlegm – particularly useful for dry, hacking coughs. By virtue of its sudorific properties, thyme also helps to increase perspiration and bring down fevers.

The relaxing benefits of thyme can also be seen in the digestive system, used to good effect for wind and colic, irritable bowel syndrome and spastic colon. The astringent tannins help to protect the gut from irritation and reduce diarrhoea, while the antiseptic oils fight infections such as gastro-enteritis and dysentery and help re-establish a normal bacterial population in the bowel. This is a great help to those taking antibiotics and those suffering with candida.

A teaspoonful of tincture half an hour before breakfast has been used traditionally with castor oil for worms. In France, thyme is used particularly as a cleansing liver tonic, stimulating the digestive system and liver function to treat indigestion, poor appetite, anaemia, liver and gall-bladder complaints, skin complaints and lethargy.

Thyme has a wonderfully pungent taste and warming properties, just right for dispelling cold in winter. Add a strong infusion to the bath or drink tea or tincture of thyme to stimulate the circulation, throw off chills and lethargy and act as an exhilarating tonic to the whole system. Its tonic action on the nervous system makes it excellent for physical and mental exhaustion, relieving tension, anxiety and general depression.

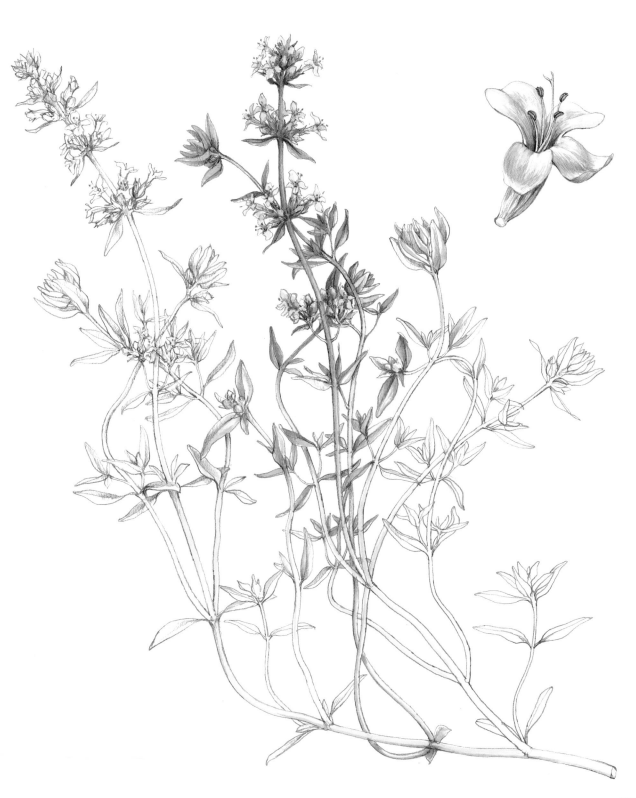

This remarkable herb has yet more to offer. As a diuretic it helps combat water retention, infections of the urinary tract, rheumatism and gout. It also acts on the reproductive system, and has been used since the Middle Ages for a variety of women's problems, particularly infections of the reproductive tract and regulating the menstrual cycle.

Recent research suggests that the volatile oils in thyme may play a vital role in the function of polyunsaturated fatty acids (PUFAs), keeping the body's cells healthy and slowing the ageing process. PUFAs build cell walls and are vital to the structure of the brain, nervous system and blood vessels. They protect against degenerative problems, heart and arterial problems, skin disease, senile dementia and cancer. The antioxidant effect of thyme oil protects the PUFAs from decay caused by oxygen, and prevents the release of free radicals – molecules that damage cells and tissues leaving behind destructive waste products in the process.

Externally, thyme oil can be used in liniments and lotions for relieving arthritis, muscular pain and itching. It disinfects cuts and grazes, wounds, sores and ulcers. An infusion or tincture of thyme makes a good gargle for sore throats, an antiseptic mouthwash and a douche for thrush and other vaginal infections. It can also be used daily for friction of the hair and as a hair lotion, giving it a healthy lustre and arresting hair fall. Thyme makes an excellent inhalant for chesty conditions, asthma, colds, catarrh and sinusitis. Vinegar of thyme is an old folk remedy used like smelling salts for nervous headaches.

Aromatherapy oil

Thyme produces several oils depending on the soil, climate and altitude in which it grows. The chemotype that contains a high level of carvarol is a powerful antiseptic, while linalol, geraniol and thujanol chemotypes have much gentler properties and are preferable for home use. Thyme linalol is the only one that is suitable for children.

The use of thyme oil in aromatherapy is very similar to that in herbal medicine. It acts as a stimulant to the circulation, warming the body and warding off illness that results from chill such as sore throats, flu, head colds and coughs. It is also stimulating to both mental and physical energy, as the ancients said. It is excellent as a tonic in debility, for depression, lethargy, when feeling nervously run down, anxious or under stress as when studying for exams. It energizes the digestion, acting as an aperitif and digestive and

calming colic and wind. In the chest thyme oil relaxes the bronchial tubes, helpful in asthma, and acts as an expectorant. Inhalations of thyme can be used for coughs, chest infections, whooping cough, emphysema and TB.

Also very helpful are thyme's powerful antiseptic properties and its ability to stimulate white blood cell production, helping the body's fight against infection. It brings down fevers, and acts as a decongestant for catarrh, colds, sinusitis and rhinitis. It acts as a diuretic and an emmenagogue and for this reason is contra-indicated in pregnancy. It is used in some parts of the world for intestinal parasites.

Homeopathic remedy: THYMUS

Both thymol, the main component of the essential oil, and the tincture of wild thyme, *Thymus serpyllum*, are homeopathic remedies. Thymol is specific for hookworms, and for genito-urinary problems. It is prescribed for sexual debility, prostate problems, priapism and nocturnal emission. The symptom picture includes low energy, unrefreshing sleep and lascivious dreams, profuse urination with burning and dribbling indicative of prostate problems, aching in the lower back and irritability. The patient wants his own way and craves the company of others.

Thymus serpyllum is used for respiratory infections particularly in children, for asthma associated with tension, for dry nervous coughs, whooping cough and sore throats. It is also prescribed for ringing in the ears, with a feeling of pressure in the head.

The flower essence

The use of thyme as a flower remedy is related to the passage of time, and its acceleration. When dabbed on to a wound or cut, or over an area of trauma or disease in the body, thyme is said to speed healing. It has an amplifying effect, increasing strength and courage, and enhancing the body's metabolic processes. It imparts greater physical stamina, making it particularly useful in the elderly. When used in combination with other flower essences, thyme acts to amplify their effects. Thyme the herb has been used since the days of the Ancient Greeks to increase energy and longevity. The flower essence similarly increases energy, enhances concentration and the ability to adapt to seasonal change and the passage of time. It is good for people struggling with time, stressed by deadlines, always trying to beat the clock; or for in old age, helping to protect mind and body from the effects of ageing.

NB Only use thyme oil in small amounts and do not use it undiluted on the skin

Dandelion

The flower of survival

Leontodons unfold
on the swath turf their ray-encircled gold,
with sol's expanding beams the flowers unclose,
And rising Hesper lights them to repose.
ERASMUS DARWIN (1731–1802)

This common weed with its cheerful flower and remarkable resilience has been respected as a healing plant for thousands of years. Said to originate in Greece and Central Asia, it was used as a medicine in Ancient Greece and was praised in herbals in the Middle Ages. It is found in folklore tradition all over the world.

There is a quaint legend about how the dandelion first appeared on the earth. In ancient days when the world was populated by fairies, elves and gnomes, the first humans to arrive caused problems as they could not see these elemental beings and so kept treading on them. Some of the sun-loving fairies dressed in bright yellow gowns had nowhere to hide, unlike the gnomes and elves who took refuge behind rocks or under the ground, so they were transformed into dandelions. If you step on a dandelion it will soon spring up again, as it is said to contain the spirit of the fairies. This accords with the almost supernatural power of the dandelion to survive – when weeded from lawns and gardens they soon reappear. The seed heads bear numerous airborne seeds, easily blown away in the wind, while their roots are long and tenaciously hold themselves in the ground in any soil. Not surprisingly, the dandelion has come to symbolize faithfulness.

The dandelion in the language of flowers also means rustic oracle. It was used as a country clock, which was fairly precise, as the flowers were said to open at five minutes past five in the morning and close at nine minutes past eight in the evening. Children prefer to tell the time by blowing at the seed heads, the number of puffs needed to blow them all off indicating the hour.

The seed head was also used to find out what your lover was thinking of you; 'he loves me' with one puff of the seed head, 'he loves me not' with the next. It was said that if you whisper the words of love to your favourite person and blow the seeds gently towards him, the seeds would carry the words

to your beloved. Children also believed that if they could blow all the seeds offa dandelion in one breath, then their wish would come true. Apparently witches said that if you rubbed yourself all over with dandelion you will be welcome everywhere and your wishes will come true.

The name Taraxacum is said to come from the Greek word *taraxo* meaning disorder, and *takos*, meaning pain or remedy, because of the dandelion's great healing ability. It is also said to come from the Arabian corruption of the Greek word *trogemon*, meaning edible. The leaves are delicious in salads or cooked like spinach, and highly nutritious, being rich in vitamins C and B, and pro-vitamin A; and minerals, particularly potassium and iron. The roots can be roasted and ground into a tasty, caffeine-free substitute for coffee. Dandelion was the food to which Hecate entertained Theseus in the Greek myths. The French name, *dent de lion* – the tooth of the lion – refers to the toothed margin of the leaves or the fact that the golden flowers resemble the colour of the royal lion and the shape of his open mouth.

Herbal remedy

Dandelion is most famous as a gently detoxifying bitter tonic, increasing elimination of toxins, wastes and pollutants through the liver and kidneys, thereby cleansing the blood.

The bitter taste of both root and leaf stimulates the bitter receptors in the mouth and by reflex this activates the whole of the digestive tract and the liver. It increases the flow of digestive juices, enhancing the appetite and easing digestion. By increasing bile production and flow, it cleanses the liver, supporting its work as the major detoxifying organ of the body. Eaten young in the spring, the leaves act as a bitter tonic to cleanse the body of wastes from the heavy clogging food and more sedentary habits of winter. Dandelion root is used in liver disease, jaundice, hepatitis, gall-bladder infections and to dissolve gallstones. It is taken for problems associated with a sluggish liver such as tiredness and irritability, headaches and skin problems. Like other herbs that work on the liver, dandelion helps to relieve emotional stagnation and enhances expression of repressed emotions such as anger, resentment and

NB The milky juice, if sucked excessively by children may lead to nausea, vomiting or diarrhoea

grief. In this sense it is cleansing or purging to the emotions as well as the body.

The stimulating effect of dandelion extends to the pancreas where it increases insulin secretion, helpful in diabetes and hypoglycaemia (low blood sugar). The root is also mildly laxative.

Dandelion, particularly the leaves, is an effective diuretic as the traditional names 'piss-a-bed' or in French *pis-en-lit* tell us, useful in water retention, cellulite conditions, urinary infections and prostate problems. While diuretic drugs leach potassium from the body and require a potassium supplement, dandelion comes complete with its high potassium content replacing that lost through increased urination. A decoction of root and leaves is a folk remedy for dissolving urinary stones and gravel.

Since dandelion leaves improve elimination of uric acid, they make a useful remedy for gout. Combined in a tea with celery seed and taken regularly they make an excellent brew for arthritis and rheumatism.

Externally, apply the white juice daily over a few weeks to cure warts. Tea of the leaves and flowers makes a good wash for ulcers and skin complaints, and a decoction makes a lotion for freckles.

Homeopathic remedy: TARAXACUM

Taraxacum is again mainly used for liver and digestive problems. It is specific for liver pain, bilious attacks, gallstones, gastric headaches, jaundiced skin and the associated debility. It is given for poor appetite, flatulence, with the sensation of bubbles bursting in the bowels, for sluggish bowels, for a bitter taste in the mouth and a sore, mapped tongue, where the tongue coating is stripped away in patches leaving sore, raw areas.

Taraxacum like the herbal remedy acts on the urinary system and is used for frequency of urination, difficulty passing water and great thirst. A Taraxacum person tends to have profuse night sweats, restless limbs which are painful to touch, and feel worse from pressure. They may have rheumatism or painful joints, tension and stiffness in the back and neck, and shooting pains in the neck muscles. There may be skin problems, such as purulent pimples on the face, with heat and redness. During a fever they may feel thirstless, or worse from drinking, the fingertips may feel cold, and they have a bitter taste in the mouth. They feel hot in the face and the toes, and sweat on falling asleep. Generally they feel worse lying down and sitting, and feel chilly after eating.

The flower essence

Dandelion suits people who have a tendency to cram far too much into their lives. They are so full of enthusiasm for life that they take on too much and become compulsive 'doers'. They overplan and overstructure their lives in an effort to fit in everything they want to do, and leave little room for relaxation or reflection, until the point is reached where they no longer know how to be quiet or relaxed. They leave little space in their lives for spiritual or emotional expression, and as they push themselves beyond the body's natural capacity, they no longer listen to the needs of their bodies. Such harsh physical demands and unexpressed inner life creates great tension, especially in the muscles of the neck and shoulders.

Dandelion helps to release this tension, allowing the body to relax and emotions to be released and expressed. It can be added to massage oils and used in body work. It enables you to listen more closely to emotional messages and bodily needs, and shifts the emphasis from being a human 'doing' to a human 'being'. Energy, activity and enthusiasm become balanced with a sense of inner ease.

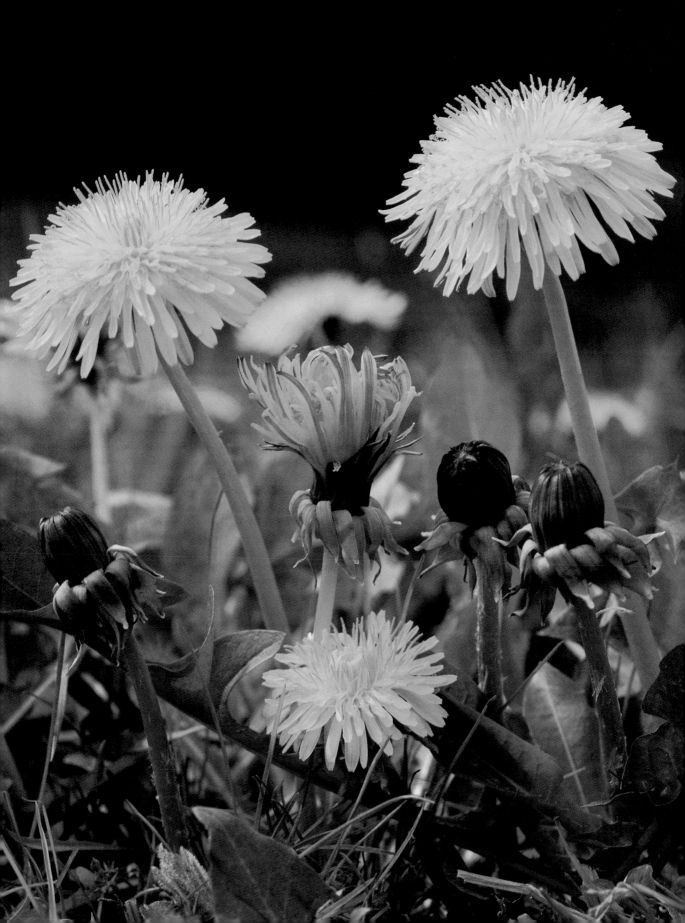

Tilia europaea

Linden, Lime

The flower of grace

The majestic linden tree that can grow to over 100 feet (30 metres) high can be found in parks and gardens all over Europe. It is planted along roads in town and countryside alike. In Greek mythology, Cronos (or Time) had an affair with Philyra, the daughter of Oceanus. He was caught in the act of love by his wife Rhea, upon which he turned himself into a stallion and galloped off. Philyra was left to bear his son, half-man, half-horse, which was Chiron, the learned centaur. Philyra was so ashamed of her offspring that she implored the gods to change her, and she was metamorphosed into the linden tree, the flowers of which were used by the Greeks as a restorative. Philyra is Greek for lime or linden tree.

Linden is a historic symbol of feminine grace, beauty, happiness, conjugal love, sweetness and peace. The tree was dedicated to Venus, while Culpeper said it was ruled by Jupiter, representing expansion, learning and wisdom.

Herbal remedy

Linden flowers make a wonderfully relaxing remedy that is delicious when taken as a tea, particularly when sitting in the shade of a linden tree. It relieves tension and anxiety, aids sleep, calms restless and excitable children and relaxes muscle tension. It makes a good remedy for conditions associated with tension including headaches, irritability, depression, period pains, neck, shoulder and back pain, dizziness, colic and cramp. These relaxant effects combined with the beneficial action of the bioflavonoids on the arteries makes linden flower an excellent remedy for reducing high blood pressure and arteriosclerosis. Having an affinity with the heart it also relaxes the coronary arteries, easing palpitations and therefore helping prevent and treat coronary heart disease. The linden tree grows slowly and steadily, and lives for centuries. It can help to prolong the lives of others through these therapeutic actions if they can learn its lesson of moderation and regular, steady progress.

Taken in hot infusion, linden flowers have a diaphoretic action, increasing blood supply to the skin and producing sweating. It is an excellent cooling remedy for reducing fevers, particularly in children, and for clearing catarrhal congestion. Taken with elderflowers it will speed colds, coughs, and flu

on their way. The mucilage has a soothing action, relieving irritating, harsh coughs and sore throats. A warm to cool infusion has a diuretic action, helping to clear fluid and toxins from the body via the urinary system, useful for oedema, rheumatism and gout, as well as inflammatory skin disease.

Externally, linden flowers can be used as a lotion for inflammatory skin problems such as boils and abscesses, for urticaria and to soothe and heal scalds and burns and sore, inflamed eyes.

Aromatherapy oil

The sweet fragrant oil from linden flowers has a similarly relaxing and antispasmodic effect. It can be added to the bath or used in massage oils to relieve many stress-related problems.

Homeopathic remedy: Tilia

Tilia is prescribed for muscular tension and weakness throughout the body, vertigo, neuralgia, headaches and migraine and to relieve pain. It is particularly recommended for toothache in children.

Tilia will relieve disturbed and restless sleep, with vivid or frightful dreams. As in herbal medicine, Tilia is given for fevers with night sweats, catarrh and colds, sore burning throats and hoarseness, and tickly irritating coughs. It is given for heart pains, palpitations, feelings of pressure in the chest, rapid pulse, and to thin the blood where there is a tendency to clotting. A Tilia person may be depressed, weepy or lovesick, irritable or reclusive and shy.

Tilia has a specific use for pelvic inflammation in women, and for post-partum infection.

The flower essence

The flower remedy is closely related to linden's historic application in healing matters of the heart, when it was a symbol of conjugal love, sweetness, peace and happiness. It is a good remedy for those who have trouble giving and receiving love and affection, because of painful experiences in the past. Linden flower helps to release emotional blocks and engenders warmth and openess. It increases awareness of our connectedness to the rest of humanity, relaxes and softens communication between people and strengthens the relationship between loved ones.

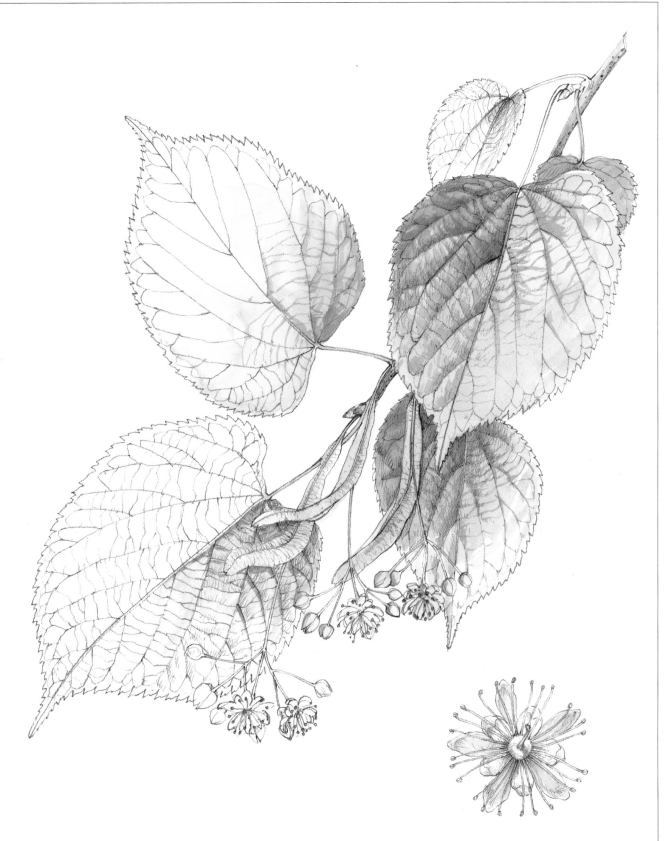

221

Red clover

The flower of good fortune

This attractive cousin of the pea can be found growing in profusion in meadows, fields and roadsides, flowering from spring to autumn. Clover is familiar to most as a good luck charm, particularly a four-leafed clover, and has been considered lucky since ancient times. It was seen as a symbol of the Holy Cross when four-leafed, and of the Trinity when three-leafed. It was believed to be especially lucky for women to whom the three-leafed clover represented the triple goddess: the maiden or young woman, the mother or fertility symbol and the crone of old age and wisdom.

Clover has also been a symbol of fertility and domestic virtue. It is rich in minerals and trace elements and contains nitrogen-fixing bacteria in the root, making it valuable as a feeding crop for cattle. The phrase 'living in clover' alludes to cattle being put to feed in rich pasture.

The Druids considered red clover to have the power to protect from danger and evil influences, including witches. It afforded psychic protection.

Herbal remedy

As a herb, the flowers are used. Red clover is first and foremost a blood cleanser, useful in deep-seated chronic conditions of toxicity. It cleanses in several ways. As a diuretic, it enhances the elimination of wastes via the urinary system. It stimulates the liver and gall-bladder, and also has a mild laxative effect. Red clover has antiviral and antifungal properties, while the sterol, beta-sitosterol, inhibits growth of tumours. It has been used for background treatment of cancer, particularly of the breast and ovaries. In folk medicine red clover has been used to thin and purify the blood. We now know that beta-sitosterol reduces the absorption of cholesterol and is therefore used in treatment of atherosclerosis.

Red clover has relaxant properties, helping to relieve stress and tension, and stress-related symptoms such as headaches and muscle spasm. In the respiratory system this relaxant effect coupled with an expectorant action soothes irritating coughs, and helps relieve asthma and bronchial problems. Since it also helps to clear the skin it is used for coughs during measles, and for children with the eczema-asthma syndrome.

Having an affinity with women, red clover can be used to treat the female reproductive system. It contains flavonoids with an oestrogenic action, and acts as a deep cleansing remedy for chronic problems such as pelvic inflammatory disease. It can be taken to relieve heavy or painful periods, and by post-menopausal women. An infusion can be used as a douche for vaginal infections, and as a wash for sore, inflamed nipples. It can also be used as a gargle for sore throats, an eyewash and a lotion for inflamed skin conditions.

Homeopathic remedy: RED CLOVER

In homeopathy also, red clover is used for cancer, and a range of respiratory symptoms: spasmodic coughs, whooping cough, coughs followed by hiccoughs, chills with a cough at night. It treats sore irritated throats, mucus in the throat with constantly wanting to clear it, and hoarseness. It is also prescribed for hay fever symptoms.

Red clover is also used for chronic skin conditions, tension and headaches, with a stiff neck and back which is relieved by heat, and confusion and headache occurring after unrefreshing sleep. It is helpful where there is constipation, great thirst and colicky pains.

The flower essence

Red clover the flower essence is also a cleansing remedy, a blood cleanser, relating to the psychic properties of the blood, where the spiritual self is said to reside. It helps to clear negativity picked up from others, and is particularly useful for those who feel susceptible to the problems of others, or to taking on the emotions of those around them. This may occur in crises, such as economic crises or natural disasters, where the reaction of fear, panic, confusion or hysteria can be highly infectious, or during political or religious rallies where crowds can become highly inflammatory, even destructive. The same may occur in emotionally charged work or family situations.

Red clover the flower essence acts as a balancer, helping one to remain centred within, despite the storms outside. It instils calmness and clarity, and enhances self-awareness.

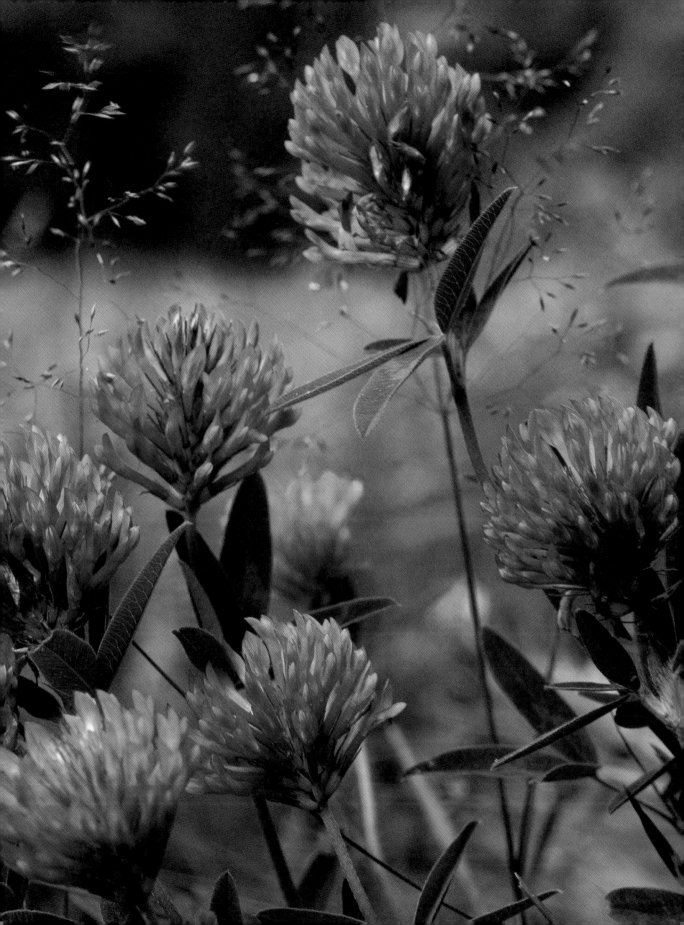

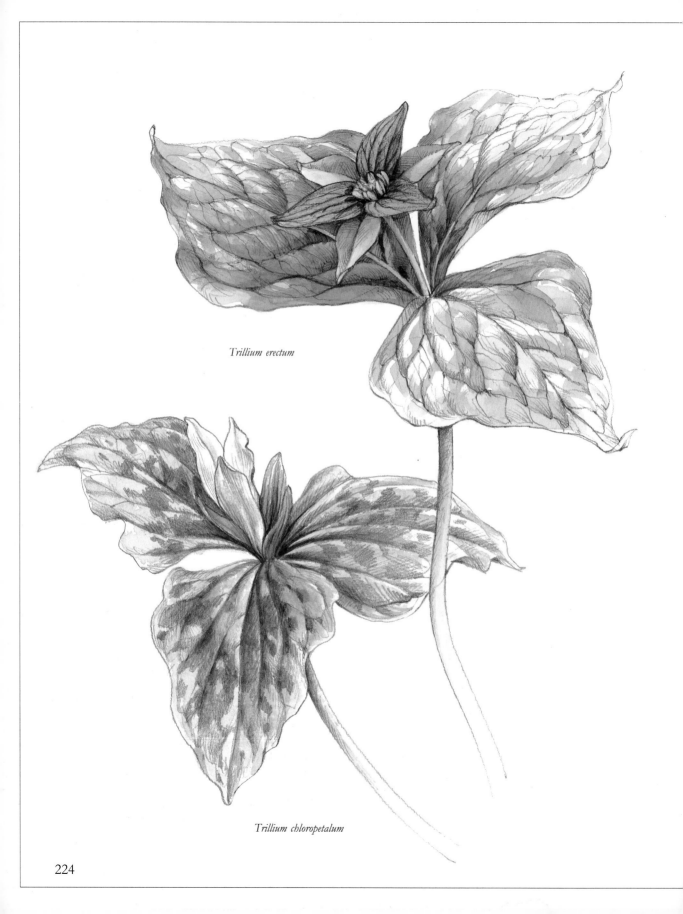

Trillium erectum

Trillium chloropetalum

Trillium erectum, T. pendulum

Beth root

The flower of modest beauty

This attractive member of the lily family is a hardy perennial found in rich, moist woodland in central and western states of America, where it is now endangered, and temperate eastern Asia. The native Americans knew it well for its use in haemorrhagic problems, but also as a love potion. The root was boiled and dropped into the food of the desired man. There is an old native American story of a beautiful young girl who fell in love with the chief's son and wanted him for her husband. She boiled the roots of trillium and took it to put on his food, but tripped on the way so it fell into an ugly old man's dish. The old man ate it and then followed her around for months, begging her to marry him.

Beth root is a symbol of modest beauty.

Herbal remedy

Beth root is a well-known native American remedy used most commonly to lessen the pain of childbirth and ease the birth by stimulating normal, effective contractions. It contains natural precursors or building blocks of female sex hormones, explaining its use for a variety of menstrual disorders. It acts as an excellent tonic for the uterus, toning up weak muscles and helping to prevent miscarriage and prolapse of the uterus. Its astringent properties are particularly useful for heavy periods, post-partum bleeding, and excessive menstruation around the menopause.

Beth root can also be used for bleeding elsewhere in the body – such as the respiratory tract, the digestive tract, the bladder, the nose and mouth. It can be used for diarrhoea and dysentery where there is blood and mucus in the stools, for bleeding from the stomach lining from gastric ulcers, and for blood in the urine. It is also used locally for nosebleeds and bleeding gums.

Externally, its antiseptic properties combined with its astringent effect make beth root useful for treating vaginal discharges and infections such as thrush and trichomonas. It will speed healing of skin problems, ulcers, bleeding, haemorrhoids and varicose veins, and soothe irritation of insect bites and stings. The native Americans used it as an effective eye medicine – they squeezed the juice directly into the eye, or soaked the root and made an eyewash from it for sore, inflamed eyes and eye infections.

Homeopathic remedy: TRILLIUM

The root and rhizome of *Trillium erectum* are used like the herbal remedy for a tendency to copious bleeding, associated with feeling faint and dizzy. The keynote for Trillium is 'flooding with fainting'. It is used for uterine haemorrhage – heavy periods, menorrhagia around menopause, heavy bleeding due to fibroids, threatened miscarriage, and post-partum bleeding. It is also given for uterine prolapse caused by weakness and pelvic muscle over-relaxation.

Trillium is also prescribed for bleeding elsewhere, be it in the lungs with TB, from the kidneys, bladder, stomach or bowels. It is good for nosebleeds, bleeding gums and copious bleeding after tooth extraction.

A Trillium person tends to be flabby with cold extremities and extreme debility from the bleeding. They look pale and have a craving for ice-cold water, and are prone to headaches and blurred vision.

The flower essence

Trillium chloropetalum, which has a greenish-white flower, is used. It is given to people who have a great need for material security and who as a result accumulate wealth and possessions, believing that the status and power these things give them are the answer to their problems. Their acquisitiveness and greed can be so powerful that it drives them to be very ambitious and selfish, overiding any concern they have for other people or their personal relationships. As they accumulate wealth around them so they accumulate weight and toxins physically.

The cause of such insecurity in Trillium people is most likely that they are cut off from their inner, spiritual strength while their awareness is limited to the physical level of existence. They seek to overcome an unconscious feeling of powerlessness, since they measure their self-worth only by material standards.

Trillium helps to give a sense of inner security and wellbeing through being more in touch with inner resources for survival rather than outer possessions. It works on the root chakra, which influences survival and earthly requirements and helps to develop sharing and co-operation with others, and concern for the common good by lending the strength to be unselfish.

Nasturtium

The flower of patriotism

Shield-like Nasturtium, too, confusedly spread,
with intermingling trefoil fills each bed –
once graceful youths, this last a Grecian swain,
The first an huntsman on the Trojan plain.
   PAUL DE RAPIN (1661–1725)

This lovely bright and colourful annual is one of the easiest and most rewarding flowers to grow from seed. Nasturtiums come from tropical South America, where they are perennial. They were among the treasures brought back from Peru by the conquistadores along with the gold of the Incas.

In 16th century England it was called 'blood flower of Peru', and Indian cress, because of its similarity to watercress (*Nasturtium officinale*) with its pungent taste and smell. The name nasturtium comes from *nasus tortus* meaning 'nose-twisting' because of its peppery smell. However, the flower was welcomed as a rare treasure in Elizabethan and Stuart England. John Evelyn recommended the seed for scurvy, 'the most effectual and powerful agents in conquering and expunging that cruel Enemy.' In one story the nasturtium is said to have arisen from the spilled blood of a Trojan warrior, the round leaves being his shield and the trumpet-shaped flower his helmet. The name Tropaeolum comes from the Greek *tropaion*, meaning trophy. In the language of flowers the nasturtium symbolizes patriotism.

All parts of the plant are edible and nutritious, being rich in iron, vitamin C, minerals and trace elements. The unripe seeds make a substitute for capers, while the flowers can be mixed in salads. The leaves add piquancy to soups, salads and sandwiches.

Herbal remedy

Like watercress, nasturtium is both pungent and bitter, making it a good blood cleanser, aiding the body's elimination of toxins. The pungency is warming and stimulating. It invigorates the digestion, improving appetite and absorption of its nutritious contents. It acts as a tonic for weak digestion and food stagnation which lead to toxicity and poor absorption. It increases the circulation, carrying the absorbed nutrients around the body to where they are needed, giving a sense of wellbeing and strength. The bitters are also detoxifying, stimulating the liver, pancreas and gall-bladder activity and the secretion of digestive enzymes. The bitters in the seeds stimulate the bowels and ensure elimination of toxins via this route. Nasturtium acts on the kidneys and bladder, increasing elimination of waste products in the urine.

Nasturtium also has antimicrobial properties. It is used particularly for chest infections, and because it also has decongestant properties it is well worth using to clear the phlegm that accompanies bronchial problems. The fresh juice or an infusion of the leaves relieves colds, catarrh, and chronic bronchial congestion. Its high vitamin C content is useful here. It can also be taken for urinary tract infections such as cystitis. As a natural antibiotic it will not destroy the normal bacterial population of the intestines.

The combination of its nourishing, detoxifying and immune-enhancing properties makes nasturtium a good tonic for those feeling depleted and run down. Being high in iron it is helpful when feeling tired because of anaemia. Its strengthening effect was used in the past as a rejuvenative and an aphrodisiac, hence its names passionflower, and flower of love.

Externally, nasturtium has an old reputation of retarding balding. The tincture of nasturtium leaves, oak bark and nettles was massaged regularly into the scalp – so nasturtium helps 'keep your hair on'.

Homeopathic remedy: NASTURTIUM
Nasturtium is used for urinary problems, including infections such as cystitis, stones and gravel.

The flower essence
Nasturtium, like the herbal remedy, is warming, rejuvenating, refreshing and revitalizing. It is particularly recommended for those who feel drained from excess mental activity, such as students and those whose careers demand concentrated intellectual work. Such people may become over-developed mentally and live too much in the head, lacking physical or emotional expression, and divorced from many of the realities of daily life. Such imbalance may predispose to illness, immune dysfunction, coughs, colds and catarrh.

Nasturtium brings balance between intellectual, emotional and physical activity. It restores emotional warmth, physical vitality and earthly practicality.

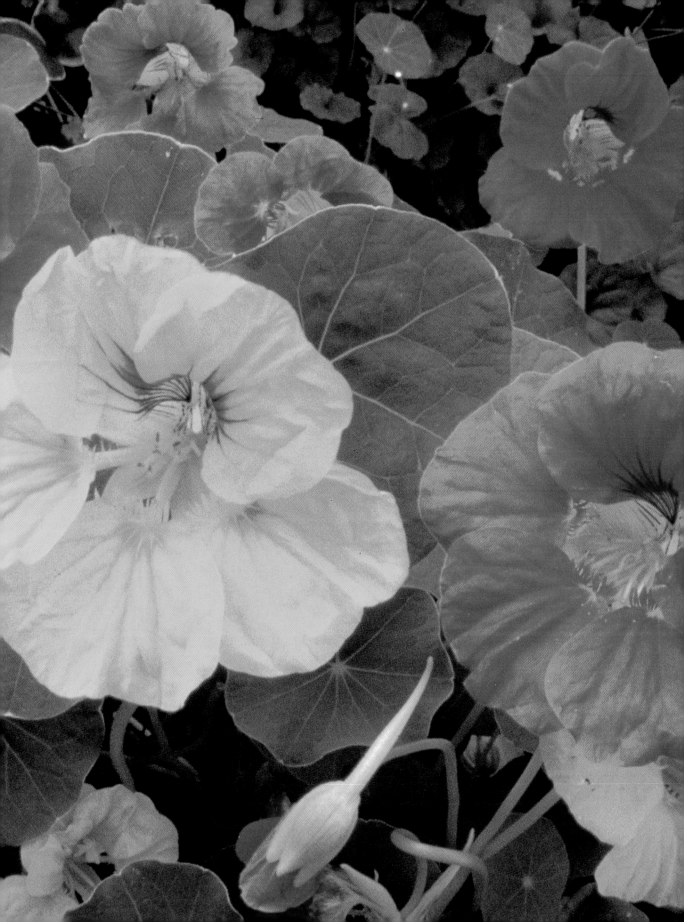

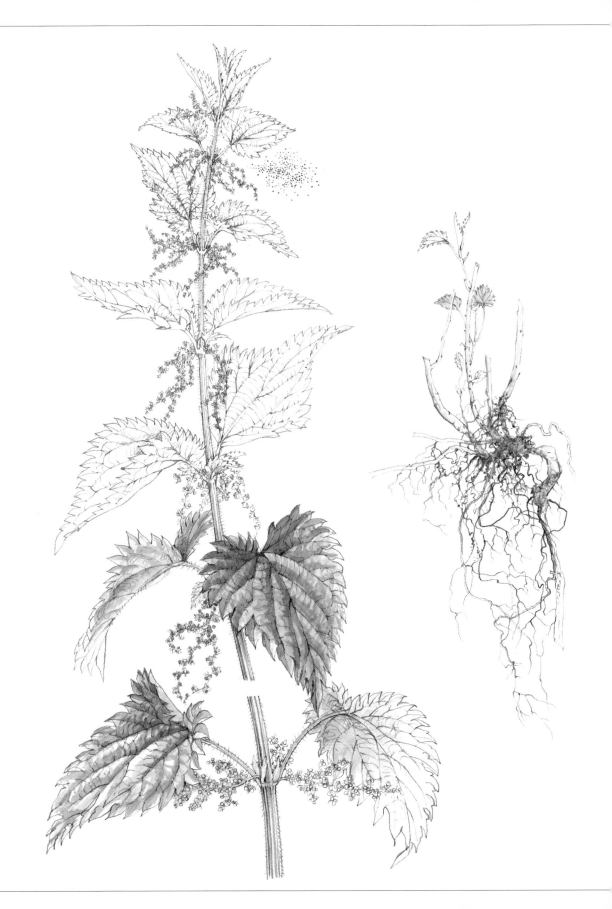

228

Nettle

The flower of spite

Tender handed stroke a nettle
And it stings you for your pains;
Grasp it like a man of mettle,
And it soft as silk remains.
  AARON HILL (1685–1750)

The common nettle, despite its cruel sting and invasive habit, has an incredible range of healing properties and practical uses. Nettles have been used in making beer and cheese, while its fibrous leaves and stalks have been made into cloth and paper.

Nettles grow in all temperate regions, and were introduced into Britain by the Romans. They brought a particularly cruel sort of nettle, *Urtica pilulifera*, with which to flog themselves warm to ward off the illnesses and infections rife in cold, damp weather. The stinging hairs of the fresh nettle contain formic acid and histamine, and have a long history of therapeutic use. It is still said that if you sting yourself regularly in the garden it will protect you from rheumatism and arthritis in later life. In South America this treatment has been used to stimulate the circulation even in serious conditions such as gangrene and threatened amputations. Galen recommended the friction of the leaves against the skin to increase the circulation and stir up 'natural heat', to stimulate desire and cure impotence. In France they apparently still suggest a young man rolls in a bed of nettles before going courting. The nettle's sting has given it a symbolic meaning of cruelty and spite.

Herbal remedy

Nettles are highly nutritious, rich in vitamins A and C, and minerals, particularly iron, silica and potassium. They have been used throughout history as a nourishing tonic for weakness and debility, convalescence and anaemia. They stimulate the liver and kidneys, cleansing the body of toxins and wastes. Nettle tops as tea, or in cooking, make a wonderful cleansing spring tonic. They help clear the skin in eczema and urticaria and restore vitality to the system.

The diuretic properties of nettles help relieve fluid retention, cystitis and urethritis. They have long been used to soften and expel kidney stones and gravel, and as a remedy for bedwetting and incontinence. They increase excretion of uric acid through the kidneys, making them an excellent remedy for gout and all other arthritic conditions.

Nettles have an astringent effect and make a stimulating tonic for external and internal bleeding. An infusion, tincture or fresh juice can be applied to cuts and wounds, haemorrhoids, the nostrils during nosebleeds and to soothe and heal burns and scalds.

In the respiratory tract, a tincture of the seeds was a traditional remedy for fevers and lung disorders. A decoction of the root was a well-known remedy for pleurisy. Fresh nettle juice is equally effective. The cleansing and astringent properties help clear catarrhal congestion and are useful in relieving allergies such as hayfever, bronchitis and asthma.

Nettles make a stimulating tonic to the digestive tract, for diarrhoea, flatulence, ulcers, phlegm and worms. They also reduce blood sugar. A tincture of the seeds raises thyroid function and reduces goitre.

Externally, nettle juice can be applied to the skin to relieve bites and stings as well as the sting of the nettle (dock, sage and rosemary are also effective for this). Made into an ointment, nettles help relieve irritating skin conditions such as eczema.

Homeopathic remedy: URTICA URENS

The dwarf stinging nettle is an excellent first aid remedy for bites and stings, with symptoms of burning, itching or stinging, minor burns and scalds. It can also be used for other skin conditions characterized by stinging, itching and burning. Urtica is a wonderful remedy for new mothers when breastfeeding. It helps to produce simply what is required by the baby. It is also helpful when weaning, to arrest milk flow and prevent engorgement of the breasts.

The flower essence

Nettle is for people who are cold and angry, prone to be cruel and spiteful, perhaps because they feel stung by others or by what life has dealt them. Nettle helps people to express and thus release their anger and through its expression to relate to others more openly. In this way nettle is cleansing of inner toxins and reduces stress. It can be used where there is anger, conflict or cruelty within a disturbed home, or at work, bringing things out into the open and helping to re-establish unity.

Mullein

The flower of inner light

By thy woodside railing, reeves
with antique mullein's flannel leaves
These, though mean, the flowers of waste,
Planted here in nature's haste
Display to the discerning eye,
Her loved, wild variety.
  JOHN CLARE (1793–1864)

The name mullein derives from the Latin *mollis* meaning soft, as this stately biennial has large soft downy leaves which are covered in little hairs. The name Verbascum is probably a corruption of the Latin *barbascum*, meaning a bearded plant. The woolly leaves were once used by poor country people to line their shoes to keep their feet warm in the winter and to protect them on rough ground, hence the other names Adam's blanket, flannel plant, velvet plant, beggar's blanket. In the language of flowers mullein symbolizes comfort. This may be because of the comfort it gave to the feet, or for the soothing nature of its action when used medicinally for irritation and inflammation in the respiratory and urinary systems, and its painkilling properties.

Mullein often grows to over 5 feet (1.5 metres) tall, and has a solitary upright stem in its second year covered with pale yellow flowers. The stem encloses a thin rod of white pith, which gave rise to such names as Aaron's rod and Jacob's staff. The down on the leaves and stem burn easily when dry and so were used as tapers or candles as far back as Roman times, when the plant was known as candelaria.

Mullein was also known to the ancients as a protective herb against evil and illness. It was grown in monastery gardens to keep out the devil and on journeys it was carried as a talisman of safety. This ability to protect against the forces of darkness was another way mullein was used to provide light, or to light one's path. Mullein was also said to be used by witches during their rituals and was called witch's candle, and Hag's taper. Hag is a word derived from Anglo-Saxon *hoege* or *hage*, meaning hedge, so the name Hag's taper may not refer to witches but simply to the fact that mullein with its stem of yellow flowers resembled a lighted taper.

In the Greek myths Ulysses took mullein to protect himself against the wiles of the witch Circe, as it was used as a safeguard against sorcery. It was also taken in love potions.

Herbal remedy

Mullein has cooling properties and helps to clear heat and congestion from the body. It makes an excellent remedy for the respiratory system. The saponins have an expectorant action, helping to produce phlegm from the chest. The mucilage is cooling and soothing, making mullein a wonderful medicine for harsh, irritating and dry coughs, sore throats, hoarseness and bronchitis. Its relaxing and painkilling effect in the chest is helpful in asthma, croup, whooping cough and pleurisy, while the mild antiseptic action of the plant is helpful for respiratory infections.

Mullein helps to clear phlegm from the system, and can be taken for chronic catarrh, sinusitis and hay fever. It has been used for centuries for pneumonia, bronchitis, and tuberculosis – in fact it used to be cultivated widely in gardens in Ireland specifically for its use in consumption (TB). The leaves used to be smoked to relieve irritating coughs. By its cleansing action in the lymphatic system it can be used to treat swollen glands and mumps.

As a soothing diuretic, mullein can be used for burning and frequency of urination in cystitis, and for fluid retention. By increasing elimination of toxins via the kidneys, it is useful in treatment of arthritis, rheumatism and gout.

The relaxant and anodyne properties, particularly of the flowers, help to encourage restful sleep, particularly for those disturbed by coughing and pain. Mullein is used for headaches and neuralgia and specifically for pain in the ears, and can be applied locally as well as taken internally for catarrhal deafness and tinnitus, ear infections, wax accumulation and head pain caused by congestion in the ears. Mullein provides comfort for earache. It will also relieve tension and anxiety, and has a history of use for nervous palpitations, heart irregularities, cramp and nervous colic. Its astringent properties are useful to treat diarrhoea, particularly when it is related to nerves. A decoction of the root was an old remedy to relieve toothache, cramps and convulsions.

Externally, a compress or poultice of mullein leaves can be applied to painful arthritic joints and

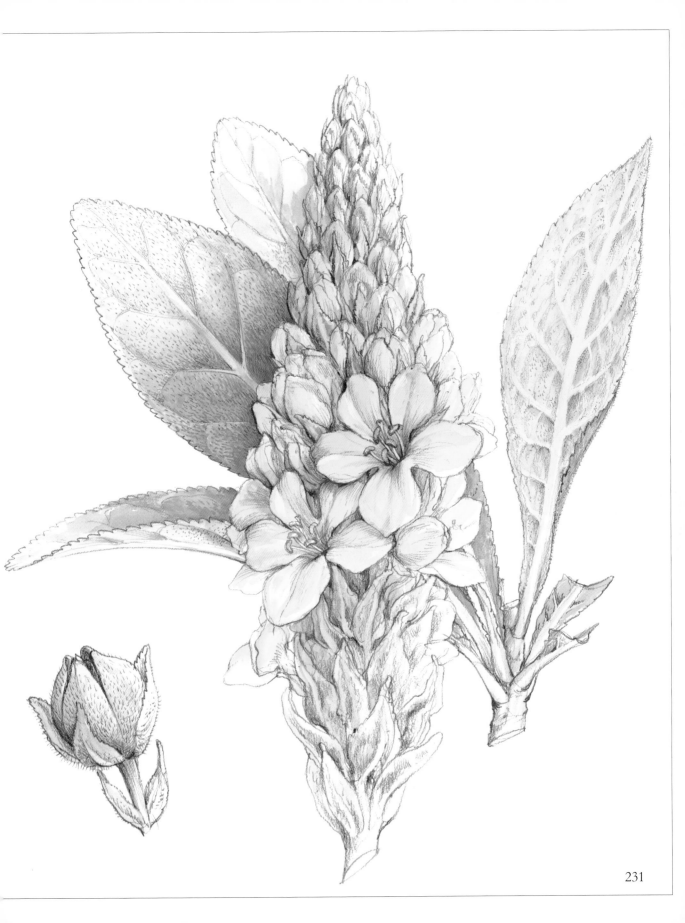

aching muscles, as well as to heal wounds, burns, sores, ulcers and piles. The flowers can be used for ringworm and other skin infections. The leaves once boiled used to be applied to the chest for asthma, to the head for headaches, and to the throat for sore throats, swollen glands and mumps. Mullein oil prepared from the flowers is excellent used as eardrops or massaged around the ears for earache, and eczema of the outer ear.

Homeopathic remedy: VERBASCUM

Mullein again has a pronounced action on the ear, the respiratory system and the urinary system. It is prescribed for deafness, as if the ear is blocked, and when getting water in the ears from swimming causes a blocked sensation. It will also relieve pain in the face (it affects the interior maxillary branch of the 5th cranial nerve), and facial neuralgia that recurs periodically, with lightning pain, as if crushed with tongs. It is also for catarrh and colds when associated with neuralgia on the left side of the face. The pain is worse with changes of temperature, pressure and motion, as in talking and sneezing.

Verbascum can also be used for hoarseness, and deep hollow coughs that sound like a trumpet, for tickling in the larynx and chest, catarrh, asthma, colds, nervous coughs, and coughing during sleep.

In the urinary system verbascum will relieve cystitis symptoms, burning and dribbling urination, frequency of urination through nervousness, and bedwetting. It can also be used effectively for piles, and irritating conditions of the genitals.

A Verbascum person may feel morose or apathetic, suffer from a poor memory, ill-humour, and be easily distracted. They also have lively imaginations.

The flower essence

Mullein again is the remedy of light, an inner light to guide us along our path. It is also a remedy for uprightness, honesty, moral conscience, particularly for those who feel weak or confused, unable to tune into their inner voice, or who are wrestling with their conscience. It is helpful when needing inner strength to withstand social pressures or trends, tempting one to lie either to oneself or to others, and to help sort out moral values. It can be taken for indecision, to clarify or hear better your inner voice, or to be guided by your inner light, and thus lead towards a greater fulfillment of your true potential. Mullein helps you to be true to yourself.

Vervain

The flower of divination

Bring your garlands, and with reverence place
The Vervain on the Altar
  'TCH' FROM MRS. LEYEL

Vervain is a modest little plant, a member of the verbena family, that is found growing wild in Britain,
central and southern Europe and Asia along
roadsides and lanes and on waste ground. It will
grow easily on most soils. Despite the inconspicuous
nature of its little lilac-blue flowers, vervain was the
foremost magical herb of antiquity. It was considered
sacred, a wizard's herb, used for casting spells and a
vital ingredient of magic potions. The Druids held it
in as high esteem as mistletoe and probably
introduced it to the Romans who used it to crown
ambassadors and similar dignitaries. The Romans
made it into bundles for ritual cleansing and to
sweep the altars to the gods, and in honour of this
sacred plant they held an annual festival called verbe-
nalia. The Druids cleansed their altars with an infusion of vervain before offering sacrifices. It was
important for spells, divination, magic medicine and
for amulets to protect against witchcraft and evil.

  With the coming of Christianity, vervain continued to be held sacred. It was said to have been discovered on Mount Calvary at the foot of the cross,
and used to staunch the bleeding from Christ's
wounds. It was called the Holy herb and was crossed
and blessed when gathered. In the Middle Ages sorcerers and magicians endowed it with miraculous
properties – it was believed to heal every wound
received in battle and bring immortality to heroes.

  At the end of the 16th century Mattiolus wrote,
'sorcerers lose their senses at the mention of the
herb. For they say that those who are rubbed with it
will obtain all they ask, and that it will cure fevers,
and cause a person to love another, and, in short,
that it cures all illness and more besides'. Clearly it
was seen as a panacea for all ills, and was used
around this time for jaundice, kidney disease, the
plague, heart disease, toothache, difficult pregnancies
and childbirth. Culpeper said it was excellent for
strengthening the womb, and that being hot and dry,
it would open all obstructions, cleansing and healing.
Culpeper also said that vervain was ruled by Venus,
and in fact the Romans had dedicated it to the

goddess Venus, calling it *Veneris Herba*, herb of
Venus. They believed it could reignite the fires of a
dying love and worked as an aphrodisiac. It was thus
picked by Roman brides to wear at their weddings. It
was dedicated also to Isis, the goddess of birth. At
New Year the Romans would exchange lucky
nosegays of vervain and they also made infusions to
sprinkle in banqueting halls to make their guests
merrier. Later in the Middle Ages it entered into the
preparation of most love philtres. A child who wore
a sprig of vervain was said to be well-behaved, lively,
good humoured and a lover of knowledge.

  Not only was vervain a sacred magical herb, and a
herb for love, but also it was a herb of protection.
Chaplets of vervain were worn by Roman heralds-
at-arms carrying messages of war, to give them
immunity from the enemy. The herald was called a
verbenarius, and vervain was believed to ensure a
peaceful settlement and used as a flag of truce
between warring factions. The physicians of Myddfai
recommended warriors when fighting to wear vervain
to protect them.

Herbal remedy

Vervain is a wonderful tonic to the nervous system,
calming the nerves and easing tension, protecting
from and increasing resistance to stress. In the past it
was famous as a remedy for nervous disorders, to
stop nightmares and for epilepsy. It can be taken to
relieve anxiety, to lift depression and for stress-related problems such as headaches, nervous coughs,
asthma, insomnia, high blood pressure and ME,
migraines and nervous exhaustion. The bitters stimulate the liver and enhance digestion, making vervain a
useful tonic for problems related to a sluggish liver,
including constipation, lethargy, depression,
headaches and irritability. It has been used for liver
disorders and gallstones, and to speed recovery and
increase energy during convalescence. In hot infusion
it acts as a diaphoretic, increasing sweating, and can
both clear toxins and bring down fevers. In cool
infusion it has a diuretic effect and is used in oedema
and for kidney stones and gravel. This also makes it
useful for fluid retention and gout. It is still used as a
woman's herb during lactation, as it increases the
flow of breastmilk. Because it brings on menstruation

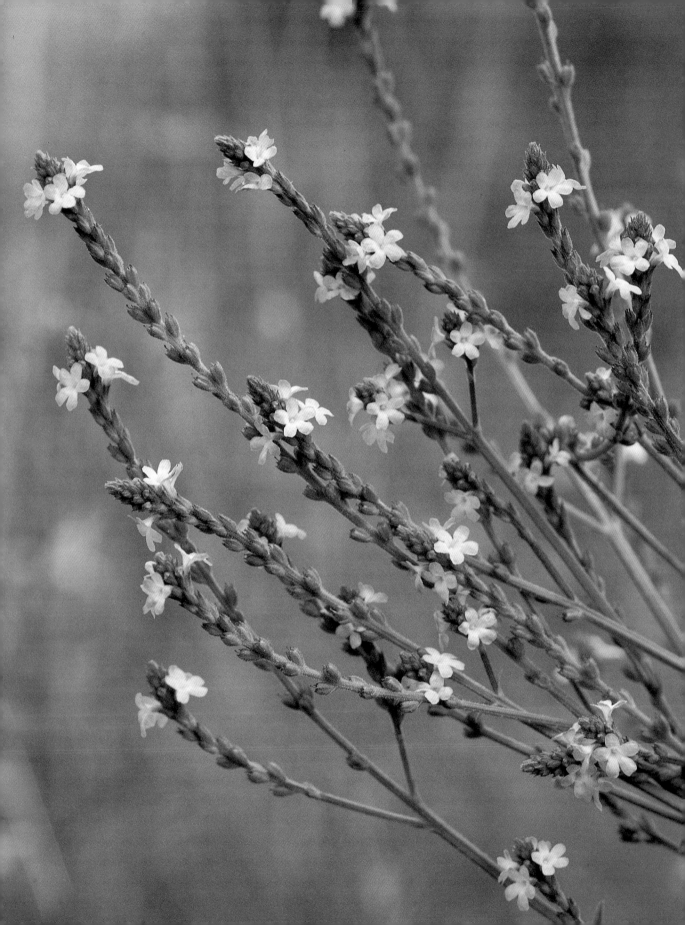

and stimulates uterine contractions is best avoided in pregnancy. Vervain makes a good remedy for menstrual migraines, and it can be used during the birth to enhance contractions.

In America, relatives of *Verbena officinalis* were used – *Verbena sticta*, wild blue vervain for upset stomachs and *Verbena hastata*, also with a blue flower, for coughs, urinary stones and gravel, worms, bruises and skin problems. The latter had tonic properties and was used for nervous problems and epilepsy.

Externally, the tannins in vervain make it a useful astringent when used as a mouthwash for bleeding gums and mouth ulcers, and as a gargle for sore throats and tonsillitis. As a skin lotion it heals sores and wounds, ulcers, burns and insect bites.

Homeopathic remedy: VERBENA

The relative of the blue vervain, *Verbena hastata*, which is indigenous to America, is employed as a tincture. It is also prescribed for nervous disorders – depression, anxiety, tension, epilepsy, muscle tension and spasm, insomnia and mental exhaustion. It helps to calm over-exciteability, and brighten mental powers in those nervously run down and exhausted.

Like the herbal remedy, verbena is used to reduce fevers and as a diuretic to clear toxins from the system which contribute to skin problems, and to aid elimination during treatment for TB. It promotes the absorption of blood, and so helps allay the pain of bruises. It is also used for rhus poisoning.

The flower essence

Vervain is a Bach Flower Remedy for charismatic people with huge resources of energy, which can be a great inspiration to others. They can be full of enthusiasm and idealism and by radiating their enormous energy they have a great capacity for leading and healing others. Vervain people tend to espouse themselves to causes, or get involved in charitable works and welfare organizations. Their commitment to their work or ideals can lead them to sacrifice all their energy and time to further their cause. It can take over their lives, and they are unable to rest or relax, feeling the need to win those around them to their viewpoint and expend all their energy in the process. They have enormous willpower and often being revolutionaries at heart are prepared to suffer for their convictions. They have great courage and are not afraid to speak out although this, combined with their over-enthusiastic, domineering, overzealous attitude, can actually be detrimental to their cause. Such people are often seen as overbearing, over-intense, even fanatical. They rarely deviate from their firm principles, convinced as they are of the rightness and urgency of their cause.

In this condition, vervain people overuse their energy resources, being constantly on the job, and never giving in to messages from their body or inner selves to rest. This can lead eventually to nervous exhaustion. They live on their nerves and become so keyed up they cannot relax even if they want to. Their tense, nervous natures often lead to digestive problems. As they are often intolerant and angry they become progressively more depleted. This may inevitably culminate in a nervous breakdown.

Vervain helps these people to use their huge resources of energy in a more natural way. Dr Bach said, 'vervain teaches us that it is by being rather than doing that great things are accomplished'. It engenders a calm and open attitude to the ideas of others, and allows their exuberance to be an inspiration to others. It helps towards a more balanced and harmonious life, treading the Middle Path.

Periwinkle

The flower of closeness

The periwinkle with its soft blue windmill-shaped flowers is a hardy evergreen plant with shining leaves making good ground cover in winter, earning its common name, joy of the ground. The two wild periwinkles grow in woodlands and banks all over Europe. They are the lesser periwinkle, *Vinca minor*, and the greater periwinkle, *Vinca major*.

The word periwinkle comes from the old Latin name *Vinca pervinca*, deriving from *pervincire*, meaning to bind closely, or from *pervincere*, to overcome. The long creeping stems of periwinkle bind together and to neighbouring plants. Culpeper said that if the leaves were eaten by a man and woman together, it will bind them closer. The whole plant was considered a vital ingredient for love philtres to guarantee a happy marriage. Culpeper said the periwinkle was ruled by Venus. The flowers were strewed on the path of the bride and groom; the blue flowers symbolized the virginity of the bride, and the evergreen leaves the everlasting love of the young couple.

In the language of flowers periwinkle means unbreakable friendship and tender memories. In Italy plaited garlands of periwinkle were placed on the coffins of dead children, and were known as 'flowers of death', symbolizing immortality, eternity and tender memories.

Periwinkle may also mean to overcome – it was once bound to the legs to overcome cramp, to the skin to stop bleeding of cuts and wounds, and when fastened around the thigh of a pregnant woman to prevent miscarriage. Medicinally, it has a binding quality, acting as an astringent, stopping diarrhoea and dysentery, as well as bleeding.

Herbal remedy

Culpeper aptly described the medicinal virtues of periwinkle when he said it is a 'great binder and stays bleeding at the mouth and nose, if it be chewed. It is a good female medicine and may be used with advantage in hysterical and other fits'. The astringent tannins in periwinkle act to curb diarrhoea and dysentery, and to protect the walls of the digestive tract from irritation and infection. They also stop bleeding. Periwinkle reduces excessive menstrual bleeding, and makes a good vaginal douche for discharges, a lotion for haemorrhoids and varicose veins, and relieves a variety of skin problems such as acne and cradle cap. It makes a mouthwash and gargle for mouth ulcers, tonsillitis and sore throats.

The leaves used to be chewed to relieve toothache and stop bleeding gums. As an astringent periwinkle will also help to clear chronic catarrh and phlegm from the chest.

Periwinkle also has a beneficial effect upon the nervous system, reducing tension and anxiety.

Another species of periwinkle, *Vinca rosea*, Madagascan periwinkle (now known as *Catharanthus roseus*) is very helpful to diabetics as it reduces blood sugar. Both the lesser and greater periwinkles have long been used by herbalists for treating diabetes as they too reduce blood sugar. The Madagascan periwinkle contains more than 70 different alkaloids, two of which are extensively used to treat malignant tumours, as well as leukaemia and Hodgkin's disease.

Homeopathic remedy: VINCA MINOR

Vinca minor is used for bleeding and haemorrhage, as in uterine bleeding, heavy periods and frequent nosebleeds. It is a good remedy for scabby eruptions and itching of the skin, often on the scalp. A Vinca person tends to feel extremely weak, as if anaemic, faint, sad and fearful of dying.

The flower essence

Periwinkle is for those who are prone to depression, nervous disorders such as anxiety, and seasonal affective disorders. It helps to clear the mind and engender a sense of inner clarity and self-knowledge which helps to dispel the depression. People who need periwinkle may feel weak and anaemic and are often prone to heavy bleeding or nosebleeds. Periwinkle helps to boost energy levels, and by healing both physical and emotional wounds from the past, it enhances regeneration.

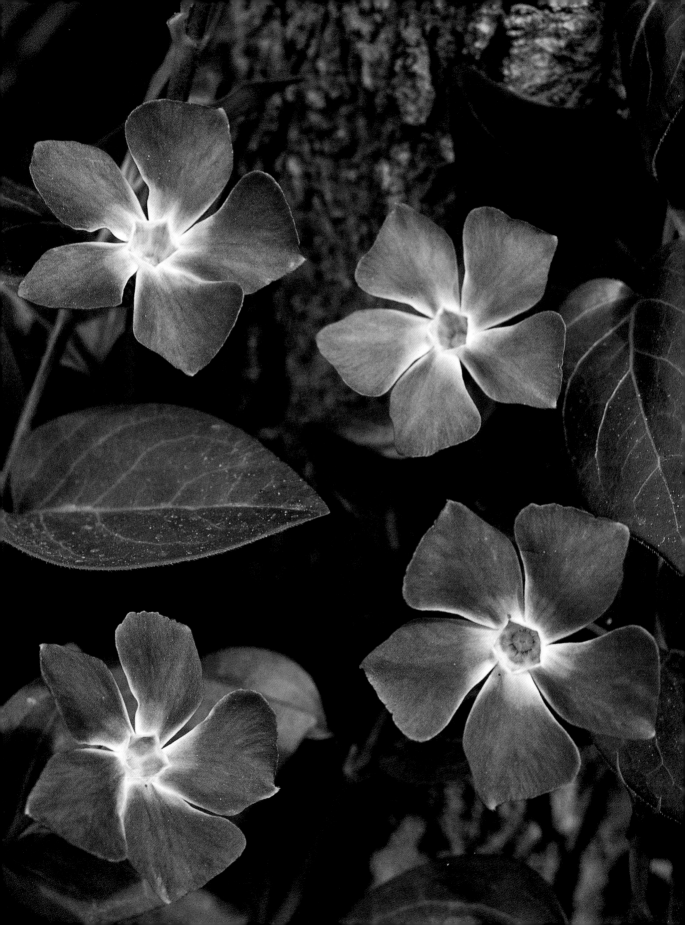

Sweet violet

The flower of shyness

Reform the errors of the Spring,
Make that tulips may have share
of sweetness, seeing they are fair,
And roses of their thorns disarm'd,
But most procure
That violets may a longer age endure.
  ANDREW MARVELL (1621–78)

The heavenly-scented sweet violet, with its pretty little flower that hides beneath the leaves, is a symbol of shyness and modesty. It flowers, but briefly, in woods, forests and hedges in spring. There are many myths and legends about the origins of the violet that may have given rise to such phrases as blushing violet or shrinking violet. One Greek myth tells how the nymph Ianthis was chased by the amorous Apollo. The frightened virgin fled to the woods and sought protection from Diana, who advised her to hide away where Apollo could not find her. Diana changed the nymph into the violet so that she could escape Apollo's importunities. Another version says that violets were created for Io, beloved of Zeus, to honour her beauty. Io's name remains in the word for the flower violet, and in Greek *io* means violet.

Violet is also the symbol for steadfastness and loyalty. Shakespeare was clearly fond of the violet and used it as a symbol of humility and constancy in love in his writings. In Medieval times violet symbolized Christ's humility. It was cultivated extensively in monastery gardens to protect against all forms of evil. Necklaces of violets were said to protect from deception and inebriation. Garlands of violets were worn by the Ancient Greeks and Romans to dispel the odours of wine and spirits and thus prevent drunkeness. Violets were also used in love potions.

Herbal remedy

Violets have been valued as medicine at least since the time of the Ancient Greeks. Hippocrates recommended them for headaches, hangovers, bad eyesight, melancholia, excess of bile and chest inflammation. Pliny said they induced sleep, strengthened the heart muscles and calmed anger. Violets were used by the Arabs for constipation, tonsillitis, insomnia and liver troubles. Modern usage reflects their ancient claims. The saponins and mucilage in violets make them an excellent soothing expectorant for relieving harsh irritating coughs, whooping cough and other chest infections. Violet syrup is a famous remedy for soothing children's coughs. It reduces fevers and feverish colds, and can be used as a gargle for sore throats and a mouthwash for inflamed gums. The mucilage also soothes the stomach and intestines and the syrup is a gentle laxative for children.

Violet's cooling properties act wherever there is heat and inflammation. It relieves headaches and migraine with a feeling of heat. The salicylates help to reduce inflammation in rheumatism and arthritis.

Externally, a poultice can be applied to hot swellings, and to soothe and heal sore cracked nipples and inflammatory skin conditions. An infusion can be used to bathe sore eyes. Violets have a reputation as a cancer remedy, particularly for tumours in the breast, lungs, throat and intestines.

Homeopathic remedy: VIOLA ODORATA

Viola is prescribed for breathlessness and spasmodic coughs, whooping cough, and breathing problems associated with anxiety. It is also for headaches, burning of the forehead, pain above the eyebrows and vertigo. It can be used for rheumatism, and pains in the bones. A Viola odorata person easily gets tense and over-excited. The brain can be very active, and a rush of ideas can cause confusion. They are bright and perceptive, can be sad or depressed, and weep constantly without knowing why. It particularly suits thin, nervous girls.

The flower essence

Violet is a flower remedy for profound shyness. It is for people who are delicate, sensitive, sweet and refined, who long to join in with group activities, but feel too nervous or timid. They appear reserved and aloof. Because of their shyness they may choose jobs or lifestyles which keep them apart from others, but this can cause isolation and loneliness. Violet helps to develop trust, so that other people do not appear so threatening, and enhances the ability to join groups without the fear of losing your identity. It engenders openness and warmth, and gives support to those unassertive people with their tendency to retreat, like the violet beneath its leaves.

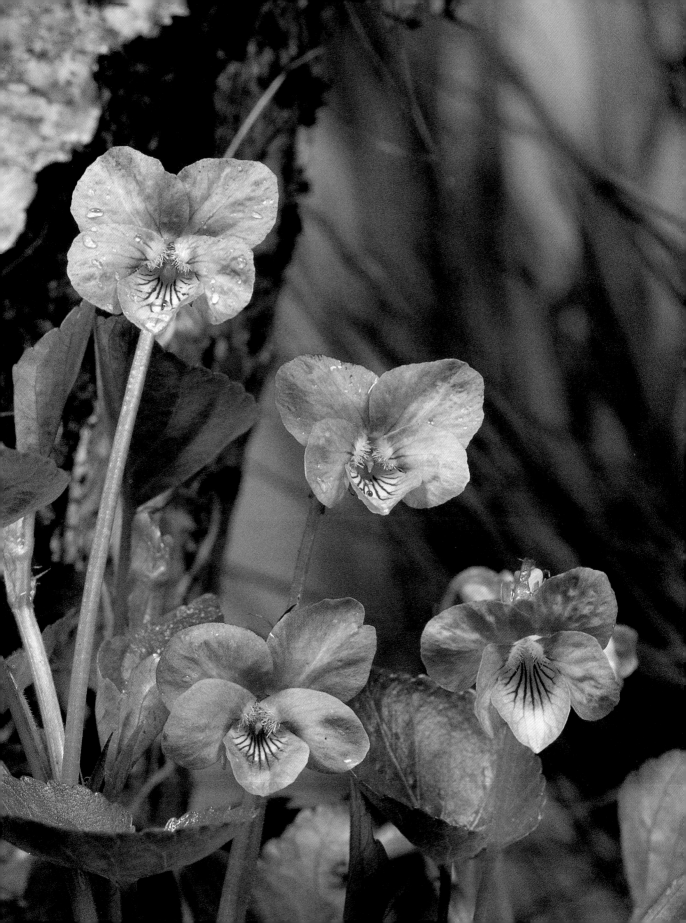

Heartsease

The flower of thoughts

What flowers are these?
The Pansie this;
Oh! That's for loving thoughts.
GEORGE CHAPMAN (1559?–1634)

Wild pansy or heartsease has close associations with affairs of the heart in myth and legend. It is so called for its ability to heal the heart, soothe the pain of separation from loved ones, and ease a broken heart. As far back as the days of Hippocrates it was used as a cordial, to lift the spirits and treat heart conditions and high blood pressure. It was used for its potency in love potions – Shakespeare had it playing an important part in *A Midsummer Night's Dream*, working as a love charm on Titania and causing her to fall for an ass. In legend, Cupid's arrow brought colour to the flower, for previously it was white.

The flower's common name pansy comes from the French *pensees* meaning thoughts. In *Hamlet* Ophelia says, 'there is pansies – that's for thoughts'. In the Victorian language of flowers heartsease means 'you are in my thoughts'. People also believed that if they carried a pansy it would ensure the love of their sweetheart.

In the French countryside heartsease is called the Trinity herb. Some say this is because each flower bears three colours, representing the Trinity, but in another legend the story is different. The pansy used to have a scent sweeter than that of its sister, the violet, and the flowers' beautiful faces dotted the cornfields with colour. People picking the pretty flowers would trample down the crops leaving little grain at harvest time. So the sad pansy prayed for help to the Holy Trinity. She begged to lose her fragrant perfume so that people would not trample down the corn to find her. Her wish came true and since then she has been known as the Trinity herb.

Heartsease is a weed of cultivated places, found mostly in garden ground and ploughed ground. It can be grown from seed in light, friable soil.

Herbal remedy

Heartsease has cooling, cleansing and anti-inflammatory properties and is excellent used internally and externally for skin problems including eczema, psoriasis and acne. It is used especially for cradle cap and eczema in babies, and other crusty skin complaints.

In the respiratory system, the mucilage in heartsease is soothing, while the saponins have an expectorant action making this herb a good remedy for harsh irritating coughs, asthma, croup and bronchitis. It reduces fevers and swollen glands, and acts as a soothing diuretic for fluid retention and cystitis.

The salicylates in heartsease relieve inflamed joints in arthritis and gout, while the rutin helps strengthen blood capillaries, and thereby stop bruising. It also reduces blood pressure and arteriosclerosis.

Homeopathic remedy: VIOLA TRICOLOR

Heartsease is used similarly for skin problems, particularly cradle cap, eczema of the scalp, impetigo and scabby skin complaints. Symptoms tend to be worse in winter and cold air. It is indicated for people with swollen cervical glands, coughs, and phlegm in the throat, for rheumatism, gout and itching eruptions around the joints. It is also prescribed for bedwetting in children who have vivid or disturbing dreams, and whose urine smells particularly strong, like a cat's. Relating back to its folk usage it is also taken for conditions relating to the heart – anxiety about the heart and palpitations on lying down. Clarke recommended it for 'sadness respecting domestic affairs', and a 'tendency to shed tears'. It is used for adults who have vivid or amorous dreams.

The flower essence

Heartsease (pansy) is used again for healing the heart. It brings comfort to those feeling hurt, rejected, lonely or broken-hearted. It is for disappointment in love, in separation, and when broken hearts cause symptoms in those previously happy and healthy.

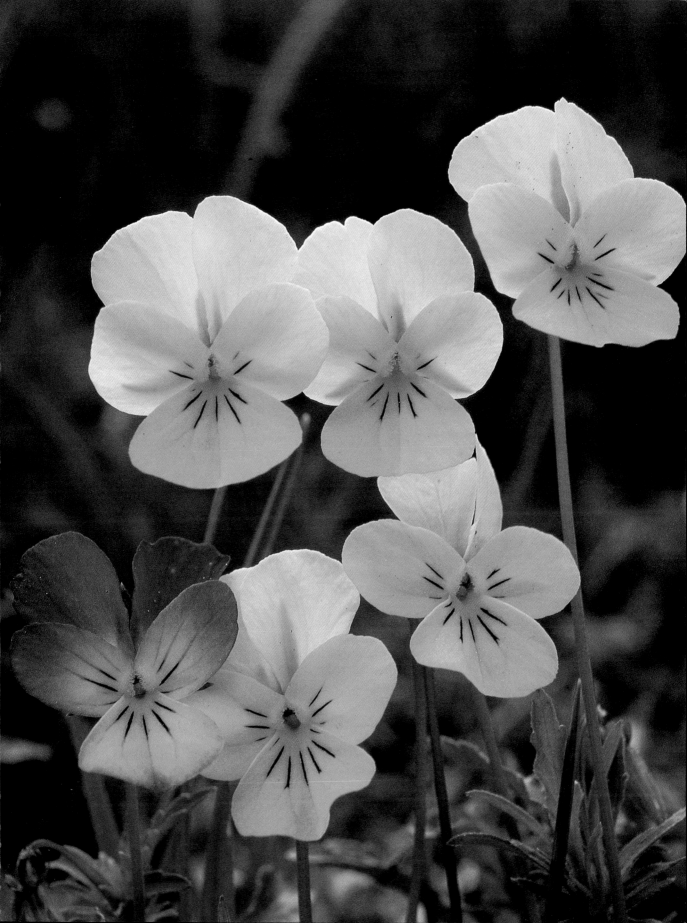

Viscum album

Mistletoe

The flower of the sacred oak

Mistletoe is an evergreen partial parasite found growing on deciduous trees in Europe and temperate Asia. It has been revered as a sacred plant by many ancient peoples of Europe and has been associated closely with magic and medicine. To the Druids mistletoe was a symbol of immortality; they regarded mistletoe as the soul of their sacred tree, the oak, and used it in their religious ceremonies. The Druids called mistletoe all-heal.

The berries are poisonous. When used medicinally it is usually taken from apple trees. The plant called mistletoe in America is *Phoradendron serotinum*, and is far more poisonous.

The custom of kissing under the mistletoe could refer to the fact that mistletoe was a symbol of fertility. In the language of flowers mistletoe means 'I surmount difficulties'.

The name mistletoe is said to come from the Anglo-Saxon word *mistilton*, indicating that it was unlike the host tree. The Latin name *viscum* (sticky) refers to the glutinous juice contained in the berries.

Herbal remedy Mistletoe has been valued as a sedative, antispasmodic and tonic to the nerves for many hundreds of years. It was used for epilepsy, convulsions, hysteria, delirium, spleen and heart problems, nervous debility and it was also used to stop bleeding. Today mistletoe is used by practising herbalists as a regulator of blood pressure, to remedy both hypertension and hypotension. It has a vasodilatory action in the arteries and is helpful where arteriosclerosis has narrowed them. Mistletoe also has a beneficial and regulatory action on the heart, normalizing a slow and unsteady pulse, and calming an over-rapid heart. It is also used for its relaxant and sedative effect on the nervous system and the muscles throughout

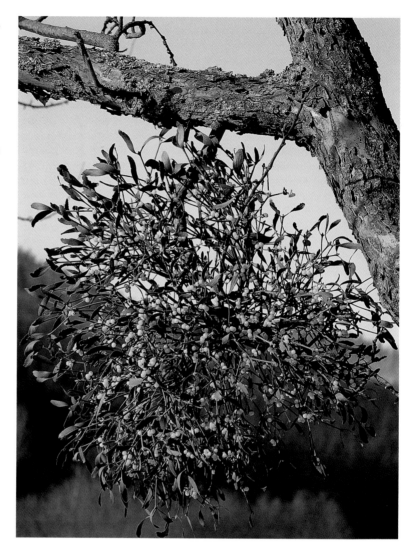

the body, so that it makes a good remedy for tense, aching muscles and cramp, nervous headaches, migraines and vertigo. There is evidence that mistletoe may have anti-tumour effects. Certainly mistletoe has been shown to have beneficial effects upon the immune system, and for this reason mistletoe is often used by people whose immunity is compromised by chronic candida, ME and HIV, and after orthodox cancer treatment.

Homeopathic remedy Viscum is prepared from the whole mistletoe plant and is used for epilepsy and convulsions, giddiness, headaches,

and spasm of the muscles. It is also prescribed for palpitations, fever, back pain, sciatica and rheumatism.

The flower essence Mistletoe is recommended for people experiencing a period of rapid change and transformation in their lives. It gives one the strength and energy to surmount all difficulties as the language of flowers tells us, and is a bringer of love and goodwill.

As a symbol of fertility mistletoe helps to bring forth the fruits of our actions, thus helping the transformation process, on both physical and psychological levels.

Ginger

The flower of paradise

The thick, tuberous roots of this reed-like plant have been used as a culinary spice and medicine since antiquity. It is native to southern Asia and widely cultivated in the tropics. It is mentioned in the writings of Confucius as early as 500BC, and in Chinese medical texts of 2,000 years ago. A large proportion of prescriptions in oriental medicine contain ginger. The Ancient Greeks used ginger after it was brought to Greece by Alexander the Great (356–352BC). Hippocrates and Dioscorides are reported to have recommended it to enhance cooking and to calm and profit the stomach and 'against all darkness of the sight'. According to the Koran, the menu served in Paradise includes ginger, as it did at the round table of King Arthur and his knights in Medieval times.

The name comes from ancient Indian Sanskrit *sringa-vera*, meaning horn body, probably referring to the root. The word was later adapted by the Greeks as *zingiberis*, leading to *gingibar* in Latin.

In Ayurvedic medicine ginger's pungent and warming properties enhance the 'fire' in the body, responsible for proper digestion, body heat, visual perception, hunger, thirst, the lustre of the skin, the softness of the body, the light in the eyes, the clarity in the mind, intelligence and determination, as well as courage. It was used by the early European herbalists as a cure for colds, colic, constipation, diarrhoea, painful and scanty periods, insomnia, kidney problems, snakebite, stomach ache, toothache, weak eyes, to strengthen the heart and as an aphrodisiac. At the medieval university of Salerno in Italy, the pioneering medical school promoted a prescription for a happy life in later years: Eat ginger and you will love and be loved as in your youth.

Herbal remedy

It is the pungent and warming properties of ginger that have made it such a valuable medicine. It has a stimulating effect on the heart and circulation, creating a feeling of warmth and wellbeing (expecially welcome on cold, damp winter days) and restoring vitality. Hot ginger tea taken at the onset of a sore throat, cold or flu, when you feel tired, chilly and aching, promotes perspiration, brings down a fever and helps to clear catarrh. It has a stimulating and expectorant action in the lungs, expelling phlegm and relieving catarrhal coughs and chest infections. In India fresh ginger tea is given to children for whooping cough.

Ginger is a wonderful warming aid to the digestion. It invigorates the stomach and intestines, stimulating the appetite and enhancing digestion by encouraging secretion of digestive enzymes. It moves stagnation of food and subsequent accumulation of toxins which has a far-reaching effect throughout the body, increasing general health and vitality and enhancing immunity.

The crystallized root can be chewed, the powdered root taken in capsules or a hot decoction drunk to prevent and relieve nausea and vomiting from most causes. It makes an excellent remedy for travel sickness; this fact was long known by sailors in the East where ginger preparations are still taken to keep seasickness at bay during long voyages in stormy seas. It also relieves sickness during pregnancy, as well as that related to an upset stomach, over-eating, nervousness and infection. It settles the stomach, soothes indigestion and calms wind. Its pain-relieving and relaxing effects in the digestive system relieve colic and spasm, abdominal pain, distension and flatulent indigestion, and help relieve griping from diarrhoea and dysentery. It is said to be a good cure for a hangover. Raw and crystallized ginger make a pleasant breath sweetener.

These warming, stimulating and relaxing properties can be seen elsewhere in the body. In the uterus it promotes menstruation, useful for delayed and scanty periods as well as clots. It relaxes spasm and painful ovulation and periods, and is recommended to invigorate the reproductive system and treat impotence caused by deficiency of vital warmth in the body. It has an ancient reputation as an aphrodisiac. It used to be considered excellent for transforming frigid women into the type of enchantress that men apparently seek in their dreams. Gerard reported that green (unripe) ginger 'is provoking to venerie and lust'. The Africans are still reputed to drink ginger tea as an aphrodisiac, while women in New Guinea eat the dried root as a contraceptive.

Recent research has found that ginger inhibits clotting and thins the blood; it lowers harmful blood cholesterol and reduces blood pressure. In the past the forehead was covered with a paste made of powdered ginger and cold water to reduce blood pressure.

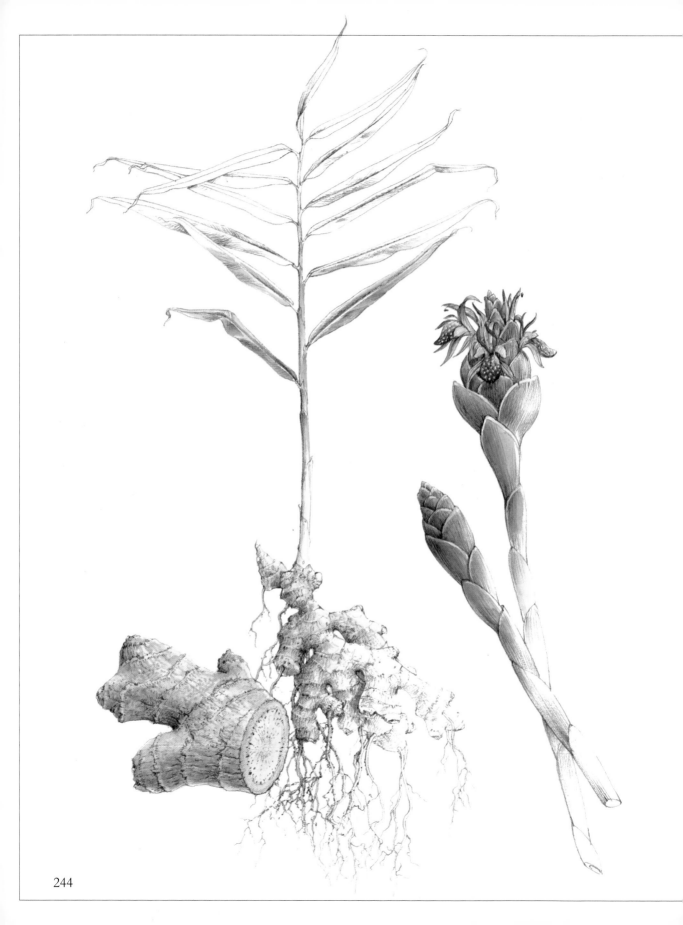

244

However, adding ginger frequently to your cooking or taking ginger tea is quite sufficient.

Ginger helps the body to fight off infections before they become entrenched by activating the circulation, producing perspiration and stimulating the digestion to eliminate toxins. The volatile oils are also antiseptic, activating immunity and dispelling bacterial and viral infections. So ginger makes a useful preventative remedy against winter chills and ills, such as tonsillitis and bronchitis, as well as infections in the digestive tract. In the East it has been used for epidemics such as cholera. Fresh ginger root is reported to be highly effective in China in treatment of rheumatism, acute bacterial dysentery, malaria and orchitis (inflammation of the testicle). Ginger has also been shown to have antioxidative properties, inhibiting free radicals in the body, and thereby further aiding immunity and the circulation. Ginger is a very useful addition to many herbal prescriptions for it has the effect of assisting them in reaching their destination and enhancing their action.

Externally, the painkilling properties of chewing fresh ginger have been used to relieve toothache. Grated or powdered ginger has been used in a paste to cover the scalp to promote hair growth and stop baldness. Dilute ginger oil has been used in massage oils and liniments for lumbago, neuralgia and painful joints made worse by cold.

Homeopathic remedy: ZINGIBER

Zingiber has a marked effect upon the digestive, urinary and respiratory systems, and is used for a state of debility in any of these areas. In a Zingiber picture digestive problems arise from eating melons, bread, and drinking impure water, and manifest as a heavy feeling like a stone in the stomach, acidity, bad breath, and a bad taste in the mouth. There is heaviness in the stomach on waking with flatulence and rumbling, great thirst, pain aggravated by eating, colic, diarrhoea, hot inflamed haemorrhoids, nausea and vomiting. There may be frequency of urination or suppression of urination, stinging and burning on passing water and fluid retention. Sexual desire is increased, though there may be a pain on erection.

In the respiratory system, symptoms indicating Zingiber include hoarseness, burning pain in the throat below the larynx, pain in the chest, a dry hacking cough, and asthma with attacks coming at night towards morning. The patient may need to sit up to breathe but despite the severity of the breathing difficulty, there is characteristically no anxiety.

A Zingiber person tends to be cheerful and good-humoured, just when the opposite might be expected. They can be forgetful and fidgety, especially in the legs and feet. They are prone to headaches, particularly after eating bread, and sensitive to light. There may be a feeling of a grain of sand in the eye, weakness in the joints, backache, cramp in the soles and palms, and fevers when they feel chilly and hot at the same time. They are generally worse at night, in damp cold air, and from motion.

Aromatherapy oil

Ginger oil is obtained from the root by steam distillation. Like the herbal remedy it has wonderfully warming qualities, increasing circulation, dispelling cold and damp, and invigorating the system. The oil can be used to enhance the immune system, increase energy and sexual vitality. It is a good nerve tonic for exhaustion and mental fatigue. It has a comforting and uplifting effect on those feeling insecure, fearful, lethargic or depressed. It improves memory and concentration. It can be used with great benefit for warming a sluggish digestion, for poor appetite, indigestion, wind, colic, nausea, and diarrhoea.

Externally, the oil can be massaged into painful arthritic joints, aching muscles, sore throats, chests to relieve bronchial congestion, and inhaled to clear phlegm in colds and catarrh.

The flower essence

Ginger has a warming and releasing effect and is particularly recommended for those who, from trauma or shock, have cut themselves off from their emotions and built a wall of invulnerability around themselves. They may appear cool, haughty, aloof, even cold.

Ginger unthaws the frozen feelings of such people, and relieves tension and fear. It increases sensitivity, magnifies perception, and enhances sensory awareness through sight, touch and hearing, bringing one into the here and now.

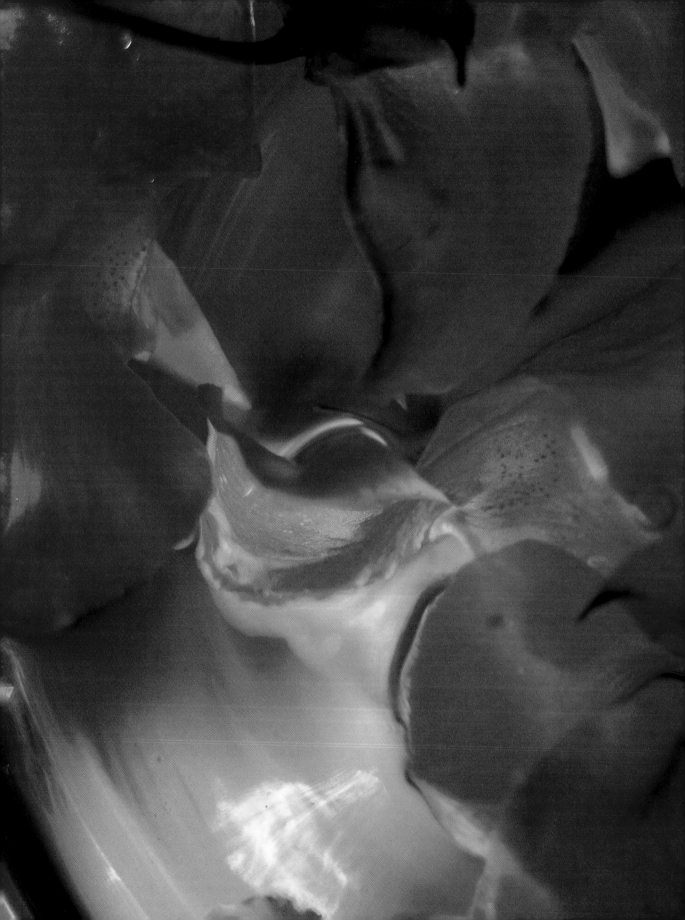

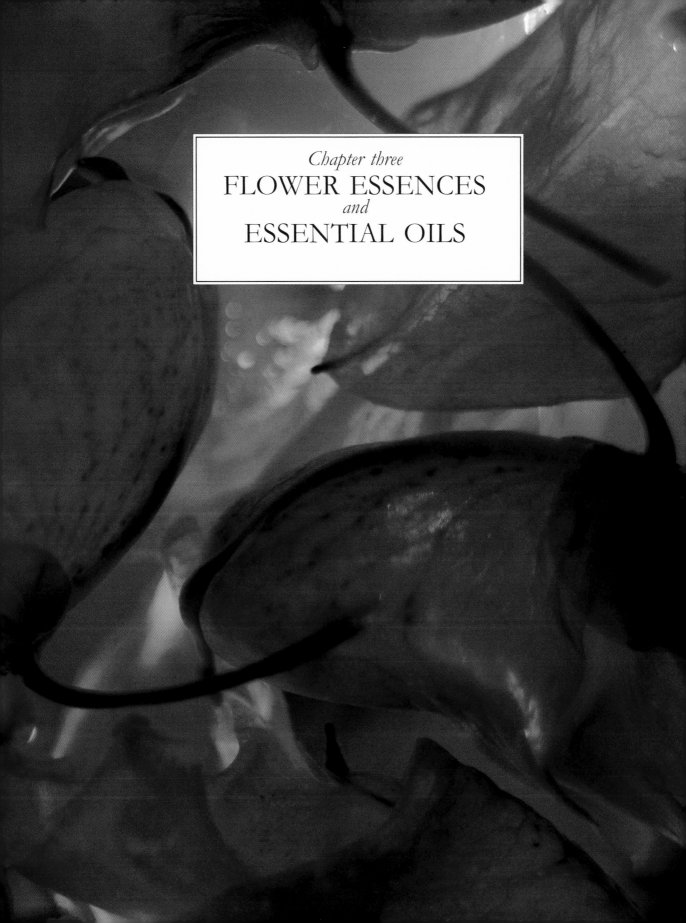

Chapter three
FLOWER ESSENCES
and
ESSENTIAL OILS

The Flower Essences

Just as God in His mercy has given us food to eat, so has He placed amongst the herbs of the fields beautiful plants to heal us when we are sick. These are there to extend a helping hand to man in those dark hours of forgetfulness when he loses sight of his Divinity, and allows the cloud of fear or pain to obscure his vision.'

Dr Edward Bach

The beautiful plants Dr Bach is referring to are his 38 flower remedies – gentle, subtle yet far-reaching remedies that are safe to use for all, from babies to adults.

Flower essences can address the disharmonies in the mind or emotions that are the underlying problems giving rise to so many physical ills. They also help us to become more aware of what it is in our nature or temperament that manifests as disharmony and disease, giving us a greater possibility of resolving such profound issues. Thus they help us to take a greater responsibility for our lives, and our well-being, and continue our voyage of self-discovery.

A full explanation of the role of the flower essences in healing, and how to choose and use them, is to be found on pages 272–273.

AGRIMONIA EUPATORIA
Agrimony
For cheerful, jovial people who hide their troubles behind their humour, not wishing to burden others with them. They will go to great lengths to avoid arguments or disharmony, and may use alcohol or drugs to stimulate themselves and help cope cheerfully with pain or anxiety. They are oversensitive to ideas and influences.

POPULUS TREMULA
Aspen
For those with vague fears of the unknown, a sense of foreboding, nightmares or terror of approaching misfortune for no apparent reason. One is often afraid to talk about these fears to other people.

FAGUS SYLVATICA
Beech
For perfectionists, who need to see more good in all around them and who are easily critical and intolerant. They tend to overlook the positive aspects of other people, over-reacting to minor details and lacking understanding of individual idiosyncrasies.

ERYTHRAEA CENTAURIUM
Centaury
For kind people who find it hard to say 'no', being over-anxious to please and serve others and tending to work harder on other people's behalf than on their own particular calling or interests. Such people are easily exploited.

CERATOSTIGMA WILLMOTTIANNA
Cerato
For uncertainty and those who doubt their ability to make decisions and judgements, and who constantly seek advice from others and are often being misguided.

THE BACH FLOWER REMEDIES

PRUNUS CERASIFERA
Cherry plum
For those fearful of being overstrained or losing control of their body, mind or emotions, such as uncontrollable anger and other impulses which may cause them to harm themselves or others, including suicidal tendencies.

AESCULUS HIPPOCASTANUM
Chestnut bud
For those who do not learn from observation and experience and constantly repeat the same experiences and make the same mistakes, before their lesson is learnt.

CICHORIUM INTYBUS
Chicory
For those who are over-concerned for the needs of others – friends, relatives or children – continually correcting them and wanting them to conform with their ideas. They are possessive, demanding and can be self-pitying.

CLEMATIS VITALBA
Clematis
For those with insufficient interest in present circumstances; for people who have a tendency to daydream, think about the future, and do not live fully in the present. They lack concentration, making little effort in everyday life, and live in hope of happier times ahead.

MALUS PUMILA OR SYLVESTRIS
Crab apple
For those who feel they need cleansing. For people who feel self-disgust or contamination, feelings of shame or low self-esteem, concentrating obsessively on one shameful aspect of themselves and ignoring others. For detoxification of the body, and cleansing of wounds, whether emotional or physical, internal or external.

ULMUS PROCERA
Elm
For diligent people, who are doing good work, often helping others, and following a vocation, but who feel overburdened or over-extended at times, which causes depression or despondency.

GENTIANA AMARELLA
Gentian
For those who are easily discouraged, in whom small setbacks can cause depression, despondency and self-doubt, even though generally they do well.

ULEX EUROPAEUS
Gorse
For those suffering from great hopelessness, feelings of despair and futility. They give up believing that any more can be done for them. If pushed or to please others, they may try various treatments with little hope of improvement.

CALLUNA VULGARIS
Heather
For lonely people who need to discuss their affairs with other people and so seek the company of anybody who will listen. They become very unhappy if they are left alone for any length of time.

ILEX AQUIFOLIUM
Holly
For people who are overcome by negative emotions such as anger, jealousy, envy and suspicion. They suffer much inside, often when there is no real cause.

LONICERA CAPRIFOLIUM
Honeysuckle
For those who live in the past, and do not expect happiness as they have enjoyed before. Such people are nostalgic, homesick, and prone to reminiscing.

CARPINUS BETULUS
Hornbeam
For those who feel they need strengthening and help physically or mentally to bear the burden life has placed upon their shoulders. For 'Monday morning' feeling, not feeling up to facing the coming day, and the pressures of everyday life.

IMPATIENS GLANDULIFERA
Impatiens
For those who think and act quickly, and so want everything done without delay. They are often happier working or being alone so that they can go at their own speed, for they are often impatient or irritated by others who do things more slowly.

LARIX DECIDUA
Larch
For despondent and despairing people who do not consider themselves as good or as capable as those around them. Even though they may be perfectly able, they lack confidence and expect failure, so that often they do not try hard enough to succeed. This becomes a self-fulfilling prophesy.

MIMULUS GUTTATUS
Mimulus
For those fearful of everyday known things, such as illness, death, old age, pain, darkness or being alone. Also for people who are very shy and afraid of others. These fears are kept inside and are not spoken of to others.

SINAPIS ARVENSIS
Mustard
For those experiencing periods of sadness, gloom or even despair, which descend for no apparent reason, making it impossible to feel happiness or joy.

QUERCUS ROBUR
Oak
For those who never give up, despite setbacks, misfortunes or illness. They keep trying one thing after another, determined to reach their goal. Never losing hope, they fight on.

OLEA EUROPAEA
Olive
For those suffering complete mental and physical exhaustion. Their daily life seems hard, without joy, and wearisome. Such people are worn out from mental or physical ordeals and suffering.

PINUS SYLVESTRIS
Pine
For despondent and despairing people who blame themselves and feel guilty. Even when they succeed, they are not satisfied with their efforts or results, and feel they could have done better. They work hard and suffer much from the faults they attach to themselves, even claiming responsibility for mistakes which are not theirs.

AESCULUS CARNEA
Red chestnut
For those overconcerned or afraid about the welfare of others, especially loved ones, during times such as illness, journeys, or when away from them. Often such people do not worry for themselves.

Rescue Remedy
This is the remedy of emergency, for calming emotions during a crisis or trauma. It is made of Impatiens, Clematis, Rock rose, Cherry plum and Star of Bethlehem.

HELIANTHEMUM NUMMULARIUM
Rock rose
For those in fear and experiencing fright, panic, terror, or hysteria. A remedy for emergencies, even when there appears to be no hope.

SCLERANTHUS ANNUUS
Scleranthus
For those who are indecisive, unable to choose between two things, and who change their minds; they have energy and mood swings. Such people are quiet and tend not to talk about their difficulties to others.

ORNITHOGALUM UMBELLATUM
Star of Bethlehem
For great distress and unhappiness following some kind of shock, such as bad news, the death of a loved one or an accident.

CASTANEA SATIVA
Sweet chestnut
For those who despair and feel that the anguish is so great it is unbearable. They have reached the limits of their endurance, and there is nothing left but dark despair.

VERBENA OFFICINALIS
Vervain
For those with strong ideas, fixed opinions, those who are always right and wish to teach and convert those around them. They can be over-enthusiastic and overpowering but, during illness, their determination helps them to struggle more than others.

VITIS VINIFERA
Vine
For strong, capable people, who are self-confident and powerful, certain they are right. They can be dictatorial and overbearing, dominating and directing others with their conviction, even during illness.

JUGLANS REGIA
Walnut
For those who need to break links with the past and to help them adjust to new phases (such as new relationships, jobs, houses), balancing emotions in transition periods (such as starting school, puberty, marriage, menopause) or even the death of a loved one. The remedy helps protect you from outside influences which may cause you to stray from your chosen path.

HOTTONIA PALUSTRIS
Water violet
For lonely and very quiet people who appear aloof, and prefer to be alone. They are independent and self-reliant, often bright and talented, and do not tend to get involved in other people's affairs. They radiate peace and tranquillity to those around them.

AESCULUS HIPPOCASTANUM
White chestnut
For those with persistent unwanted thoughts and ideas, which, though thrown out, return when there is not sufficient interest in the present fully to occupy the mind. For those with mental arguments, preoccupation, obsessive thoughts which cause mental torture, and an inability to relax or concentrate fully on work or leisure in the day.

BROMUS RAMOSUS
Wild oat
For those who feel dissatisfied in their way of life, but have difficulty in determining what path to follow, though their ambition is strong.

ROSA CANINA
Wild rose
For those with little interest in the present, who resign themselves to their present circumstances, and make little effort to find joy or happiness. For uncomplaining apathy.

SALIX VITELLINA
Willow
For those who feel bitter or resentful about their misfortune, and, as a result, take less interest in the things in life they used to enjoy doing. They are despondent and feel that life is unjust and unfair.

THE CALIFORNIAN FLOWER ESSENCES
(The F.E.S. Quintessentials)

ALOE VERA
Aloe vera
For those fiery and creative people who have over-extended themselves and are feeling burnt out or exhausted. It restores energy and vitality and helps to balance creative activity with rest.

LILIUM PARVUM
Alpine lily
For women who idealize femininity in an abstract way and find it hard to come to terms with their physical female attributes and sexuality, as well as physical changes such as occur in pregnancy and menstruation. It helps acceptance of all aspects of womanhood, physical as well as emotional and spiritual.

ANGELICA ARCHANGELICA
Angelica
For those who feel spiritually bereft and isolated, who live predominantly in a materialistic or over-intellectual world. It enables a connection to the Higher Self and a feeling of protection and guidance, particularly when needed at times of change and challenge such as birth, death, marriage or divorce.

DATURA SPP
Angel's trumpet
For those approaching death, or a profound transformation in their lives, who are deeply fearful of letting go of their physical body, and the known. It allows surrender to whatever awaits us, and transforms fear of the unknown into joyful awareness of one's spiritual self and its purpose.

ARNICA MOLLIS
Arnica
Speeds healing after an accident, injury or trauma, particularly where shock prevents full recovery. It re-establishes connections to parts of oneself which may have been blocked off because of shock or trauma.

NEMOPHILA MENZIESII
Baby blue eyes
For those who feel insecure, defensive and distrustful of others. This may spring from insecurity during childhood and lack of a strong protective father figure to impart a feeling of safety. Lack of trust spreads to the spiritual world leading to a sense of spiritual isolation. It helps to engender a feeling of safety and security, trust of others and a connection to the spiritual self.

OCIMUM BASILICUM
Basil
For those who feel unable to integrate their sexual and spiritual lives. Sex is often seen as secret or wrong, impure in relation to the purity of the spirit. It helps to integrate sexuality and spirituality and resolve conflicts in relationships which arise because of polarization.

CIMICIFUGA RACEMOSA
Black cohosh
For those who tend to be intense, brooding, prone to dark, morbid thoughts, often caught up in destructive relationships in which they feel powerless. This may manifest in physical illness, particularly related to the reproductive system. It helps to enhance inner strength and power to transform negative, threatening circumstances.

RUDBECKIA HIRTA
Black-eyed Susan
For those who avoid or do not acknowledge the darker side of themselves, for blocking off parts of the personality or traumatic events from the past. It helps one to confront buried emotions and the shadow side and integrate it into oneself. It helps to raise self-esteem and release blockages to great resources of energy.

RUBUS URSINUS
Blackberry
For those with high ideals and lofty intentions but who have difficulty translating them into action, giving rise to frustration and confusion. It helps to increase the will to carry through ideas into action and provide the energy and inspiration to overcome inertia.

DICENTRA FORMOSA
Bleeding heart
For those who pour too much of themselves into their relationships with others, who are emotionally over-dependent, causing their partner to back away. For the pain and anguish caused by needing someone too much. It helps to enhance inner peace and strength, and the ability to give rather than need love through greater nourishment of the inner self.

BORAGO OFFICINALIS
Borage
For those with a heavy heart, who feel disheartened, discouraged or disappointed. It helps to lift the spirits, give courage and restore enthusiasm.

RANUNCULUS OCCIDENTALIS
Buttercup
For those who undervalue themselves or their career or vocation, who see themselves as small and unremarkable to the outside world. It increases self-worth and the ability to recognize inner value rather than outer achievement.

CALENDULA OFFICINALIS
Calendula
For those whose words tend to be cutting, and who are argumentative and unreceptive to the needs of others. It increases the ability to listen receptively, engenders warmth and consideration for the feelings of others.

DARLINGTONIA CALIFORNICA
California pitcher plant
For those who feel weak, lacking in vitality and tend to suffer from weak digestion. They are cut off from their instinctive desires and their physical and sexual feelings. It helps to integrate the earthy physical and 'lower' sides of ourselves, with the 'higher' self.

ESCHSCHOLZIA CALIFORNICA
California poppy
For those who seek spiritual 'highs' outside of themselves, attracted to the glamour and brightness of psychedelic drugs, charismatic teachers or occult rituals. It helps to develop a more solid inner life, awakens the light within and enhances self-reliance.

ROSA CALIFORNICA
California wild rose
For those who feel lacking in enthusiasm and warmth towards others: they are apathetic, often withdrawn, alienated from others, particularly at certain phases of life such as adolescence and old age. It restores enthusiasm for life and the ability to throw yourself wholeheartedly into whatever you are doing.

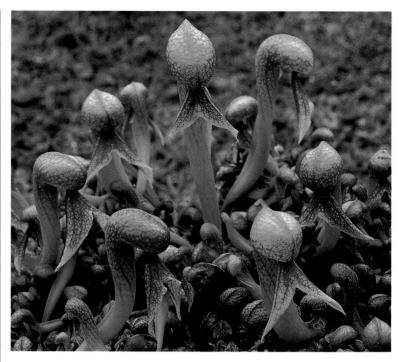

California pitcher plant

ZANTEDESCHIA AETHIOPICA
Calla lily
For those who feel troubled and confused about their sexual identity and gender, and do not feel at home in their bodies. It helps to integrate the masculine and feminine qualities within ourselves, allowing acceptance and clarity of sexual identity.

DUDLEYA CYMOSA
Canyon dudleya
For those who need the stimulation of dramatic psychic or emotional experiences, often attracted to mediumship, occult experimentation and psychic fantasies. It helps people to be grounded, to derive satisfaction from daily activities and to gain nourishment from quiet times and disciplined spiritual practices.

CAPSICUM ANNUUM
Cayenne
For those who feel sluggish, uninspired, and who are experiencing a period of stagnation in their inner or outer lives. They may feel resistant to change, or immobilized by procrastination and lack of direction. It increases fire and its transforming energy which are required for overcoming blocks to growth.

MATRICARIA CHAMOMILLA
Chamomile
For those who are moody, changeable, upset and tense about little things, children who are 'sunshine and showers'. Tension accumulates around the solar plexus leading to digestive problems. It helps to release tension and resolve inner conflict, enabling inner quiet and serenity.

LARREA TRIDENTATA
Chaparral
For the overburdening of the senses and psyche by the bombardment of chaotic and violent images of the modern world, particularly from city life and the media. It helps to pro-

tect and cleanse the psyche and is useful for detoxification after using medical and psychiatric drugs.

CHRYSANTHEMUM MORIFOLIUM
Chrysanthemum

For those immersed deeply in the material world, seeking fame and fortune to make their mark, and living in fear of death. It helps dissolve blockages to the spiritual self and connect with less ephemeral aspects of life.

ZEA MAYS
Corn

For those who need to live close to nature unrestricted by the constraints of the modern world. It helps people to deal with urban, technological or confined living conditions when necessary, and despite physical limitations, to continue to evolve spiritually.

COSMOS BIPINNATUS
Cosmos

For those who find it hard to express their thoughts and emotions, which may come out jumbled and disorganized. It improves clarity of thought and articulation, and enables communication of inner wisdom through the personality.

TARAXACUM OFFICINALE
Dandelion

For those with great enthusiasm for life but who try to cram too much activity into their lives. They over-structure their time and leave little room for rest and relaxation and as a result become very tense and stressed. It helps one to relax, release tension and repressed emotions stored in tense muscles.

CEANOTHUS INTEGERRINUS
Deerbrush

For self-deception regarding our motives and lack of honesty and openness in relationships. It helps awareness of underlying and unconscious motivating forces so that one can be more honest and open and outer actions can then reflect inner truth and integrity.

ANETHUM GRAVEOLENS
Dill

For those who feel overwhelmed by the bombardment of the senses in the busy modern world in which we live, contributing to psychic indigestion and nervousness. It reduces overstimulation and allows us to use the senses in a way conducive to spiritual growth.

CORNUS NUTTALLII
Dogwood

For those who are physically tense, who may be storing repressed emotions or trauma deep within the body; they may have been physically abused in the past or work in harsh physical conditions. It helps to restore grace and harmony in the body and warmth and softness to the emotions despite living in adversity.

LILIUM LONGIFLORUM
Easter lily

For those who feel that their sexuality is impure, unclean, thereby inhibiting their spiritual growth. It helps to reconcile sexuality and spirituality and to allow sexual energy to enhance spiritual development.

ECHINACEA PURPUREA
Echinacea

For those who lack a sense of identity because of the anonymity of modern life, or who, because of physical or emotional trauma, feel as if they are 'falling apart'. Such threats to the sense of self may underlie many immune-related illnesses. It strengthens the sense of self and engenders a feeling of wholeness.

OENOTHERA HOOKERI
Evening primrose

For those lacking in emotional nurture in infancy, who did not bond properly with their mother and now suffer from feeling rejected and unwanted. They avoid close emotional contact and committed relationships and often have an aversion to sexuality. It helps to heal feelings of rejection, being unlovable, and enables one to open emotionally to form deep relationships.

CALOCHORTUS ALBUS
Fairy lantern

For those whose emotional development in childhood was restricted or arrested, resulting in childlike behaviour during adulthood. They are immature, dependent and unable to take on responsibilities. It helps one to move through such blocks to development and mature into responsible adults.

ERYTHRONIUM PURPURASCENS
Fawn lily

For those attracted to an isolated spiritual life, where meditation and contemplation is not threatened by the fast pace and distractions of modern life. It helps them to integrate themselves more into society and to share their gifts and wisdom with others, thereby drawing energy from the physical world.

ERODIUM CICUTARIUM
Filaree

For those who are too involved in the minutiae of life, who worry excessively about mundane events, unable to keep things in a broader perspective. It helps to contain such wastage of energy, so that there is plenty in reserve for more productive activities, and fulfilment of one's higher potential.

MYOSOTIS SYLVATICA
Forget-me-not

For those grieving over the loss of a loved one, and for unresolved sadness from loss in the family in childhood. It increases possibility of relationships beyond the earthly realms and resolves feelings of isolation associated with grief.

FUCHSIA HYBRIDA
Fuchsia

For those with repressed emotions who avoid confronting inner problems by masking them with over-emotionality and psychosomatic symptoms such as frequent minor stomach aches and headaches. It facilitates greater awareness of emotions such as anger and grief, often through initial catharsis, and subsequent release.

ALLIUM SATIVUM
Garlic

For those who are easily influenced, drained of energy by others, leaving them feeling fearful, weak and uncentred. They may be prone to infection and problems of immunity. It imparts strength and resistance to outside influences, restoring a feeling of wholeness.

DICENTRA CHRYSANTHA
Golden ear drops

For those who block out the memory of painful events in their childhood, causing them emotional problems in the present which they do not understand. It helps them to contact and release trauma and unhappiness often through crying, so that they can gain wisdom and insight from such experience.

SOLIDAGO CALIFORNICA
Golden rod

For those without a clear sense of their identity, who are easily influenced by family or social mores, feeling the need to conform to gain acceptance and approval. It helps establish a sense of identity and allow one to remain true to oneself while interacting with others.

ACHILLEA FILIPENDULINA
Golden yarrow

For people who are particularly sensitive to and influenced by their environment and other people, who may isolate themselves and blunt their sensitivity as a form of protection. It helps to protect one from

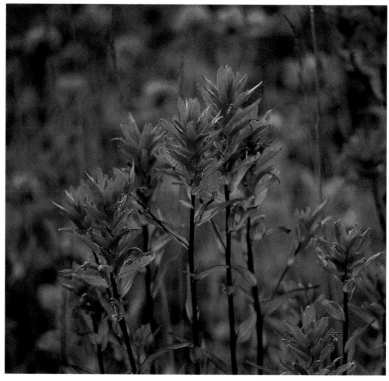

Indian paintbrush

oversensitivity while allowing openness and active involvement with others.

HIBISCUS ROSA-SINENSIS
Hibiscus

For those affected by exploitation of female sexuality in the media or by past sexual trauma, so that their sexuality is separated off from deeper feelings of love and affection. It helps connect sexuality to love and caring and to resolve fear of intimacy and allow sex to be an expression of warmth and affection.

CYNOGLOSSUM GRANDE
Hound's tongue

For those intellectual and analytical people who tend to perceive nature and the cosmos in purely materialistic terms, denying a spiritual perspective. It awakens a sense of wonder and awe, and a clearer perception of the spiritual dimensions of life.

CASTILLEJA MINIATA
Indian paintbrush

For those highly creative people who have trouble staying grounded and deriving the energy they need from balanced physical forces in the body. It helps dispel lethargy and exhaustion by integrating the use of creative and physical energy and maintaining a sense of groundedness.

SILENE CALIFORNICA
Indian pink

For those people who live life to the full, doing many things at the same time, and find it hard to find a still centre within themselves amid their busy lives. They can be tense and over-emotional and deplete their reserves of energy through lack of quietness and relaxation. It helps one to remain centred amid activity and derive health and energy from inner peace and calm.

IRIS VERSICOLOR/IRIS DOUGLASIANA
Iris
For those who lack inspiration, whose creativity feels stifled or blocked, whose 'feet of clay' weigh them down in the mundane world. It releases blocks to creativity, allows one to draw on inspiration from without and within to become more fully alive.

CYPRIPEDIUM PARVIFLORUM/ CYPRIPEDIUM REGINAE
Lady's slipper
For those who are unable to draw upon their inner wisdom and strength to guide them and provide energy for their daily life and work. They may suffer from nervous exhaustion and sexual debility. It acts as a tonic to the nervous system, enabling you to contact your inner strength and calm, bringing you in touch with inherent gifts and abilities to use in daily life.

DELPHINIUM NUTTALLIANUM
Larkspur
For those in positions of responsibility and leadership who become overburdened by a sense of duty, or inflated with power and self-importance. It helps to develop positive leadership qualities and charisma, to replace self-aggrandisement with generosity and altruism and thereby inspire and motivate others.

LAVANDULA OFFICINALIS
Lavender
For sensitive and mentally active people, drawn to development of their spiritual lives and to practices such as meditation. They tend to be easily wound up and tense. It acts to calm the mind, to relax the body and to balance sensitivity with groundedness, thereby enabling the stillness required for meditation and inner calm.

NELUMBO NUCIFERA
Lotus
A sacred symbol for over 5000 years, used as a flower essence for all phases of spiritual development and spiritual studies. It reduces the tendency to spiritual pride and spiritual materialism and enhances higher consciousness and meditative insight.

AMARANTHUS CANDATUS
Love-lies-bleeding
For those suffering from physical pain or mental anguish, which can become intensified through identification with the pain or agony and allowing it to take over one's life. It helps you to derive meaning and purpose from such intense experience, by seeing it in broader perspective, as part of a larger experience of the human condition, and thereby know love and compassion for the suffering of others.

MADIA ELEGANS
Madia
For those whose energy is easily scattered, their concentration dispersed, who feel distracted and uncentred. It helps you to direct your energy and focus attention and through such discipline to develop your greater potential.

SIDALACEA GLAUSCENS
Mallow
For those who feel blocked emotionally and unable to reach out to others because of mistrust. It helps to open the feelings and enable giving and receiving of love and affection.

ARCTOSTAPHYLOS VISCIDA
Manzanita
For those who feel negative about their body and the physical or earthly realm, perhaps because of their religious beliefs. They may impose strict disciplines upon the body, strict dietary regimens and exercises. It helps you to see the body not as something corrupt and ugly but as the temple of the soul, to be cherished and respected.

CALOCHORTUS LEICHTLINII
Mariposa lily
For those who feel alienated from others, unwanted and unloved, often because of feelings of rejection or trauma at an early age, problems with maternal bonding as an infant, or lack of proper nurture as a child. It helps one to come to terms with painful experience in the past and to increase receptivity to human and divine love from others and within oneself.

ASCLEPIAS CORDIFOLIA
Milkweed
For those who are over-dependent on others, who have never properly grown up, perhaps because of disturbances during childhood. They may become addicted to drugs or tranquilizers, illness or extreme spiritual disciplines to escape from the realities of adult life and its responsibilities. It increases self-reliance and independence through strengthening the sense of Self, and realizing the importance of the Self.

IPOMOEA PURPUREA
Morning glory
For those attracted to late night activities, erratic eating and sleeping patterns, whose energy becomes depleted, causing them to crave stimulants such as caffeine or drugs such as cocaine. It helps you to adjust to rhythms in life that are more akin to the cycles of nature, thereby increasing vitality and enhancing health and wellbeing.

MONARDELLA ADORATISSIMA
Mountain pennyroyal
For those whose thoughts are clouded by negativity, and who are easily affected by the negative thoughts and feelings of others. It helps to expel negativity and cleanse the psyche, increasing vitality and mental clarity.

PENSTEMON NEWBERRYI
Mountain pride
For those who find it hard to stand up for themselves or their beliefs, who withdraw in the face of challenge, and opt for a quiet life. It lends strength and assertiveness, positive masculine energy and activity, helping to transform passivity or disillusionment. It enhances the spiritual warrior in us.

ARTEMISIA DOUGLASIANA
Mugwort
For those who are dreamy, 'moony', out of touch with the world of physical reality because of an overactive psychic life. It enhances the receptivity of the psyche and awareness of dreams while helping you to remain grounded in practical affairs of the world.

VERBASCUM THAPSUS
Mullein
For those facing challenges in life when they must wrestle with their conscience, who may resort to dishonesty or deception because of weakness or pressure from others. It helps to develop an inner sense of morality, an ability to listen to inner guidance, allowing you to be true to yourself, upright and strong in the face of adversity.

TROPAEOLUM MAJUS
Nasturtium
For those who tend to live too much in their heads, for intellectuals who neglect their emotional and physical lives, for students or those in phases of life demanding strong mental activity, whose vitality and health is depleted. It connects you to the body and emotions, restoring vitality and warmth and balancing intellect with experience.

NICOTIANA ALATA
Nicotiana
For those whose feelings are blunted, even hardened, to enable them to adapt and thrive in the harsh modern world. They may employ tobacco or other stimulants to deaden their emotions and help them to cope. It helps to reconnect us to our real feelings, and to the Earth and all who live here, and to enhance appreciation of finer more subtle things in life, thereby enabling true peace.

BERBERIS AQUIFOLIUM
Oregon grape
For those who mistrust others, who see the world as hostile and threatening, perhaps because of bad experience in the past or lack of proper nurture as a child. It helps to dispel fear and paranoia, suspicion and hostility and to see the positive side of other people, thus enabling situations in which warmth and goodwill can be shared.

PENSTEMON DAVIDSONII
Penstemon
For those who feel that life has been unfair to them because of unfortunate circumstances that have befallen them; they feel persecuted, victimized and self-pitying. It helps you to tap resources of courage and resilience and to be able to perceive difficult circumstances as opportunities for growth and transformation.

MENTHA PIPERITA
Peppermint
For those who feel sluggish, lethargic, and mentally cloudy or apathetic, often related to digestive or metabolic imbalances. They may crave the stimulation of food which then makes them feel sluggish or sleepy afterwards. It improves digestion, and frees energy, keeping the mind alert and clear for higher purposes.

RHUS DIVERSILOBA
Poison oak
For those who find it hard to show their feelings and their vulnerability. They erect a protective wall around themselves and project themselves as being tough and insensitive. It helps you dispel fear of openness and intimacy and accept the soft, vulnerable side of yourself.

PUNICA GRANATUM
Pomegranate
For women who feel torn between their home life and nurturing their children, and developing their career. When trying to balance the two simultaneously they may feel exhausted and unfulfilled in both roles. It helps to relieve such conflict and enhance energy and creativity to support women in their nurturing role, whether at home or at work.

TRITELEIA IXIOIDES
Pretty face
For those who are overconcerned by their physical appearance, who judge themselves or others by their exterior beauty rather than their inner attributes, and fear ageing. It helps you to see yourself and others beyond the 'mask' or the physical form and see the beauty that radiates from within.

MIMULUS KELLOGGII
Purple monkeyflower
For those whose need for safety and security makes them dependent on conventional social or religious institutions and ignore any calling from within to follow a different path. It helps to dispel fear of spiritual experiences and inner guidance and lend courage and calm to find your own way in life.

BRIZA MAXIMA
Quaking grass
For members of a group or family where there is conflict or jousting for power. It helps to improve negotiating skills and awareness of others, by allowing those with forceful personalities or big egos to see themselves within the context of the group and thus bring about harmony.

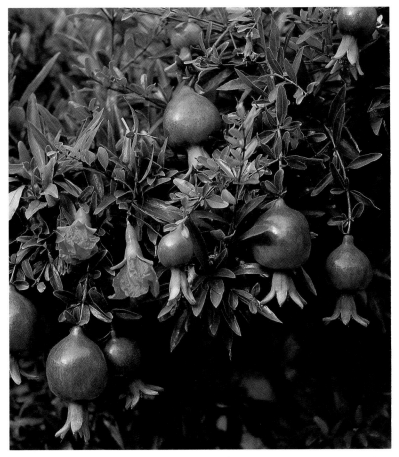

Pomegranate

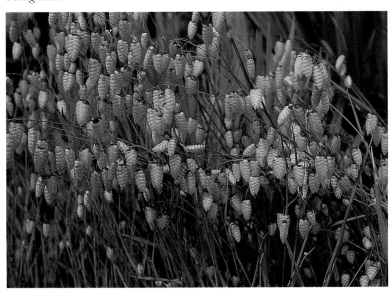

Quaking grass

DAUCUS CAROTA
Queen Anne's lace

For those seeking the spiritual path and whose clarity and perception is clouded by unresolved emotional or sexual problems. It helps to harmonize 'higher' and 'lower' centres and while remaining grounded, increasing spiritual insight and clarity.

CHAENOMELES SPECIOSA
Quince

For those, particularly women, who feel torn between the need to be loving and nurturing and the need for power and strength. Such conflict arises in parenthood when gentleness and affection as well as discipline and objectivity are required. It helps to reconcile these apparent opposites and demonstrate that real power or strength can also be love and vice versa.

CHRYSOTHAMNUS NAUSEOSUS
Rabbit brush

For those whose attention gets caught up in detail and minutiae of life, and cannot see life in broader perspective. The chaos of such detail and events, such as in a busy office, can seem overwhelming and draining. It helps you to cope with the challenges of such everyday occurrences by seeing them within a larger picture of organization, thus enhancing energy and flexibility.

TRIFOLIUM PRATENSE
Red clover

For those who get caught up in other people's problems, or mass hysteria in emergencies or emotionally charged family problems. It helps to maintain a sense of individuality and detachment, and the ability to stay calm and centred during a crisis.

ROSMARINUS OFFICINALIS
Rosemary

For those who tend to be forgetful, absent-minded, dreamy, and not grounded in their physical body.

257

They may feel insecure, and lacking in warmth and vital energy. It increases warmth, vitality and confidence physically and emotionally and awakens the mind.

SALVIA OFFICINALIS
Sage
For those, particularly in later years, who see their lives as ill-fated and ill-deserved, and are unable to perceive their meaning or higher purpose. It helps you to gain wisdom from the experience of the years so that you can teach and counsel others.

ARTEMISIA TRIDENTATA
Sagebrush
For those attached to false images of themselves, or of the world, clinging hard to the security of the material world with its possessions, lifestyle and social pressures, and out of touch with the real Self. It helps you to let go of such images and attachments and be true to the Self, thereby allowing the possibility of transformation.

CEREUS GIGANTEUS
Saguaro
For those who have problems with authority and want to escape from the confines of the culture or society in which they live and their ancient traditions. It is particularly recommended for rebellious teenagers. It helps to clarify relationships to those in authority and appreciate the wisdom of spiritual elders and ancient traditions.

HYPERICUM PERFORATUM
St John's wort
For those who are oversensitive to sunlight, the environment, the effect of others around them and psychic influences, causing them to be fearful and vulnerable, with disturbed sleep and dreams. It provides strength and protection from a variety of influences, and allows light in your life to serve to illumine rather than threaten.

MIMULUS CARDINALIS
Scarlet monkeyflower
For those who fear their emotions, their 'shadow side', and try to keep it well hidden, suppressing unpleasant emotions and thereby causing great tension and inner pressure. It lends courage to acknowledge and confront such feelings so that they do not grow out of real proportion. It enables honesty and greater vitality through release of tension.

CYTISUS SCOPARIUS
Scotch broom
For those who feel anxious, despairing or depressed about their lives, the state of the world and the future of the planet. It helps you to be more positive and optimistic, and to see obstacles and challenges as opportunities for growth and service to the world.

PRUNELLA VULGARIS
Self-heal
For those who despair of ever getting well, who have lost faith in their own innate healing abilities and hand over the responsibility of their health to others. It enhances the power of self-healing and the confidence in yourself, enabling greater self-reliance and involvement in your healing journey.

CHRYSANTHEMUM MAXIMUM
Shasta daisy
For those whose restless search for knowledge leads them to study one thing, then another, over-intellectualizing or analysing and causing mental or spiritual 'indigestion'. It helps to synthesize knowledge gained from diverse sources into a greater wholeness and thereby derive greater insight and understanding.

DODECATHEON HENDERSONII
Shooting star
For those who feel profoundly alienated, not at home in their bodies, their families or on this planet, out of touch with the warmth of relationship to others. It helps to overcome alienation and to perceive the purpose of their incarnation in a human form.

ANTIRRHINUM MAJUS
Snapdragon
For powerful people with strong wills and high energy, who misuse their energy through verbal aggression and criticism. It helps to redirect 'lower' energy to be expressed through its natural channels, such as through sex and digestion, releasing tension and allowing greater creativity.

CENTAUREA SOLSTITIALIS
Star thistle
For those lacking a deep sense of security, who look for safety and security in material possessions, and have difficulty sharing either their things or themselves. It reduces dependence on outer things by engendering an inner sense of security and inner abundance. It allows greater sharing and generosity.

CALOCHORTUS TOLMIEI
Star tulip
For those who feel out of touch with their inner selves, unable to meditate or pray, or find a place of inner calm. Also for those who deny their softer, more feminine side, and build a hard protective shell around themselves. It helps you to be more aware of inner guidance, opens and softens the emotions, enables inner peace and security.

MIMULUS AURANTIACUS
Sticky monkeyflower
For those who fear intimacy, and close relationships through fear of exposing themselves to others. They may repress their sexuality or

mask their feelings of vulnerability by involvement in numerous super-ficial sexual encounters. It helps to release fear about the closeness of contact possible through sex and allows relationships to be deep and meaningful, guided by love and not by fear.

HELIANTHUS ANNUUS
Sunflower

For those afflicted by low self-esteem and lack of confidence in themselves, who hide their light under a bushel. For others who shine too brightly, full of their own self-glory. It helps to balance the masculine side of your nature, enabling the sun-like qualities to shine forth, healing others with its warmth.

LATHYRUS LATIFOLIUS
Sweet pea

For those who find it hard to put down roots, to become involved in their community or their surroundings; they feel homeless, and like an outsider, as they never really belong anywhere. It helps you to feel connected to a place or a community, to develop a sense of your place on this earth and to make commitments.

TANACETUM VULGARE
Tansy

For those who feel sluggish and lethargic, who tend to be indecisive or indifferent, often as a way of avoiding pressure or challenging sit-uations, which relates back to patterns established in childhood. It helps you to confront difficulties or negative emotions, and learn to cope with them by connecting with inner strength and direction.

LILIUM HUMBOLDTII
Tiger lily

For those who are overly aggressive, competitive, striving against others in a yang, masculine way, or for those women who find it hard to connect with their

masculine, assertive side. It helps to balance masculine with feminine qualities to bring feminine nurturing values into the hostile world, as in business and politics, to help people work together for the common good instead of for themselves.

TRILLIUM CHLOROPETALUM
Trillium

For those who measure their self-worth by material standards, being caught up in the physical plane of existence where possessions and social power are all-important. They need to accumulate wealth to feel strong as they are cut off from their source of spiritual strength. It connects you to higher powers, helping your personal desires to be overridden by altruistic actions, through awareness of inner riches.

CAMPSIS TAGLIABUANA
Trumpet vine

For those who find it hard to express themselves adequately through the spoken word, perhaps because of a speech impediment such as stuttering or feelings of shyness or dullness. It helps to bring interest and vitality to the voice, and allows creativity to be expressed through the voice by letting go of concern about how others are judging you.

VIOLA ODORATA
Violet

For those who are shy, and appear cool and aloof but actually feel fear-ful and lonely. They long to join in with others, and develop close relationships or become part of a group but are worried by lack of trust and fear of losing their sense of identity. It helps to engender warmth and trust in relationships, and to allow sharing of yourself with others, without losing your identity and remaining true to yourself.

ACHILLEA MILLEFOLIUM
Yarrow

For those who are easily affected and depleted by their surroundings and the influence of others, and tend to be prone to environmental illnesses, allergies and psycho-somatic problems. It helps to shield from outside influences and reduce leakage of energy and absorption of negative influences.

CALOCHORTUS MONOPHYLLUS
Yellow star tulip

For those who lack sensitivity, compassion, awareness of others' feelings and whose relationships suffer because of lack of awareness of the effect of their actions on others. It increases receptivity towards others, sensitivity and com-passion for the suffering of others, enabling greater responsibility and empathy within relationships.

ERIODYCTION CALIFORNICUM
Yerba santa

For unresolved grief and sadness, buried in the heart and causing depression and melancholy that per-vades life. Breathing problems such as asthma or pneumonia may be caused by congestion in the chest. It promotes release of unresolved emotions and restores life and joy to the heart, enabling the free-flow of natural feelings again and breath-ing without constriction.

ZINNIA ELEGANS
Zinnia

For those who take themselves and life too seriously, who tend to work too hard and feel overburdened by their responsibilities. It enables you to step outside yourself and bring a refreshing sense of humour and joy into your life, thereby balancing work with playfulness and serious-ness with light-heartedness.

AUSTRALIAN BUSH FLOWER ESSENCES

PROSTANTHERA CUNEATA
Alpine mint bush
For those who spend much time listening to others' problems and doing their best to help and to heal them. The weight of responsibility and the draining nature of their work can lead to exhaustion and dispiritedness. It refreshes and revitalizes depleted energy, renews joy in your work and the ability to carry on helping others.

LOBELIA GIBBOSA
Angelsword
For those who are influenced by thoughts and ideas of other people and feel confused, particularly about spiritual truths. It protects you from outside influences so that you can listen to the inner self and inner guidance both from past experience and the present.

LYSIPHYLLUM CUNNINGHAMII
Bauhinia
For those rigid people who resist change and close their minds to new ideas and activities, feeling threatened by things that are new. It engenders open-mindedness, acceptance and appreciation of others and their lifestyles and ideas.

PLANCHONIA CAREYA
Billy goat plum
For those who are repelled by sex and their own bodies and their sexuality. For those feeling self-loathing and disgust, perhaps relating to skin problems or abnormal secretions and a feeling of being dirty. It helps you accept your physical and sexual self, and enjoy sensuality and sex.

TETRATHECA ERICIFOLIA
Black-eyed Susan
For those who are constantly active, rushing around, overworked and stressed, who find it hard to let go and relax. They are quick-thinking and can be impatient if others don't move as fast as they do. It enables relaxation and enhances ability to look to your inner life and experience stillness and peace. This is the remedy for stress.

WAHLENBERGIA SPP
Bluebell
For those who are insecure, and are materialistic and acquisitive in an attempt to make themselves feel safe. They are greedy and fearful of losing all they have acquired. It increases inner confidence and security, and enhances the ability to share happily with others. It increases warmth towards others.

ADANSONIA GREGORII
Boab
For those caught in negative patterns of their ancestors, their families or a group to which they belong, and for people who tend to repeat the same mistakes again and again, or one lifetime after another. It helps to free one from negative energy of others, releases deeply held beliefs, prejudices, negative emotions and thought patterns. It heals the collective unconscious.

BORONIA LEDIFOLIA
Boronia
For those who are prone to obsessions and obsessive thoughts about events or situations, or about loved ones, or who pine after a breakdown of a relationship, suffering from a broken heart. They may suffer from insomnia because of constant unwanted thoughts. It helps to calm the mind and the heart, and engender serenity and detachment.

CALLISTEMON LINEARIS
Bottlebrush
For those going through transitional phases in their life, such as puberty, pregnancy, menopause, retirement and feeling unable to cope with such enormous change. For those holding on to the past and fear of things to come. It helps acceptance of life in the present, and the ability to let go, engendering confidence and calm.

EPACRIS LONGIFLORA
Bush fuchsia
For those who have difficulties learning and projecting themselves. They may suffer from dyslexia or stuttering, and may be cut off from their inner wisdom. It helps to resolve such learning problems, integrates the right and left sides of the brain, enhances development of intuition and guidance from within.

GARDENIA MEGASPERMA
Bush gardenia
For those who get caught up in their own life interests and career, and lose contact with those close to them, often taking them for granted. It helps to reopen channels of communication and increases interest in other people's lives. It resparks attraction in relationships.

PATERSONIA LONGIFOLIA
Bush iris
For those grounded in material life, and cut off from their higher selves; for lack of belief or spirituality, and fear of death, for over-indulgence in the physical side of life. It stimulates awakening of the spirit, insight and opening of the inner doors of perception.

CROWEA SALIGNA
Crowea
For those who feel uncentred, out of sorts, and anxious, often for no apparent reason. It helps one to feel calm, balanced and well, and increases energy and vitality. This is a good remedy for worry.

HAKEA TERETIFOLIA
Dagger hakea

For bitterness, anger and resentment between family or those close to each other. A good remedy for those who hold grudges and harbour intense anger behind a sweet-natured face. It helps openness, communication and resolution of conflict. This is the remedy of forgiveness.

BANERA RUBIOIDES
Dog rose

For those who feel insecure, lacking in confidence with others, fearful and shy. Niggling fears suppress the life force and reduce vital energy, and block the flow of warmth and love between people. It increases self-confidence, energy, self-worth, inner courage and assurity.

BAUERA SESSILIFLORA
Dog rose of the wild forces

For those whose emotions are so intense that they fear losing control. They may suffer from physical symptoms, particularly pain, with no apparent physical cause. It helps to balance the emotions, calm the mind, and remain sane in the face of great challenges, thus enabling inner growth.

STYPHELIA TRIFLORA
Five corners

For those who lack self-worth, feel insecure and who dislike their body or physical appearance and lack self-expression as a result. It helps self-acceptance, recognition of your beauty, and increases self-esteem and expression.

ACTINOTUS HELIANTHI
Flannel flower

For those, particularly men, who shy away from physical contact and activity, for fear of intimacy and lack of sensitivity often related to past trauma or hurt. It engenders emotional trust, confidence in intimacy and sensuality and increases sensitivity and feeling.

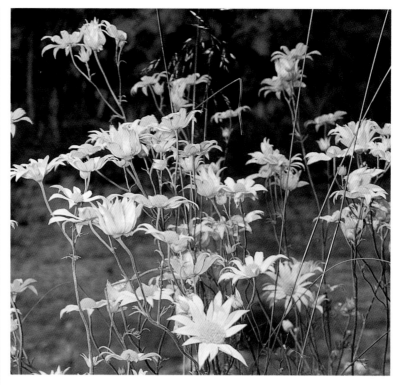

Flannel flower

THYSANOTUS TUBEROSUS
Fringed violet

For those suffering the effects of trauma, shock, grief, sexual abuse or physical injury, and fearful of such experience being repeated. It heals damage to the aura, helps reintegration of the physical and etheric bodies, and affords psychic protection for those working with psychic skills.

CALANDENIA DILATATO
Green spider orchid

For those who are aspiring to deeper and higher levels of knowledge and insight within themselves, and for those in the position of teaching and passing on such knowledge. It allows assimilation of knowledge by helping you to guard information about spiritual matters and not dissipate its energy or use it for gaining respect or acceptance. It also releases fear and nightmares associated with the past.

GREVILLEA BUXIFOLIA
Grey spider flower

For fear and panic in emergencies or traumatic situations, or simply in everyday life when challenged, for example, by taking exams, giving a lecture, making a speech, or being interviewed for a job. It engenders calmness and confidence in your ability, and allows you to perform at your best.

DORYANTHES EXCELSA
Gymea lily

For powerful people who tend to be dominating and demanding, proud and arrogant, charismatic and used to getting their own way. It reduces the need for status, recognition, glamour and being in control, and helps you to be more humble and appreciative of others.

HIBBERTIA PENDUNCULATA

Hibbertia

For those who constantly feel the need to improve themselves, and increase their knowledge. For perfectionists who discipline themselves excessively and become fanatical or addicted to acquiring knowledge. It helps you to trust more to your innate wisdom and knowledge gained from experience, to accept yourself as you are and relax from needing to feel better than others.

BRACHYCHITON ACERIFOLIUS

Illawarra flame tree

For those who feel left out, rejected, like an outsider, partly because of an inability to commit to the responsibility of relationships, and low self-esteem. They may be aware of their abilities but feel overwhelmed by the responsibility of using them. It engenders confidence, self-worth, strength and interdependence.

ISOPOGON ANETHIFOLIUS

Isopogon

For those who are cut off from their feelings and tend to be ruled by their heads; for needing to control others. For those unable to draw lessons from past experience, with poor memory and signs of senility. It helps you to connect to your emotions and to forgotten parts of yourself, and helps you learn from experience.

JACARANDA MIMOSAEFOLIA

Jacaranda

For those unable to think clearly and lacking single-mindedness and direction. They tend to dither, change their minds, and scatter their energy by aimless activity. It helps clarity of mind, decisiveness and purpose, enabling the transformation of ideas into actions and completed projects.

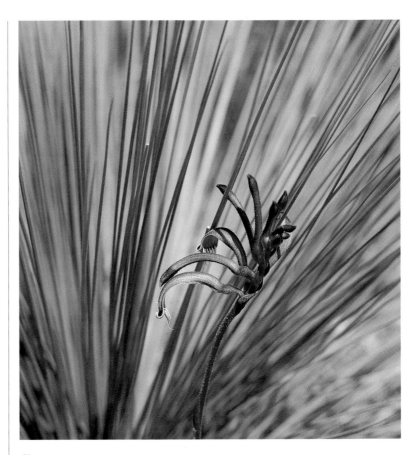

Kangaroo paw

ANIGOZANTHOS MANGLESII

Kangaroo paw

For those who lack sensitivity towards others, who tend to be thoughtless, tactless, socially inept and gauche in company. It helps you to recognize the needs of others, and enjoy their company. It improves communication skills.

COCHLOSPERMUM FRASERI

Kapok bush

For those who lack perseverance, who give up trying too easily as they are quickly discouraged. They tend to be prone to feelings of apathy and resignation. It helps self-confidence in your abilities to apply yourself and get things done, and encourages perseverance.

ACTINOTUS MINOR

Little flannel flower

For people who take life very seriously, lacking a sense of fun and joy. For children who behave more like adults, taking on the troubles of the world. It helps people to connect with their inner child, and engenders playfulness, love of fun, spontaneity and a sense of humour.

EUCALYPTUS MACROCARPA

Macrocarpa

For those who have over-extended themselves or are suffering the effects of stress, who are burnt out and have a lowered resistance to disease. By enhancing the function of the adrenal gland, it helps to increase resistance to stress and increase energy and vitality.

PROSTANTHERA STRIATIFLORA
Mint bush
For those experiencing the 'dark night of the soul', feeling they are being tested often to the limits of their endurance. For those facing major challenges in their lives, and who feel surrounded by confusion and complexity, unable to see the way forward. It increases the ability to cope with such trials and tribulations and to see a way through, helping you to emerge from darkness into light, ready to move on.

LAMBERTIA FORMOSA
Mountain devil
For those who suffer from jealousy, anger, suspicion, resentment and hatred and are being poisoned by such negative emotions leading to a variety of chronic illnesses. It helps them to let go of such feelings and engenders warmth and affection, forgiveness, openness, and dissolving barriers to love.

PTILOTUS ATRIPICIFOLIUS
Mulla mulla
For fear of fire, heat, hot objects and the sun's rays, often because of past trauma associated with fire. It helps to resolve fear from the past and to feel comfortable with the rejuvenating energy of the sun, thereby increasing health and vitality.

BANKSIA SERRATA
Old man banksia
For those who feel heavy, lethargic, with sluggish energy and metabolism, often related to an underactive thyroid. They lack enthusiasm and interest in life and are easily disheartened. It increases energy and enthusiasm, restores interest in life and *joie de vivre*.

CARICA PAPAYA
Paw paw
For those who feel overwhelmed and burdened by problems that seem unsurmountable, decisions that appear unresolvable, or infor-

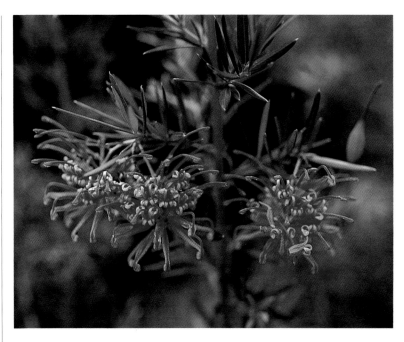

Red grevillea

mation that seems too much to take in. It increases the ability to take on challenges, assimilate information, and to solve problems.

LEPTOSPERMUM SQUARROSUM
Peach flowered tea tree
For those who have trouble committing themselves to projects and activities and sustaining their interest. They are easily bored and discouraged and prone to mood swings. They tend to suffer from hypochondria and energy highs and lows, possibly related to imbalanced pancreatic function. It acts to balance mood and health and energy, increasing the ability to sustain activity and interest and thereby complete projects and attain goals.

PHILOTHECA SALSOLIFOLIA
Philotheca
For those who have low opinions of themselves and so do not easily accept praise or acknowledgement of their talents or successes. They are better at giving out than taking in. It helps you to accept gifts or praise from others and to allow others to acknowledge your gifts and successes.

PTILOTUS EXALTUS
Pink mulla mulla
For those suffering pain and feeling hurt from experiences in the past, and fearful of being hurt again. They build a wall of invulnerability around themselves, a hard shell and withdraw from close contact with others. It helps to release pain from the past and dissolve blockages to warmth and intimacy with others; relieves the constant suspicion of others and fear of being hurt.

GREVILLEA SPECIOSA
Red grevillea
For those who feel in a rut, knowing what they want to do, but not how to go about it. They tend to be over-dependent on other people and easily affected by criticism by others. It helps you to be more independent, unaffected by the opinions of others. It gives courage and dynamic energy to bring about required changes.

CORYBAS DILATATUS
Red helmet orchid
For those who have unresolved issues around father figures, and this may manifest as rebelliousness, or disregard of authority. It helps men to bond to their children and allow themselves time to share with their families. It enhances sensitivity towards others and respect for authority.

NELUMBO NUCIFERA
Red lily
For those who feel vague, uncentred, their energy and concentration scattered and who tend to go about in a dream. Helps spiritual practices such as meditation by aiding concentration and the ability to live in the present in a grounded and focused way.

SUNEIRIA RUBRA
Red suva frangipani
For those going through difficult times in a relationship or partnership, in the middle of a marital breakdown or experiencing the shock of the loss of someone close. It imparts the strength to cope with the raw emotions at such a time with equanimity, engenders calmness and a sense of being supported and nurtured rather than torn apart.

TRICHODESMA ZEYLANICUM
Rough bluebell
For those with a great need for love and affection but are not able to give it back. They tend to be underhand and manipulative, aware of the needs of others and yet uncaring, preferring to use people, play the role of martyr and make others feel obligated to them. It helps you to be more generous and loving, and engender sensitivity and compassion for others.

CASUARINA GLAUCA
She oak
For women whose emotional problems affect their fertility and who are unable to conceive. There may be feelings of inadequacy, lack of self-confidence, fears about coping with pregnancy and bringing up children that contribute to hormonal imbalances and infertility. It helps to release your emotional blocks preventing conception and increases confidence in your feminine creativity.

EUCALYPTUS CAESIA
Silver princess
For those who feel as if at a crossroads in their lives, unsure of which direction to take. Also for people who have reached one important goal and now that they are there they feel flat and unfulfilled. It helps show direction, a glimpse of where to go and enhances enjoyment of the journey while striving for the goal.

PIMELEA LINIFOLIA
Slender rice flower
For those who are narrow-minded, opinionated, prejudiced or racist, who criticize others and their lifestyles and beliefs. It helps you to stop judging others and other religious or national groups detrimentally, and to perceive the connection between all human beings. It brings about group harmony and co-operation, enabling people to work together towards the common good.

XANTHOSIA ROTUNDIFOLIA
Southern cross
For those who are bitter and resentful, feeling that life has been unfair to them, and that they are hard done by. It helps you to see that much of life is what you create for yourself, and that you can change your life simply by transforming a negative attitude into a positive outlook.

TRIODIA SPP
Spinifex
For those who feel victims of their bodies, with no control over their physical symptoms, especially if they are recurrent or chronic. It helps to increase confidence in your inherent self-healing ability and to resolve emotional causes of lowered immunity leading to infections such as candidiasis, herpes and chlamydia.

CLIANTHUS FORMOSUS
Sturt desert pea
For unresolved grief and sadness, suppressed emotions causing depression and constriction of the lungs. It helps to bring emotions to the surface and to allow their expression through crying, thus releasing much tension from the body, particularly around the heart and lung area.

GOSSYPIUM STURTIANUM
Sturt desert rose
For guilt and low self-esteem related to past actions or behaviour, regret and self-criticism that weighs you down. It helps you to accept what happened in the past and move on, with a sense of conviction, invulnerable to pressure from others. It increases inner strength and personal integrity.

BANKSIA ROBUR
Swamp banksia
For those dynamic, active people who have lost their energy, drive and *joie de vivre* because of stress, setbacks, overwork, ill-health or trauma. It helps to rekindle their abundant energy and enthusiasm for life, and wash away frustration and negativity.

DROSERA SPATHULATA
Sundew
For those who are vague, uncentred, indecisive and tend to daydream, especially when there is work to be done. It helps to keep you focused and in the present, increases motivation and attention to detail, and reduces the need to withdraw or escape from the realities of your life.

ACACIA TERMINALIS
Sunshine wattle

For those who have suffered in the past and bring their negativity from their experiences into the present. They view life as a struggle and their outlook is bleak. It helps you to see the present for what it is, unclouded by the past, and allows beauty and joy back into your life, and excitement about the future.

SENECIA MAGNIFICUS
Tall yellow top

For those who live in their heads, cut off from their true feelings. They also feel cut off from their roots and unconnected to family, workplace or country. They feel lonely, alienated and unloved, and long to belong, to go 'home'. It brings a sense of connection and commitment to family, work or a place. It helps you to put down roots, open your heart and connect to others.

CALYTRIX EXSTIPULATA
Turkey bush

For those who lack confidence in their creative abilities, for creative blocks and discouragement in the beginner as well as the artist. It enhances the desire to be creative and release blocks to free-flowing inspiration, thereby renewing confidence in yourself and your abilities.

TELOPEA SPECIOSISSIMA
Waratah

For crises and emergencies, for blackness, depression and despair, and inability to cope with challenges in life. It helps to bring out survival skills and give courage and strength to deal with crises. It enhances positive transformation for those going through the 'black night of the soul'.

RICINOCARPUS PINIFOLIUS
Wedding bush

For those who have problems with commitment, whether to jobs, relationships or activities. They flit

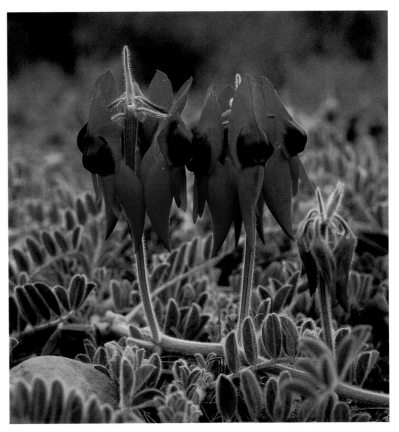

Sturt desert pea

from one thing to another, losing interest after the initial attraction wears off, never establishing close relationships. It helps to develop discipline and commitment, so that it is possible to derive fulfilment from dedication to a task, or a relationship.

SOLANUM QUADRILOCULATUM
Wild potato bush

For those who feel imprisoned by their physical bodies often through handicap or paralysis, unable to progress in life because of their physical limitations. It helps you to engender a positive feeling about your body, and to feel freer of its limitations and filled with renewed energy and enthusiasm.

WISTERIA SINENSIS
Wisteria

For women who have problems with their femininity and sexuality, and for men who deny the softer, feminine part of themselves. It helps women to relax and enjoy sex, often through letting go of negative past experiences. It relieves fear of intimacy and softness in both men and women.

CALADENIA FLAVA
Yellow cowslip orchid

For those intellectual, analytical people who are cut off from their feelings and tend to be over-critical and judgmental, as well as aloof and withdrawn. It engenders an open and inquisitive mind, and warmth and acceptance of others. It connects you to your emotions, balancing head and heart.

265

THE ESSENTIAL OILS

The exotic perfumes of flowers and leaves, and the wonderful aroma and taste of culinary herbs derive their taste and smell from volatile oils. These oils possess a wealth of therapeutic virtues.

Essential oils have an important role in healing, and details of how to use them are to be found on pages 271–272. Listed here are the oils most commonly used in the practice of aromatherapy, and the conditions relieved by them.

Caution: Never take essential oils internally.

Basil
Migraine, headaches, aches, chest infections, digestive problems, colic, colds, catarrh, fevers. Poor concentration, fainting, disorganization, mental fatigue, nervous exhaustion. Low libido, depression, painful or scanty periods, tension, engorged breasts, PMS.

Note: Avoid in early pregnancy

Bergamot
Coughs, fevers, urinary tract infections, vaginal infections or discharge. Poor appetite and eating problems, acne, boils, cold sores and other herpes infections including chickenpox and shingles. Cuts and wounds. Depression, tension, anxiety, lack of self-confidence.

Note: Increases photosensitivity; avoid use before exposure to sun or a sunbed

Black pepper
Constipation, colds, flu, weakness, poor concentration, depression, feeling of powerlessness. Poor circulation, weak digestion, colic, wind, abdominal pain, muscular pain, stiffness, fatigue, rheumatic and arthritic pain.

Note: Dilute well as it can irritate the skin

Cajeput
Colds, flu, catarrh, sinusitis, sore throats, headaches. Arthritis, gout, rheumatism, toothache. Indecision, lack of direction or understanding.

Note: Dilute well as it can irritate skin and mucous membranes

Chamomile
Colic, gastritis, indigestion, peptic ulcers, diarrhoea. PMS, period pains, irritable bladder, fluid retention, cystitis, eczema, boils, skin infections, allergies. Headaches, migraine, children's fevers, teething, earaches. Menopause symptoms, muscular pain, inflamed joints, sprains, burns. Tension, anxiety, depression, over-excitement, restlessness, insomnia, irritability.

Cinnamon
Poor circulation, colds, flu, depression, lethargy. Rheumatism, arthritis, muscle pain. Weak digestion, colic, wind, nausea, indigestion.

Note: Avoid in early pregnancy

Clary sage
Muscle tension, PMS, depression, exhaustion, anxiety, tension, nervousness. Uterine tension in childbirth, period pain, asthma, migraine, abdominal pain, digestive problems. Night sweats, acne, low libido, sore throats, aches and pains.
Caution: In early pregnancy, avoid when taking alcohol

Clove
Toothache, headaches, weak contractions in childbirth. Bronchitis, colds, flu, diarrhoea, arthritis, rheumatism.

Caution: Avoid during pregnancy, and on sensitive skin

Coriander
Tiredness, weakness, poor circulation, poor appetite, lack of motivation. Digestive problems, wind, neuralgia, rheumatic pain, flu, nervousness, pain.

Cypress
Painful periods, heavy periods. Excessive perspiration (e.g. night sweats, hot flushes, sweaty feet), greasy skin, incontinence, poor circulation, oedema, piles, varicose veins. Asthma, repelling insects, cuts and wounds, rheumatism and arthritis, muscular aches, colds, chest infections, nervous tension.

Note: Avoid in early pregnancy

Citronella
Repelling insects, weakness, fatigue.

Dill
Colic, crying and sleeplessness in babies. Poor circulation in the limbs, tension in the muscles and pains in the joints.

Eucalyptus
Colds, flu, catarrh, sinusitis, fevers, bacterial and viral infections, bronchitis, diseases of childhood (measles and chickenpox), epidemics, repelling insects. Urinary infections, fluid retention, cuts and wounds, skin infections, cold sores, burns, shingles. Rheumatism, arthritis, muscular aches and pains.

Fennel

Gout, toxic conditions, inflamed joints, alcoholism, wind, colic, hiccoughs, nausea, indigestion, constipation, excessive appetite. Kidney stones, fluid retention, urinary infections, irregular periods, painful periods, PMS, menopausal symptoms, poor milk flow, obesity.

Note: Avoid in epilepsy and for children under six. Avoid in early pregnancy

Frankincense

Respiratory infections, catarrh, laryngitis, asthma, fevers. Urinary infections, heavy periods, anxiety, tension, hyperventilation, poor concentration, ageing skin, fear, insecurity, lack of self-confidence. Eczema, scarring, sores, wounds.

Geranium

Depression, urinary and respiratory infections, sore throats. Greasy skin, eczema, menopausal problems, PMS, irregular periods, fluid retention. Anxiety, over-excitement, mood swings, nervous tension, diarrhoea, kidney stones, neuralgia, circulatory problems, repelling insects.

Ginger

Catarrh, sinusitis, colds, flu, chest infections, tiredness, depression, low libido. Diarrhoea, rheumatism, arthritis, poor circulation, weak digestion, colic, nausea, stomach cramps, period pain, muscular pain and tension, sprains.

Hops

Tense muscles, sleeplessness. Pain from headaches and arthritis. Tension, anxiety, irritability and restlessness. Calms sexual desire in men, enhances women's libido, relieves menopausal symptoms.

Hyssop

Viral infections, chest infections, catarrh, sinusitis, sore throats, bruises, rheumatism, arthritis. Skin problems, poor concentration, mental fatigue, circulatory problems, nervous tension, asthma.

Note: Avoid in early pregnancy, and in cases of epilepsy or high blood pressure

Jasmine

Period pain, pain and tension in childbirth, retained placenta, postnatal weakness or depression, low libido, frigidity, tension, anxiety, especially around sexuality, depression, fear, muscle tension, lethargy, lack of confidence, grief. Sore throats, coughs, catarrh, chest infections, sensitive dry skin.

Note: Avoid in early pregnancy

Juniper

Toxic conditions, fluid retention, cystitis, vaginal discharge, scanty or irregular periods, piles, acne, infections, convalescence, lethargy, poor appetite, rheumatism, gout, arthritis. Exhaustion, hangovers, liver problems, obesity, chest infections.

Note: Avoid in early pregnancy, and in cases of kidney infection

Lavender

Depression, anxiety, tension, nervousness, restlessness, insomnia, mood swings, PMS, menopause. Infections, colds, flu, coughs, catarrh, sinusitis, burns, skin problems, infections such as athlete's foot. Injuries, cuts and wounds. Ulcers, migraine, headaches, muscular pain and tension. Rheumatism, sciatica, arthritis, period pain, scanty periods, vaginal discharge and infection. During childbirth to relieve pain and strengthen contractions, retained placenta. Children's ailments – colic, infections, irritability, insomnia. Palpitations, high blood pressure. Repelling insects, stings and bites. Nausea, asthma.

Lemon

Infections, fevers, lowered immunity, chest infections, colds, flu, catarrh, sinusitis, sore throats, ear infections and earaches. Cuts and wounds, nosebleeds. Stomach and bowel infections, diarrhoea, acid stomach, gastritis, peptic ulcers, gallstones. Rheumatism, gout, arthritis, varicose veins, high blood pressure, arteriosclerosis. Greasy skin, boils and spots, verrucas, warts. Lethargy, tiredness, nervous tension, anxiety.

Linden

Stress-related problems – nervous indigestion, headaches, muscular stiffness, weakness, cramps and pain, insomnia, restlessness, irritability, depression.

Marjoram

Chest infections, coughs, colds, flu, asthma, catarrh, sinusitis. Insomnia, headaches, nerve pain. High blood pressure, poor circulation, muscle tension and pain. Rheumatism, arthritis, sprains, bruises. Digestive problems, colic, constipation, period pain, cramp. Grief, loneliness, anxiety, tension, depression, excess libido, insomnia.

Note: Avoid in early pregnancy

Melissa

Skin problems, allergies, eczema, asthma, coughs. Menstrual irregularities, period pain, infertility. High blood pressure, hyperventilation, palpitations. Shock, depression, anxiety, tension, lethargy, bereavement, insomnia. Repelling insects. Stress headaches, digestive problems, indigestion, colic, diarrhoea. Herpes, bacterial and fungal infections.

Myrrh

Chest infections, colds, flu, catarrh, sinusitis. Sore throats, mouth infections, ulcers, bleeding gums. Digestive problems, diarrhoea, poor appetite. To stimulate contractions during childbirth, vaginal infections, thrush. Cuts and wounds, ulcers, infections, eczema, athlete's foot, lowered immunity, candidiasis.

Note: Avoid in early pregnancy

Neroli

Depression, insomnia, anxiety, tension, stress, low libido, shock, sexual problems, fear. Skin problems, scarring, dry skin, ageing skin. Digestive problems, colic, diarrhoea, period pains, menopausal problems, palpitations.

Nutmeg

Rheumatic pain, arthritis, poor circulation. Nervousness, weakness, insomnia, lethargy, depression, muscle pain, nausea, vomiting.

Note: Use only in low doses. Avoid in early pregnancy

Orange

Depression, insomnia, lethargy, anxiety, nervousness. Digestive problems – colic, stomach aches, constipation, chronic diarrhoea, poor circulation, bleeding gums. Period pains, muscular spasm.

Oregano

Bronchitis, viral infections, fungal infections, thrush. Rheumatism, arthritis, muscular aches and pains. Digestive problems. Irregular, scanty periods.

Note: Avoid in early pregnancy when it may irritate the skin

Peppermint

Liver and digestive problems, indigestion, colic, wind, diarrhoea, heartburn, nausea, vomiting, travel sickness. Infections, colds, flu, poor circulation, lethargy, depression, fevers, catarrh, sinusitis, skin problems and infections. Headaches, migraine, nerve pain, poor concentration, mental fatigue, tiredness, shock. Arthritis.

Pine

Chest infections, catarrh, colds, flu, sore throats. Poor circulation, tiredness, weakness, rheumatic pain. Muscular pain and tension. Bladder and kidney infections, fluid retention.

Rose Maroc, or Bulgar

Irregular periods, period pain, PMS, prolapse, tendency to miscarriage, gynaecological problems, heavy periods, infertility. Depression, grief, emotional problems related to sexuality, low libido, frigidity, anxiety, postnatal depression, heartbreak, lack of confidence, bereavement, menopausal problems. Poor circulation, allergies, tiredness, debility. Dry, sensitive, ageing skin.

Note: Avoid in early pregnancy

Rose geranium

Stress related disorders – headaches, stomach aches, menstrual cramps, debility, tension, melancholy, depression. Mood swings, PMS, menopausal problems. Lax muscles, diarrhoea, heavy periods. Grazes and cuts, pimples, greasy skin, acne. Piles, varicose veins, chilblains, burns, eczema, cellulite. Boils, abscesses, head lice. Repelling insects, perspiration. Engorgement of the breasts, mastitis.

Rosemary

Lethargy, exhaustion, poor concentration, poor memory, mental dullness and fatigue, migraine, fainting, headaches, depression, tension, anxiety. Raised cholesterol, liver problems, constipation. Chest infections, colds, flu, catarrh, sinusitis, asthma. Gout, rheumatism, arthritis, muscle tension and pain, sprains. Skin problems, ageing skin, problem hair, poor circulation. Pain.

Rosewood

Headaches, tiredness, lethargy, nausea, nervousness, poor concentration, mental fatigue, depression, restlessness.

Sage

Inhale for coughs, colds and catarrh. In massage for men warms the muscles.

Caution: Never use in pregnancy

Sandalwood

Urinary infections, vaginal infections and discharge, chest infections, sore throats, catarrh. Skin problems – sensitive skin, acne, rashes, skin infections, fungal and bacterial infections. Low libido, nervousness, anxiety, fear, lethargy, insecurity, lack of self confidence, over-sensitivity, depression, menstrual problems.

Thyme

Digestive problems, weak digestion, wind, poor appetite, stomach and bowel infections, diarrhoea, worms. Colds, coughs, flu, catarrh, sinusitis, sore throats, asthma, chest infections, mouth and gum infections, lowered immunity, thrush, urinary infections, fluid retention. Poor circulation, fatigue, convalescence, depression, poor concentration and memory, mental dullness, insomnia. Cuts and wounds, rheumatism, arthritis. Insect bites and stings.

Note: Avoid in early pregnancy

Ti-Tree (TEA-TREE)

Lowered immunity, bacterial, viral and fungal infections. Colds, flu, childhood infections, fevers, cold sores, shingles, chickenpox. Verrucas, warts, acne, spots and boils, ringworm, burns, athlete's foot, thrush, candidiasis, glandular fever.

Note: Dilute well – may irritate sensitive skins

Yarrow

Arthritis and gout. Cramp, colic, painful periods. Poor circulation and digestion, heavy and prolonged periods.

Ylang-ylang

Hyperventilation, palpitations, shock, stress, anxiety, nervousness, anger, depression, high blood pressure, insomnia, low libido, skin problems, tension, sexual problems, lack of self confidence.

FLOWERS FOR COMMON AILMENTS

How to use herbal remedies

Herbs exert their beneficial influence on us in many ways. Simply being amongst them in a fragrant herb garden, or picking wild herbs in a country lane in summer, is enough for us to feel their wonderful effects. The easiest way to take herbs is of course to eat them, which many of us do daily. We use parsley in salads, dill with fish, marjoram with pizza, mint with lamb, horseradish with beef, basil with pasta, and garlic with everything. The active ingredients of the herbs are absorbed from the digestive tract into the bloodstream and circulate around the body.

Preparations for internal use
Apart from culinary use, herbs can be taken internally as teas, also called infusions, as tinctures, or as tablets.

Infusions These are made in the same way as a cup of tea using the soft parts of plants – the leaves, stems and flowers. The standard dose is 1 oz (25 g) of dried herb, or 2 oz (50 g) of fresh herb to 1 pint (600 ml) of boiling water. You can vary this according to taste – it is important to make your herb teas palatable so that when you need to drink them you do so regularly. Put the herbs in a warmed teapot, pour on boiling water, leave covered to infuse for ten minutes and then strain. A cupful is generally taken three times daily for chronic conditions, and six times daily or more in acute illness. An infusion will keep for up to two days in a refrigerator.

Some herbs, particularly those with a high mucilage content, need to be prepared in the same way but with cold water. Where this is the case, it is mentioned in the relevant flower profile in Chapter 2. Most infusions are taken hot, except when treating the urinary system, when they need to be drunk lukewarm to cold.
When making infusions you can blend several herbs together, either to combine the effects of different herbs or to make the brew tastier. Several aromatic herbs are recommended to add to herbal infusions, which can otherwise be bitter. These include mint, lemon balm, lemon verbena, fennel, lavender and licorice. All make delicious drinks on their own or in combination.

Decoctions These are similar to infusions but prepared from the hard woody parts of plants, such as the bark, seeds, roots, rhizomes and nuts. These parts require greater heat to impart their constituents to the water. Break or hammer them first with a pestle and mortar, or chop them if fresh, then place in a pan with the water, bring to the boil, cover and simmer for ten minutes and strain. Use a little more than a pint of water per ounce of herb to make up for any lost in the simmering. The dosage is the same as for infusions.

Using infusions and decoctions
As well as drinking infusions and decoctions, you can use them in eyebaths, gargles, mouthwashes and lotions, generally two to three times daily for chronic problems and every two hours in acute cases.

Syrups These sweet liquids are often preferred by children. Give one dessertspoon (two for adults) three or four times daily in chronic problems and twice as much in acute illness.

You can use an infusion or decoction to make a syrup by mixing 12 oz (325 g) sugar into a pint (600 ml) of the liquid and heat until the sugar dissolves. Store the syrup in a refrigerator. Alternatively, you can weigh your infusion or decoction and add to it a teaspoon of honey for every 4 oz (100 g) of its weight. Heat this slowly and stir as it thickens, skimming off any scum that forms on the surface.

Another way to make syrup is to pour a pint (600 ml) of boiling water over 2½ lb (1.25 kg) of soft brown sugar and stir over a low heat until the sugar is dissolved and the solution starts to boil. Remove from the heat. Add one part herbal tincture (see below) to three parts syrup and this will keep indefinitely.

Tinctures These are concentrated extracts of herbs. A mixture of water and alcohol is generally used to extract the constituents of the remedy and act as a preservative. The ratio of alcohol to water varies from one remedy to another; 25 per cent alcohol is used for simple glycosides and tannins, while 90 per cent alcohol is needed for resins and gums.

To make a tincture, use dried herbs at a ratio of one part herb to five parts of liquid, or fresh herbs at a ratio of one part herb to two of liquid. Place the herb in a large jar and pour the alcohol and water mixture over it. Leave to macerate, shaking daily for two weeks. Then, using a wine press, press out the liquid and discard the herb – which makes very good compost. Store in labelled, dark bottles or glass jars, away from heat and light.

When making tinctures at home you can use undiluted alcohol such as brandy, gin or vodka. Alternatively you can use glycerol (glycerine), which gives a sweet taste to the extracts and makes them more palatable. Use equal parts of water and glycerol for dried herbs, and 80 per cent glycerol for watery, fresh herbs such as borage to ensure they do not deteriorate or become contaminated by infection.

Using tinctures A standard dose is one teaspoon of tincture diluted with a little water three times daily with or after food in chronic conditions, and every two hours in acute illness. Children should be given half dosages, and babies a quarter of the adult dose.

Tinctures generally keep well for about two years, and although more time-consuming to prepare than teas, they have the advantage of being easy to store and only requiring to be taken in small amounts.

Tinctures can also be used to make gargles and mouthwashes, lotions and douches. Use half to one teaspoon in a cupful of water two or three times daily in chronic problems and every two hours for acute conditions.

Suppositories Both local and systemic problems can be treated quickly and simply by this method. Suppositories bypass the alimentary canal and are absorbed quickly into the system. The herbal remedy is absorbed directly into the bloodstream through the mucosa of the rectum.

You can prepare suppositories easily at home by adding finely powdered dried herbs to a base of melted cocoa butter. Pour this into moulds made in the required shape from aluminium foil, and allow to cool. Store in a refrigerator. It is a good idea to make a row of suppositories in the foil at one time.

Tablets and capsules Herbs in tablet or capsule form can often be bought from herb suppliers or health food shops. You can also make capsules at home using gelatine capsules filled with powdered mixtures of the herbs you require. The process is made easier by using a capsule maker, which enables you to make up a large quantity at a time. The two standard capsule sizes are 0 and 00. Size 0 holds about 0.35 g of powder, so that three capsules should be taken three times daily to achieve the standard dose. Size 00 holds about 0.5 g of powder, requiring two capsules to be taken three times daily.

Preparations for external use

The skin is highly absorbent; constituents of any herbal preparation applied to it will be carried by tiny capillaries under the skin surface into the bloodstream and then around the body. There are various ways in which you can employ this pathway into the body.

Herbal baths A fragrant warm bath is a wonderfully luxurious and relaxing way to take herbal medicines and a very easy way to treat babies and children. You can hang a muslin bag filled with fresh or dried herbs under the hot tap. Alternatively you can add strong herb infusions into the bathwater. Soak in the water for 15–30 minutes. You can also add a few drops of your chosen essential oil to the bathwater – always dilute the oils first for babies and children, or if you have a sensitive skin.

In a herbal bath the plant constituents are absorbed through the skin's pores, which are opened by the warmth of the water. Volatile oils are carried on the steam to be inhaled through the nose and mouth into the lungs and from there into the bloodstream. From the nose, the oils send messages via nerve receptors to the brain and have a rapidly relaxing and soothing effect, easing mental and emotional strain. Lavender, chamomile and ylang ylang are wonderfully relaxing and smell lovely, while rosemary is also relaxing but has a stimulating edge, sending blood to the brain and enhancing alertness.

Hand and footbaths Our hands and feet are very sensitive areas, with plenty of nerve endings. Despite some thickening of the skin from use, herbal constituents pass easily from these areas into the bloodstream. Mustard footbaths are an old English remedy for all afflictions of cold and damp, from colds and flu to poor circulation and arthritis. The famous French herbalist Maurice Messegue advocates this therapeutic pathway for the use of herbs in his several books on herbal medicine and recommends footbaths for eight minutes in the evening and handbath for eight minutes in the morning. Hand and footbaths are excellent ways to treat babies and children who only need to keep still for half the time recommended for adults – four

minutes morning and evening.

Ointments and creams To make a simple ointment, herbs are macerated in oil. Put 16 oz (450 ml) of olive oil and 2 oz (50 g) of beeswax into a heatproof dish, add as much of the herb as the mixture will cover, and let it heat gently for a few hours in a bain-marie. This allows time for the constituents of the remedy to be absorbed into the oil. Press out through a muslin bag, discard the herb, and pour the warm oil into jars, where it will quickly solidify.

You can also make up creams very easily by stirring tinctures, infusions, decoctions or a few drops of essential oil into a base of aqueous cream from the pharmacist.

Poultices A poultice is a soft, damp mixture applied to part of the body. You can use fresh or dried herbs as a poultice, placed between two pieces of gauze. When using fresh leaves, stems or roots, make sure to bruise or crush them first. When using dried herbs, add a little hot water to the powdered or finely chopped herbs to make a paste to spread over the gauze. Then bind the gauze poultice to the affected part using a light cotton bandage and keep it warm with a hot water bottle. You can use cabbage leaves in this way for painful, arthritic joints or tender, engorged breasts, while a bran poultice will ease mastitis.

Compresses Take a clean cloth or flannel, and soak it either in a hot or cold herbal infusion or decoction, or in water to which a few drops of essential oil have been added. Then wring it out and apply to the affected area, such as the site of a headache, period pain, backache, inflamed joints, or varicose veins. Repeat several times for good effect.

Liniments Also called embrocations, liniments are rubbing oils used in massage to relax or stimulate muscles and ligaments, or soothe away pain from inflammation or injury. They consist of extracts of herbs in an oil or alcohol base, or a mixture of herbal oils and alcohol tinctures of herbs. They are intended to be absorbed quickly through the skin to the affected part and for this reason often contain stimulating oils or cayenne which help to increase local circulation.

Oils Essential oils are extracted from aromatic plants by a process of steam distillation and so cannot be prepared at home. You can buy them from many different sources including health food shops and mail order companies.

You can easily make herbal oils, however, by infusing finely chopped herbs in a pure vegetable oil such as almond, sunflower or olive oil, for about two weeks. Place the herbs in a glass jar with a tight-fitting lid and cover them with oil. Place the jar on a sunny windowsill and shake it daily. Gradually the oil will take up the constituents of the remedy you use. After two weeks or more, filter the oil and press the remainder out of the herb through a muslin bag. Store in an airtight dark bottle.

Oils can be used for massage, and are a particularly easy way to give herbs to children. A few drops of herbal oil can be diluted in a base oil (2 drops per 5 ml) and also used for massage. You can also put five to ten drops into a bowl of hot water for inhalations, into a little water to use as an aromatic or disinfectant room spray, or in a facial steamer for cleaning the skin.

How to use aromatherapy oils

The therapeutic action of oils

The volatile oils which give aromatic herbs their wonderful smell and taste are composed of a wide variety of chemical compounds. The different combinations of these in plants give us the wonderful variation in their aromas and therapeutic effects. Up to 50 different chemical constituents have been identified in some oils. All volatile oils are antiseptic, and enhance the function of the immune system in warding off bacterial, viral or fungal infection. Many oils have anti-inflammatory and antispasmodic properties. Those in chamomile, for example, are particularly applicable for the relief of inflamed and irritated conditions of the digestive tract, while those in dill relax spasm and colicky pain in the digestive system. Some oils have an expectorant action such as in thyme and hyssop, and aid the clearing of phlegm from the chest, while others are diuretic, useful in relief of fluid retention and urinary infections. While they exert their beneficial effects on the physical body, they also reach the brain and nervous system, meaning that aromatherapy has a wide range of applications in treatment in the realm of the emotions (see p. 274–277).

How oils act on the body

Volatile oils can be taken into the body in a variety of ways in order to exert their beneficial influences. They can simply be taken as aromatic herbs in foods and drinks, which many of us do every day. Diluted, the oil can be rubbed on to the skin or inhaled through the nose. When we breathe in their aromas we stimulate certain nerve endings situated in the upper part of the nose (olfactory receptor cells) and these carry nerve impulses or messages to the brain, especially the limbic system, the area that relates to instinctual responses, emotions, sex drive and memory. As the oils are inhaled, tiny molecules are also taken into the lungs and absorbed into the bloodstream and thence around the body, through the alveoli in the lungs.

When oils are rubbed onto the skin, or absorbed through the skin by bathing with aromatic oils in the water, the oils stimulate nerve endings in the skin. Messages are relayed to the underlying tissues, muscles, blood and lymphatic vessels, and also via the nervous system to the pituitary gland, the master gland that regulates the action of all other endocrine glands, including the adrenals. These effects make aromatherapy of enormous benefit in treating hormonal problems, relieving stress and enhancing relaxation. Rose oil, for example, is a wonderful oil that has a particular affinity for women. It helps to alleviate tension and anxiety and symptoms related to the reproductive system, such as menstrual problems, PMS, anxiety after childbirth, emotional problems concerning sexuality and postnatal depression. Volatile oils can be absorbed in as little as 30 minutes but their therapeutic effect can last for many hours. Once in the bloodstream, volatile oils are dispersed throughout the body, influencing the various organs or systems according to the specific properties of the oils. Once they have exerted their beneficial action, they are excreted from the body via the skin, the lungs and the urine.

Volatile oils act upon the limbic system, which, as well as being concerned with our emotions, deals with memory. For this reason, aromas can trigger memories of places, people and events in the past. The smell of eucalyptus for me is evocative of Colombia, where the leaves and seed pods are burnt to purify the atmosphere. When selecting oils for your use, it is important to choose the fragrances that you like, since these will probably be best suited to your physical and emotional needs. Your choice may well be inspired by pleasant associations from the past.

Using the oils

Massage Aromatherapy oils are powerful because they are concentrates of what exists in a more dilute form in nature. All oils therefore need to be diluted in a base oil, such as sweet almond oil, before being applied to the skin. Massage is the most luxurious way to use oils – you can make a massage oil with:

50 ml of base oil (almond, apricot kernel, avocado, soya, grapeseed) (50 ml = 1.75 fluid ounces)
25 drops of essential oil

The essential oil you use can be composed of a mixture of two or three oils of your choice. Use 12 drops of essential oil per base of 50 ml if your skin is particularly sensitive, if you are pregnant, or when massaging children over six years old. For babies, use 2–3 drops per 50 ml. The only exception to this rule is lavender, which is safe enough to apply directly to the skin for treating, for example, a cut or burn. Tea-tree oil can also be applied neat. Store your massage oil in a bottle made of dark glass with a well-fitting lid, to reduce deterioration of the oil.

Baths Fragrant baths are easy to make – just sprinkle 5–10 drops of essential oil into the water, swish the water around a little to disperse the oils, and enjoy a good soaking for about 15 minutes. They can help you relax, and release tender, aching or tense muscles after a long day. They can also invigorate you ready to start again in the morning. Add 2–5 drops of oil to sitz baths to treat pelvic infections such as cystitis or thrush, and to hand and footbaths. When using oils in the bath for children and babies it is best to dilute them first, 2–5 drops in 10ml base oil.

Vaporizers and steam inhalation

A few drops (5–10) of oil can be put into a vaporizer and the oils will evaporate into the atmosphere, affecting you as well as those around you. This is very restful method to employ in the room of a baby or child at night, as the oils will help clear the airways and enhance the battle against infection. It is also well worth putting a vaporizer in your place of work. Oils such as rosemary will aid concentration and alertness while lavender will help to relax you if over-tense. In the same way, oils can be dropped on to a handkerchief, a radiator, a (cold) light bulb, or even a wood-burning stove to fragrance the room.

Steam inhalation, using 2–4 drops in a bowl of hot (not boiling) water with a towel over the head is excellent for clearing catarrh from the head and chest during respiratory infections. You will need to inhale deeply for about 3–5 minutes for best effects.

Gargles and mouthwashes

Essential oils can also be used to make gargles or mouthwashes for adults. Mix 2–3 drops in a drop of alcohol in a glass and fill it up with water. Do not swallow.

Compresses and room sprays

Essential oils make useful compresses, either hot or cold. Disperse 3–6 drops of oil in medium-sized bowl of water. Place a clean washrag or cloth on the surface of the water to pick up the oil and apply repeatedly to the area. Use cold water for swellings of burns, bruises and knocks, and hot water for arthritis and period pain.

For room sprays to fumigate a sick-room, or to make an insect repellent, place 10 drops of an oil such as lavender or eucalyptus in a spray container and shake it vigorously before spraying.

CAUTION WHEN USING AROMATHERAPY OILS

It is important to keep all oils away from children as they are powerful concentrates. Avoid using them near the eyes, or undiluted, and do not take them internally. If you have a sensitive skin it is best to try the oils you wish to use on a small patch of skin a couple of times before applying them over the body or adding them to baths.

Some oils can increase the skin's sensitivity to sunlight or ultraviolet light. These include bergamot, lemon, lemon verbena, orange and lime.

It is particularly important to use oils under the guidance of a qualified practitioner if you suffer from high blood pressure, epilepsy or a nervous disorder. If you are pregnant, certain oils should be avoided as they may set off bleeding or possibly miscarriage. Such oils bear a warning note or caution where they appear in Chapters 2 and 3.

How to use flower essences

How the remedies are made

Dr Bach's original 38 flower remedies, described in Chapter 3, were made from the early morning dew that settles on the petals of flowers and which takes up the healing energy of the flower. Because this is not available to everyone Dr Bach devised simple methods of extracting the subtle healing properties of the flowers using water and sunlight, which was easy enough for anyone to employ.

The sun method involved placing the flower heads, picked carefully so as not to damage them, into a thin, clear glass or crystal bowl, filled with spring water, to float on top. The bowl is then placed on the ground near the parent plants and left in the sun for a few hours, during which time the healing energy from the flowers should be transferred to the water. The flowers are then taken carefully out of the water with a twig or a leaf, and the essence is poured into bottles half full of brandy, which acts as a preservative.

The boiling method was devised by Dr Bach for some of the flower remedies including willow, elm and star-of-Bethlehem. The flowers are placed in an enamel pan of spring water and this is simmered for half an hour, covered and left to cool. Then the essence is filtered and preserved in equal parts of brandy. These essences are then called mother tinctures, and are further diluted in brandy and called stock bottle, the concentrate in which the remedy is generally sold.

The flowers used for flower essences should be in best condition, at the height of their vitality, newly-flowered and not about to go over. If picked wild they should be found growing as far away as possible from sprayed fields or pollution from traffic or factories.

Taking the remedies

The three major collections of flower remedies are listed in Chapter 3. Many others appear in Chapter 2. Advice on choosing flower essences suited to you is given below. Having chosen the flower remedies that are best suited to your needs, select four or five of those that seem particularly appropriate at the time of choosing. It may be necessary to change your prescription at a later date as some problems begin to resolve and others may come to light.

Take 2 drops of each remedy chosen from the stock bottle, and mix them in a 30ml amber dropper bottle (available from pharmacists or suppliers) shaking the bottle vigorously. Then fill the bottle almost to the top with spring water and shake vigorously again. To preserve your remedy add 1 teaspoonful of brandy (or cider vinegar if you want to avoid alcohol). Take 4 drops four times daily; in crisis situations you may wish to take it more frequently than this.

The Australian Bush Flower Essences are taken seven at a time and twice daily, morning and night. Normally flower essences are dropped under the tongue to make for speedy absorption, but it is important to avoid the dropper touching your mouth in case it causes bacterial infection of the essence.

The drops can also be added to water, fruit juice or herbal teas. Equally they can be applied to the skin, on the wrists, the forehead, temples or even the feet – sometimes it is not possible to give drops by mouth, if someone is asleep, unconscious or in a state of shock. However essences can also be added to bathwater, or to washing water to splash on to your face in the morning. It helps to drop 7 drops of essence into the water in a bowl and leave it in the sun for few hours before using it. Flower essences can be dropped on to the pillow of someone who is sick, suffering from insomnia or nightmares, or added to water in a plant spray and used as an atomizer to spray around the room. It is best to keep your bottle of flower essence where you have it to hand when you need it. Try to keep it away from other medications, and electrical appliances such as radios, televisions or computers.

How do flower essences work?

Flower remedies do not work like drugs with an immediate physical or mental effect, but have a more gentle effect by their influence on the subtle energy structures. These are similar to the acupuncture meridians used in Chinese medicine, or the chakras, familiar in Ayurvedic philosophy. In this way flower essences have the ability to benefit us on a subtle level, through our thoughts and emotions, but since these energy systems also influence us on a biochemical level in the cells, they also benefit us physically.

Choosing flower remedies

There are literally thousands of flower remedies to choose from, to address your own individual needs, each one having its own unique properties and healing affinities. Faced with such choices, it can feel something of a challenge to decide which four or five to start with. Time spent in reflection or meditation will help to develop a clearer picture of yourself and your essential needs. You could write down facets of your nature or temperament that come to mind, so that you start to build a case history for yourself. Add these notes to details of the type of physical illnesses to which you may be prone, which may further serve to indicate imbalances underlying them by forming some kind of pattern.

Once a clearer picture of yourself begins to form, you can read through the flower essences and see which ones jump out of the page at you. Inevitably you will find many that you will immediately recognize that could benefit you. To narrow down your choice underline the ones that feel most appropriate at the time of choosing. Some people find dowsing greatly helpful – using a pendulum, which can be anything from a stone, crystal or ring on a piece of string, is actually very simple. By asking the pendulum whether specific remedies are appropriate, you will find that it will swing one way for yes and the other for no. Other people use kinesiology or muscle testing to select their flower remedies. To do this, test the strength of the right arm muscle by asking someone to attempt to push the arm downwards when you hold your arm outstretched horizontally. Then hold a stock bottle in the left hand and test the strength of the other arm when held outstretched again. If it remains as strong it indicates the flower remedy is suitable. If the arm gives way under little pressure, the flower essence is not right at the moment.

The course of treatment

Once you start to take the flower remedies on a regular basis, your self-awareness should naturally increase. You may find that for a short time the very mental or emotional states that indicated your choice of remedy actually feel worse, particularly if you have been unable to express them, and you may become painfully aware of your inner disharmony. It is better to let go and cry or shout if you want to, than hold in your feelings.

The reaction of some people to flower essences is often more subtle, and changes within are noticed very gradually. The heightened awareness of oneself can act as a great tool of transformation as it creates the impetus to change the emotions or attitudes that give rise to your pain. You can thereby work along with the flower essences to affect your inner development and resolution of discomfort and disease. It may be that after a while other emotions become more apparent, and this may indicate the time to change your selection or choose a new set of flower remedies.

Some people gradually forget to take their remedies and this generally indicates that they feel better, and do not require more remedies for the time being. It is generally best to take the same prescription for about six to eight weeks, unless another remedy becomes strongly indicated or your circumstances change.

EMOTIONAL PROBLEMS

These are the recommended remedies for common emotional problems.
See pages 269–273 for advice on taking the remedies.

Acquisitiveness
Flower essence
Beth root

Addiction
Herbal remedies
Passionflower
California poppy

Flower essences
Skullcap
Self-heal
Agrimony

Aggression
Flower essences
Hawthorn
Tiger lily

Ambition
Flower essences
Beth root
Vervain
Tiger lily

Anger
Herbal remedies
Passionflower
Sweet violet
Dandelion
Feverfew
Rose

Flower essences
Nettle
Blue flag
Chamomile

Anxiety
Herbal remedies
California poppy
Chamomile
Hops
Lady's slipper
Lavender
Lemon balm
Linden
Marjoram
Passionflower
Pine
Rosemary
Skullcap
Sweet marjoram
Vervain
Wood betony

Aromatherapy oils
Chamomile
Clary sage
Lavender
Lemon balm
Melissa
Rose geranium
Rosemary
Basil
Sweet marjoram

Flower essences
Garlic
Skullcap
Rosemary
Aspen
Periwinkle
Lemon balm
Chamomile
White chestnut
Gentian

Argumentativeness
Flower essences
Marigold
Nettle
Lavender

Arrogance
Flower essence
Sunflower

Bereavement
Flower essence
Honeysuckle

Bitterness
Flower essences
Hawthorn
Willow
Oregon grape
Gentian

Changeability
Flower essence
Anemone

Childhood trauma
Flower essence
Alchemilla

Coldness
Herbal remedies
Angelica
Ginger
Passionflower

Flower essences
Mallow
Hawthorn
Nasturtium
Ginger
Marigold
Linden
Nettle
Evening primrose

Compulsion
Flower essence
Dandelion

Confusion
Herbal remedies
Sage
Hawthorn
Hops

Flower essences
Angelica
Greater celandine
Mullein
Wood betony
Rosemary
Periwinkle
Geranium
Datura
Eyebright

Constraint
Flower essences
Eucalyptus
Wood betony

Cruelty
Flower essences
Marigold
Nettle

Debility
Herbal remedies
Ginger
Clary sage
Lavender
Ginseng

Aromatherapy oils
Lemon balm
Clary sage
Lavender
Pine
Rose geranium

Flower essence
Geranium

Defensiveness
Flower essence
Blessed thistle

Dependence
Flower essence
Sweet marjoram

Depletion
Herbal remedies
Pasque flower
Ginger
Blessed thistle
Pine
Lady's slipper

Flower essences
Anemone
Olive
Echinacea
Ginseng
Elder
Periwinkle
Mistletoe
Lemon balm
Lady's slipper

Depression
Herbal remedies
Cayenne
Clary sage
Cowslip
Lady's slipper
Lemon balm
Marjoram
Pasque flower
Rose
Rosemary
Skullcap
St John's wort
Sweet marjoram
Thyme
Vervain
Wood betony

Aromatherapy oils
Clary sage
Geranium
Ginger
Hyssop
Jasmine
Lemon balm
Linden
Rose
Rose geranium
Rosemary

Sweet marjoram
Thyme

Flower essences
Borage
Mustard
Rosemary
Sunflower
Larch
Lavender
Periwinkle
Lemon balm
Chamomile
Geranium
Gentian
White chestnut
Yerba santa
Black cohosh

Despair
Flower essences
Mustard
Sweet chestnut

Despondency
Flower essences
Gentian
Borage

Disappointment
Flower essences
Heartsease
Hawthorn
Datura

Disorganization
Flower essence
Daisy

Disorientation
Flower essences
Datura
Ginseng
Alchemilla
Echinacea

Distress
Flower essence
Olive

Domineeringness
Flower essence
Chicory

Effects of ageing
Herbal remedies
Sage
Thyme
Cayenne
Rosemary
Sweet marjoram
Ginseng

Aromatherapy oils
Sweet marjoram
Rosemary

Flower essence
Thyme

Emotional blocking
Herbal remedy
Sage

Flower essences
Hawthorn
Linden
Blue flag

Emotional depletion
Flower essence
Garlic

Emotional imbalance
Flower essence
Rosemary

Emotional suppression
Herbal remedy
Dandelion

Flower essences
Primrose
Dandelion

Emotional stress
Flower essence
Lavender

Envy
Flower essence
Holly

Escapism
Flower essences
Poppy
Agrimony
Chestnut bud
Drosera
California poppy

Exhaustion
Herbal remedies
Pasque flower
Angelica
Vervain

Thyme
Skullcap
Rosemary
Clary sage

Aromatherapy oils
Rosemary
Thyme
Hyssop
Clary sage
Pine

Flower essences
Aloe
Olive
Yarrow
Sweet chestnut

Fanaticism
Flower essence
Vervain

Fear
Flower essences
Poppy
Mallow
Garlic
Ginger
Sweet marjoram
Peony
Aspen
Elder
Water lily
St John's wort
Evening primrose
Basil
Datura

Fear of change
Flower essence
Alchemilla
Hops

Fear of loneliness
Flower essence
Eucalyptus

Forgetfulness
Herbal remedies
Sage
Hawthorn
Ginger
Lemon balm
Rosemary
Blessed thistle
Sweet marjoram

Aromatherapy oils
Rosemary
Sweet marjoram

Frustration
Flower essence
Blue flag

Greed
Flower essence
Beth root

Grief
Herbal remedies
Sweet violet
Dandelion
Borage
Rose

Flower essences
Forget-me-not
Sweet marjoram

Guilt
Flower essences
Borage
Hyssop
Pine

Hatred
Flower essence
Holly

Heartbreak
Herbal remedy
Sweet marjoram

Aromatherapy oil
Sweet marjoram

Flower essences
Heartsease
Hawthorn
Borage

Helplessness
Flower essences
Skullcap
Mustard
Mistletoe

Hyperactivity
Herbal remedies
Linden
Lemon balm
Lavender
Chamomile
Lady's slipper

Aromatherapy oils
Lavender
Chamomile

Flower essence
Chamomile

Hysteria
Herbal remedies
Cowslip
Lemon balm
Skullcap
Feverfew

Flower essences
Mugwort
Red clover

Immaturity
Flower essence
Sage

Impatience
Flower essence
Chamomile

Impotence
Herbal remedy
Ginger

Aromatherapy oil
Jasmine

Flower essence
Larch

Impracticality
Flower essence
Mugwort

Inability to cope
Flower essence
Rock rose

Inactivity
Flower essence
Castor oil

Indecision
Flower essences
Mullein
Cayenne
Drosera

Inner disharmony
Herbal remedy
Lavender

Aromatherapy oil
Lavender

Flower essences
Lavender
California poppy

Insecurity
Flower essences
Anemone
Mallow
Beth root
Chicory
Sweet marjoram
Chickweed
Oregon grape
Blue flag
Holly
Evening primrose

Insensitivity
Flower essences
Beth root
Marigold
Eyebright

Intolerance
Flower essence
Vervain

Intransigence
Flower essences
Sage
Greater celandine
Cayenne
Oak
Mistletoe
Walnut

Irrationality
Flower essence
Mugwort

Irresolution
Flower essence
Mistletoe

Irritability
Herbal remedies
Pasque flower
Passionflower
Elder
Linden
Cowslip
Blessed thistle
Rose
Hops

Flower essence
Chamomile

Isolation
Flower essences
Mallow
Viola odorata
Greater celandine
Ginger
Mustard
Willow
Linden

Jealousy
Flower essence
Holly

Lack of confidence
Aromatherapy oil
Clary sage

Flower essences
Wallflower
Sunflower
Self-heal
Water lily
Gentian

Flowers for common ailments

Lack of focus
Flower essences
Drosera
Daisy

Lack of fulfilment
Flower essence
Lemon balm

Lack of inspiration
Herbal remedy
Peppermint

Aromatherapy oil
Peppermint

Flower essences
Angelica
Olive
Blue flag

Lack of motivation/ purpose
Aromatherapy oil
Rose geranium

Flower essences
Sage
Geranium
Drosera

Lack of self-forgiveness
Flower essences
Hyssop
Pine

Laziness
Flower essences
Castor oil
Peppermint
Drosera

Lethargy
Herbal remedies
Thyme
Cayenne
Rosemary
Blessed thistle
Lavender
Sweet marjoram

Aromatherapy oils
Lavender
Rosemary
Thyme
Sweet marjoram

Flower essences
Aloe
Yarrow
Castor oil
Thyme
Peppermint

Libidinousness
Herbal remedy
Sweet marjoram

Aromatherapy oil
Sweet marjoram

Flower essence
Wood betony

Loneliness
Herbal remedies
Sweet marjoram
Rose

Aromatherapy oils
Sweet marjoram
Rose

Flower essences
Forget-me-not
Datura

Low self-esteem
Flower essences
Anemone
Mallow
Heartsease
Viola odorata
Skullcap
Sunflower
Larch
Blessed thistle
Elder

Lunacy
Flower essences
Peony
Datura

Malice
Flower essence
Holly

Manipulation
Flower essence
Chicory

Martyrdom
Flower essences
Pine
Centaury

Melancholy
Flower essence
Larch

Mental confusion
Herbal remedy
Sage

Flower essence
Daisy

Mental overwork
Flower essences
Nasturtium
Dandelion

Moodiness
Flower essence
Chamomile

Mental sluggishness
Flower essences
Jasmine
Eyebright

Moral confusion
Flower essences
Mullein
Wood betony

Morbidity
Flower essences
Aspen
Black cohosh

Negativity
Herbal remedy
Cowslip

Aromatherapy oil
Jasmine

Flower essences
Wallflower
Red clover
Willow
Blue flag
Gentian
Black cohosh

Nervousness
Herbal remedies
Vervain
Lemon balm
Skullcap
Rosemary
Lavender
Chamomile
Basil

Aromatherapy oils
Rosemary
Lemon balm
Lavender
Chamomile
Basil

Flower essences
Dill
Viola odorata
Centaury

Nostalgia
Flower essence
Honeysuckle

Over-active dreaming
Herbal remedy
Catnip

Flower essences
Mugwort
Peony
St John's wort
Chamomile

Over-dependence
Flower essence
Self-heal

Over-emotionalism
Flower essence
Mugwort

Over-independence
Flower essence
Eucalyptus

Over-sensitivity
Herbal remedy
Feverfew

Flower essences
Yarrow
Viola odorata
Red clover
St John's wort
Centaury

Over-stimulation
Flower essence
Dill

Over-concern for others
Flower essence
Lemon balm

Panic
Flower essences
Sweet chestnut
Rock rose

Paranoia
Flower essence
Oregon grape

Perfectionism
Flower essences
Pine
Oregon grape
Blue flag

Persistent unwanted thoughts
Herbal remedy
Passionflower

Flower essence
White chestnut

Poor concentration
Flower essences
Greater celandine
Thyme
Peppermint
Chamomile
Daisy

Possessiveness
Flower essence
Chicory

Powerlessness
Flower essence
Black cohosh

Problems learning from life
Flower essences
Chamomile
Honeysuckle
Chestnut bud

Regret
Flower essences
Honeysuckle
Chestnut bud

Rejection
Flower essence
Heartsease

Repression
Flower essences
Poppy
Primrose

Resentment
Flower essences
Sage
Willow
Nettle
Holly

Restlessness
Herbal remedies
Passionflower
Hawthorn
Hops
Lady's slipper

Flower essence
Passionflower

Self-criticism
Flower essences
Aloe
Wallflower
Larch
Pine
Oregon grape

Emotional problems

Self-delusion
Flower essence
Mullein

Self-demand
Flower essences
Witch hazel
Dandelion
Oak

Self-destruction
Flower essence
Willow

Self-disgust
Flower essences
Rose
Basil

Aromatherapy oil
Jasmine

Self-isolation
Flower essences
Eucalyptus
Arnica

Self-pity
Flower essence
Chicory

Self-punishment
Flower essence
Pine

Self-sacrifice
Flower essences
Witch hazel
Centaury

Selfishness
Flower essences
Beth root
Chicory
Sunflower

Sexual debility
Herbal remedies
Hops (for women)
Ginseng
Black cohosh

Aromatherapy oils
Clary sage
Rose

Flower essence
Lady's slipper

Sexual inhibition
Aromatherapy oils
Clary sage
Rose
Jasmine

Flower essence
Water lily

Sexual insecurity
Aromatherapy oils
Clary sage
Rose
Jasmine

Flower essence
Rose

Sexual/spiritual disjunction
Flower essences
Wood betony
Basil

Shame
Aromatherapy oil
Rose

Flower essence
Rose

Shock
Herbal remedies
Arnica
Daisy

Flower essences
Ginger
Arnica

Shyness
Flower essences
Viola odorata
Rose
Water lily

Sorrow
Flower essence
Sweet marjoram

Spiritual blocks
Flower essences
Passionflower
Angelica
Beth root
Echinacea
Oak
Ginseng
Gentian
Agrimony
Lady's slipper
Lavender

Spiritual closure
Flower essence
Passionflower

Spiritual confusion
Herbal remedy
Passionflower

Flower essence
Jasmine

Stagnation
Flower essences
Alchemilla
Cayenne
Larch
Oak
Walnut
Honeysuckle

Stress
Herbal remedies
Pasque flower
Skullcap
Borage
Ginseng
California poppy

Aromatherapy oils
Hyssop
Clary sage
Pine

Flower essences
Dill
Olive
Echinacea
Ginseng
Thyme
Mistletoe
Lemon balm

Stubbornness
Flower essence
Greater celandine

Terror
Flower essence
Rock rose

Thrill-seeking
Flower essence
California poppy

Trauma
Herbal remedy
Arnica

Flower essences
Echinacea
Arnica

Troubledness
Flower essence
Mullein

Unassertiveness
Flower essence
Poppy

Uncentredness
Flower essence
Drosera

Uncertainty
Flower essence
Angelica

Unconscious fear
Flower essence
Aspen

Uncreativeness
Flower essences
Cayenne
Rosemary
Oak
Blue flag

Ungroundedness
Flower essences
Poppy
Nasturtium
Mugwort
California poppy

Unresolved emotions
Flower essences
Forget-me-not
Hyssop
Chickweed
Linden
Periwinkle
Walnut
Evening primrose
Agrimony
Chestnut bud
Yerba santa

Vagueness
Flower essence
Drosera

Vanity
Flower essence
Sunflower

Vulnerability
Herbal remedy
Daisy

Flower essences
Yarrow
Anemone
Viola odorata
Garlic
Red clover
Blessed thistle
Sweet marjoram
Peony
Aspen
Elder
Tiger lily
Holly
Walnut
Centaury
Black cohosh

Weakness
Herbal remedy
Nasturtium

Flower essences
Mullein
Echinacea
Geranium

Work-obsession
Flower essences
Aloe
Vervain
Oak

PHYSICAL AILMENTS

These are the recommended remedies for common physical ailments, arranged according to the systems of the body. See pages 270–274 for advice on taking the remedies.

IMMUNE SYSTEM

Fevers
Herbal remedies
Yarrow
Garlic
Linden
Lemon balm
Chamomile

Aromatherapy oils
Eucalyptus
Lavender
Pine
Thyme
Chamomile
Marjoram

Infections
Herbal remedies
Garlic
Thyme
Ginger
Echinacea
Lavender
St John's wort

Aromatherapy oils
Eucalyptus
Lavender
Pine
Thyme
Chamomile
Marjoram

Allergies
Herbal remedies
Lemon balm
Borage
Echinacea
Chamomile
Evening primrose
Ginseng
Nettles

Aromatherapy oil
Melissa
Chamomile

Low immunity
Herbal remedies
Sage
Garlic
Thyme
Ginger
Cayenne

Hyssop
Calendula
Echinacea
Ginseng
Rose

Aromatherapy oils
Ginger
Hyssop
Thyme
Sweet basil
Rose
Jasmine

Flower essences
Garlic
Nasturtium
Eucalyptus

Candidiasis
Herbal remedies
Aloe juice
Garlic
Thyme
Echinacea
Chamomile

ME/Post viral syndrome
Herbal remedies
Garlic
Vervain
Echinacea
Centaury
St John's wort

Herpes
Herbal remedies
Aloe gel
Lemon balm
Hyssop
Calendula
Marjoram
Peppermint

Aromatherapy oil
Jasmine

NERVOUS SYSTEM

Tension
Herbal remedies
Basil
California poppy
Cowslip
Dill

Hops
Linden
Passionflower
Skullcap
St John's wort
Thyme
Wood betony

Aromatherapy oils
Basil
Geranium
Hops
Hyssop
Lemon balm
Peppermint
Sweet basil
Thyme

Flower essences
Blue flag
Chickweed
Dandelion
Ginger
Hyssop
Passionflower
Peony
Skullcap
Tiger lily

Insomnia, hyperactivity
Herbal remedies
Pasque flower
Passionflower
Linden
Vervain
Cowslip
Skullcap
Hops
Lavender
Marjoram

Aromatherapy oils
Clary sage
Hops
Lavender
Linden
Chamomile
Rose

Sluggishness
Herbal remedies
Eucalyptus
Dandelion

Flower essence
Peppermint

Headaches
Herbal remedies
Pasque flower
Passionflower
Vervain
Skullcap
Rosemary
Feverfew
Lavender
Black cohosh
Peppermint

Aromatherapy oils
Melissa
Clary sage
Lavender
Linden
Geranium
Peppermint

Migraine
Herbal remedies
Wood betony
Vervain
Cayenne
Rosemary
Feverfew
Lavender

Aromatherapy oils
Lavender
Chamomile

Tiredness, exhaustion
Herbal remedies
Vervain

Aromatherapy oils
Hyssop
Clary sage
Pine
Rose

Flower essences
Vervain
Skullcap
Rosemary
Rose

Seasonal Affective Disorder
Herbal remedies
Thyme
Periwinkle
Primrose
St John's wort

Neuralgia, sciatica
Herbal remedies
Pasque flower
Passionflower
Mustard
Lavender
Chamomile
Black cohosh
St John's wort
California poppy

Aromatherapy oils
Rosemary
Lavender
Chamomile
Peppermint

RESPIRATORY SYSTEM

Colds and flu
Herbal remedies
Yarrow
Elder
Catnip
Linden
Eucalyptus
Thyme

Aromatherapy oils
Lavender
Pine
Eucalyptus
Thyme

Flower essences
Eucalyptus
Ginger
Rosemary
Sunflower
Hyssop
Calendula
Lavender
Pine

Catarrh and sinusitis
Herbal remedies
Yarrow
Catnip
Garlic
Thyme
Ginger
Mustard
Cayenne
Feverfew
Sweet basil
Peppermint

Physical ailments

Aromatherapy oils
Pine
Eucalyptus
Peppermint

Flower essence
Eucalyptus

Earache
Herbal remedies
Eucalyptus
Mullein
Chamomile
Peppermint

Sore throat
Herbal remedies
Sage
Thyme
Garlic
Ginger
Mullein
Hyssop

Aromatherapy oil
Thyme

Asthma
Herbal remedies
Drosera
Eucalyptus
Thyme
Red clover
Mullein
Hyssop
Pine
Evening primrose
Black cohosh

Aromatherapy oils
Lavender
Eucalyptus
Thyme
Chamomile
Peppermint

Coughs, bronchitis, whooping cough
Herbal remedies
Pasque flower
Catnip
Garlic
Eucalyptus
Thyme
Mullein
Hyssop
Pine
Holly
Drosera

Aromatherapy oils
Lavender
Pine
Eucalyptus
Thyme

Flower essence
Eucalyptus

Laryngitis, croup
Herbal remedies
Elder
Eucalyptus
Witch hazel
Chickweed
Lavender
Honeysuckle

Aromatherapy oils
Lavender
Thyme

DIGESTIVE SYSTEM
Constipation
Dandelion
Aloe juice
Castor oil
Olive oil
Walnut

Diarrhoea
Herbal remedies
Alchemilla
Oak
Chamomile
Geranium
Ginger

Aromatherapy oil
Chamomile

Nausea, vomiting
Herbal remedies
Dill
Angelica
Lemon balm
Lavender
Peppermint

Aromatherapy oils
Lavender
Sweet basil
Peppermint

Heartburn, indigestion
Herbal remedies
Yarrow
Dill
Marshmallow
Lemon balm
Meadowsweet
Gentian
Chamomile
Peppermint

Aromatherapy oils
Melissa
Lavender
Chamomile
Peppermint

Bowel problems
Herbal remedies
Aloe gel
Aloe juice
Catnip
Garlic
Nasturtium
Borage
Self-heal

Gastritis, peptic ulcers
Herbal remedies
Aloe juice
Marshmallow
Lemon balm
Meadowsweet
Chamomile
Agrimony

Aromatherapy oil
Chamomile

Liver and gall-bladder problems
Herbal remedies
Dandelion
Chicory
Centaury
Agrimony
Oregon grape

Worms
Herbal remedies
Sage
Garlic
Mugwort
Gentian
Walnut

Colic
Herbal remedies
Dill
Catnip
Lemon balm
Ginger
Lavender
Chamomile

Aromatherapy oils
Melissa
Lavender
Yarrow
Dill
Chamomile
Sweet basil
Peppermint

URINARY SYSTEM
Cystitis, urethritis
Herbal remedies
Alchemilla
Marshmallow
Nasturtium

Meadowsweet
Chamomile

Aromatherapy oils
Pine
Eucalyptus
Chamomile

Kidney infections, stones
Herbal remedies
Alchemilla
Marshmallow
Dandelion
Meadowsweet
Rose

Water retention
Herbal remedies
Vervain
Dandelion
Borage
Chickweed
Meadowsweet

Bedwetting
Herbal remedies
Olive oil
St John's wort

CIRCULATORY SYSTEM
Anaemia
Herbal remedies
Periwinkle
Angelica
Centaury
Oregon grape

Poor circulation, chilblains
Herbal remedies
Yarrow
Angelica
Mustard
Walnut

Aromatherapy oils
Geranium
Marjoram

Cramps
Herbal remedies
Passionflower
Garlic
Chamomile

Aromatherapy oils
Yarrow
Linden
Chamomile

Arteriosclerosis
Herbal remedies
Garlic
Linden

Thyme
Rosemary
Olive oil
Evening primrose

High blood pressure
Herbal remedies
Yarrow
Passionflower
Garlic
Hawthorn
Linden

Varicose veins, haemorrhoids
Herbal remedies
Geranium
Witch hazel
Yarrow
Self-heal
Calendula
Oak
Horse chestnut

Aromatherapy oil
Geranium

Varicose ulcers
Witch hazel
Chamomile
Calendula
Oak
Chamomile

Aromatherapy oil
Eucalyptus

BONES, JOINTS AND MUSCLES
Arthritis and gout
Herbal remedies
Aloe juice
Heartsease
Sweet violet
Cowslip
Thyme
Borage
Rosemary
Echinacea
Meadowsweet
Evening primrose
Willow

Aromatherapy oils
Marjoram
Lavender
Rosemary
Pine
Yarrow
Eucalyptus
Chamomile

Rheumatism
Herbal remedies
Sweet violet
Thyme
Black cohosh
Meadowsweet
Oregon grape
Willow

Aromatherapy oils
Eucalyptus
Lavender
Rosemary

SKIN AND EYES
Eczema, cradle cap
Herbal remedies
Aloe juice
Heartsease
Red clover
Borage
Olive oil
Melissa
Calendula
Echinacea
Chickweed
Evening primrose
Nettles

Aromatherapy oil
Geranium

Abscesses, boils
Herbal remedies
Aloe juice
Heartsease
Dandelion root
Sweet violet
Echinacea
Blue flag

Aromatherapy oils
Eucalyptus
Rose

Warts and verrucae
Herbal remedies
Garlic
Greater celandine

Infections, infestations
Herbal remedies
Sage
Eucalyptus
Rosemary
Echinacea
Thyme
Ginger
Mullein
Pine
Sweet basil
Peppermint

Aromatherapy oils
Pine
Thyme
Geranium
Peppermint

Psoriasis
Herbal remedies
Dandelion root
Echinacea
Heartsease
Red clover
Larch
Oregon grape

Conjunctivitis, blephoritis
Herbal remedies
Aloe juice
Elder
Witch hazel
Greater celandine
Self-heal
Eyebright

Eyestrain, tired eyes
Herbal remedies
Yarrow
Greater celandine
Meadowsweet
Chamomile
Eyebright

Styes and pimples
Herbal remedies
Elder
Chamomile
Echinacea
Heartsease
Calendula
Lavender
Blue flag
Eyebright

REPRODUC-TIVE SYSTEM
Pre-menstrual syn-drome
Herbal remedies
Pasque flower
Lemon balm
Skullcap
Chamomile
Evening primrose
Rose
Jasmine

Aromatherapy oils
Clary sage
Chamomile
Geranium
Rose

Painful, heavy periods
Herbal remedies
Yarrow
Sage
Rose
Alchemilla
Mugwort
Beth root
Geranium
Black cohosh
Jasmine

Aromatherapy oils
Yarrow
Geranium

Vaginal infections
Herbal remedies
Sage
Alchemilla
Garlic
Mugwort
Beth root
Calendula
Echinacea
Oak

Menopausal problems
Herbal remedies
Sage
Mugwort
Blessed thistle
Hops
Ginseng
Evening primrose
Black cohosh
St John's wort

Aromatherapy oils
Clary sage
Hops
Chamomile
Geranium
Jasmine

Low libido, impotence
Herbal remedies
Ginger
Hops
Ginseng
Rose
Black cohosh

Aromatherapy oils
Ginger
Clary sage
Hops
Rose
Jasmine

Prostate problems
Herbal remedies
Dandelion
Aspen

PREGNANCY AND CHILDBIRTH
Morning sickness
Herbal remedies
Ginger
Chamomile
Tiger lily

Childbirth
Herbal remedies
Pasque flower
Alchemilla
Mugwort
Beth root
Chamomile
Black cohosh
Jasmine

Postnatal depression
Herbal remedies
Pasque flower
Jasmine

Aromatherapy oils
Pasque flower
Clary sage
Jasmine

Breastfeeding problems
Herbal remedies
Vervain
Borage
Blessed thistle
Nettles

FIRST AID
Nosebleeds
Herbal remedies
Witch hazel
Beth root
Oak
Nettles
Periwinkle

Bruises
Herbal remedies
Yarrow
Arnica
Witch hazel
Calendula
Lavender

Cuts and wounds
Herbal remedies
Yarrow
Aloe juice

Witch hazel
Calendula
Lavender
Geranium

Aromatherapy oils
Lavender
Chamomile
Peppermint

Minor burns and scalds
Herbal remedies
Lavender
Aloe juice
Yarrow
Witch hazel
Olive oil

Travel sickness
Herbal remedies
Ginger
Calendula
Chickweed
Lavender
Sweet basil
Peppermint

Sprains and strains
Herbal remedies
Marshmallow,
Hollyhock
Witch hazel
Hyssop
Calendula
Wood betony
Lavender

Insect bites and stings
Herbal remedies
Garlic
Witch hazel
Self-heal
Calendula
Lavender

Fainting and shock
Herbal remedies
Arnica

Flower essence
Arnica

Glossary

adaptogenic helping to restore balance within the body
alkaloid chemical compound containing a nitrogen atom which in plants has effects including killing pain, poisoning, and causing hallucinations
alterative producing gradually beneficial effects through detoxification and improving nutrition
analgesic pain relieving
antacid a substance which reduces stomach acid
antibacterial destroying or stopping the growth of bacterial infestations
antibiotic destroying or stopping the growth of bacteria
antifungal treating fungal infections
antihistamine neutralizing the effects of histamine in an allergic response
antiseptic preventing putrefaction
antispasmodic preventing or relieving spasms or cramps
antiviral destroying or stopping the growth of viral infections
astringent contracting tissue, reducing secretions or discharges
bitters chemicals which stimulate appetite and promote digestion; some are anti-inflammatory, others relaxant
carminative easing cramping pains and expelling flatulence
demulcent soothing irritated tissues, especially mucous membranes
diaphoretic promoting perspiration
diuretic promoting the flow of urine
emetic causing vomiting
emmenagogue promoting menstrual flow, and therefore to be avoided in pregnancy
emollient soothing and healing the skin
expectorant promoting expulsion of mucus from the respiratory tract
febrifuge reducing fever
flavonoid glycosides chemicals consisting of molecules made up of two sections, one of which is a sugar; some have a strong effect on the heart, and some are purgative
hypoglycaemic lowering of blood sugar
laxative promoting evacuation of the bowels
mucilage gel-like substance with molecules made up of long chains of sugar units; they soothe inflamed tissues
narcotic inducing sleep or unconsciousness
oestrogenic having similar properties to female oestrogen hormones
phenol basic building-block of many plant constituents; phenolic compounds include salicylic acid, which is often combined with a sugar to form a glycoside that is antiseptic
purgative producing vigorous emptying of the bowels
rubefacient gently irritating, producing redness of the skin
saponin glycoside which forms a soap-like lather when shaken with water; steroidal saponins mimic the precursors of female sex hormones, while tri-terpenoid saponins mimic the adrenal hormone ACTH
sudorific promoting perspiration
vasodilator widening blood vessels, lowering blood pressure
volatile oil complex compound of hydrocarbons and alcohols lending many herbs their characteristic taste and flavour; they can be antiseptic, antifungal or aromatic

Bibliography

Aburrow, Yvonne *The Enchanted Forest* CAPALL BANN, 1993
Allardice, P and Gee, M *The Ausralian Natural Health Directory* HODDER & STOUGHTON, Sydney 1995
Aubin, M and Picard, P *Homeopathy for Doctor and Patient* ASHGROVE PRESS, UK 1993
Balkam, Jan *Aromatherapy* BLITZ EDS, BOOKMART, UK 1994
Baumann, Hellmut *Greek Wild Flowers* HERBERT PRESS, 1993
Beyerl, Paul *Master Book of Herbalism* PHOENIX, US 1984
Boericke *Materica Medica,* JAIN PUBLISHERS, NEW DELHI 1927
Bown, D *Ornamental Herbs for Your Garden* HARPERCOLLINS, 1993
Brooke, E *A Woman's Book of Herbs,* WOMAN'S PRESS, 1992
Cameron, E *A Floral ABC,* WEBB & BOWER LTD, UK 1982
Castro, M *The Complete Homeopathy Handbook,* PAPERMAC, 1990
Chancellor, P *Handbook of the Bach Flower Remedies* C W DANIEL, UK 1971
Coley, Hilda *The Romance of Garden Flowers* MACLEHOSE & CO, GLASGOW 1948
Culpepers Complete Herbal, FOULSHAM
Cunningham, D *Flower Remedies Handbook* STERLING, US 1992
Davies, M *The Magical Lore of Herbs* CAPALL BANN, 1994
Ewart, Neil *The Lore of Flowers* BLANDFORD PRESS, 1982
Fernie, W T *Herbal Simples* WRIGHT & SONS, 1914
Fielder, M *Plant Medicine and Folklore* WINCHESTER, US 1975
Foster, Steven *Herbal Renaissance* GIBBS-SMITH, US 1984
Furnell, Dennis *Health from the Hedgerow,* BATSFORD, 1985
Goodrick-Clarke, N *Paracelsus Essential Readings* CRUCIBLE, 1990
Gordon, Lesley *A Country Herbal* PEERAGE BOOKS, 1980
Grieve, Mrs M *A Modern Herbal* PENGUIN BOOKS, 1976
Gurudas *Flower Essences and Vibrational Healing* CASSANDRA PRESS, US 1983
Haddon, Celia *Lovely is the Rose* MICHAEL JOSEPH, 1995
Harvey, C & Cochrane, A *The Encyclopaedia of Flower Essences* THORSONS, 1995
Hutchens, Alma *Indian Herbology of North America,* Shambhala, US 1973
Kaminski, P & Katz, R *Flower Essence Repertory* FLOWER ESSENCE SOCIETY, US 1994
Kerr, John *Understanding Aromatherapy* JOHN AND GILLIAN KERR BOOKS, Sydney 1995
Koehn, Alfred *A Gift of Japanese Flowers* CHARLES E TUTTLE CO RUTLAND, VERMONT & TOKYO, JAPAN 1992
Lad, Dr Vasant & Frawley, David *The Yoga of Herbs* LOTUS PRESS, US 1986
Lawless, J *Aromatherapy and the Mind* THORSONS, 1994
Leyel, Mrs C F *Elixirs of Life* FABER, 1947
Leyel, Mrs C F *Green Medicine* FABER
Leyel, Mrs C F *HeartsEase* FABER, 1948
Leyel, Mrs C F *Herbal Delights* FABER
Mabey, R (ed) *The New Herbal* GAIA BOOKS, 1988
Macleod, Dawn *A Book of Herbs* DUCKWORTH, LONDON, 1968
Magic and Medicine of Plants READER'S DIGEST, Sydney 1994
Marsh, Jean *The Illuminated Language of Flowers* HOLT, RINEHART & WINSTON, 1978
McIntyre, Anne *The Complete Woman's Herbal* HODDER & STOUGHTON, Sydney 1995
McIntyre, Michael *Herbal Medicine for Everyone* PENGUIN, 1988

Mowrey, D *Herbal Tonic Therapies* KEATS PUBLISHING, US 1993

Nagy, Liza *The Natural Choice Guide to Aromatherapy* HODDER & STOUGHTON, Sydney 1995

Palaiseul, Jean *Grandmother's Secrets* PENGUIN, 1976

Patnaik, Naveen *The Garden of Life* AQUARIAN, LONDON 1993

Pickles, Sheila *The Language of Flowers* PAVILION, 1995

Pickles, Sheila *The Language of Wild Flowers* PAVILION, 1995

Purchon, N *Aromatherapy* HODDER & STOUGHTON, Sydney 1994

Purchon, N *Herbcraft* HODDER & STOUGHTON, Sydney 1995

Scheffer, M *Bach Flower Therapy* THORSONS, 1990

Schultes, R & Hofman, A *Plants of the Gods* HUTCHINSON, 1980

Swahn, J O *The Lore of Spices* GRANGE BOOKS LONDON, 1991

Thiele, Ray *The Natural Choice Guide to Herbalism* HODDER & STOUGHTON, Sydney 1995

Vlamis, G *Flowers to the Rescue* THORSONS, 1986

Wells, Mark *The Bach Flowers Today* AUTONOMY BOOKS, Melbourne 1993

White, Ian *Australian Bush Flower Remedies*, BANTAM BOOKS, Sydney 1991

White, Ian *Bush Flower Essences* FINDHORN PRESS, 1993

Willard, Terry *Textbook of Modern Herbology* WILD ROSE COLLEGE, ALBERTA 1993

INDEX

To assist the reader to locate specific subjects more rapidly, the index has been divided into four sections: Flower and Plant Names; Ailments and Conditions; Plant Properties, Preparations and Treatments; General.

Ailments and Conditions

Bold page numbers indicate main entries in the Appendix.

Plant Properties, Preparations and Treatments

Bold page references indicate preparation methods.